The Evidence-Based Guide to

ANTIPSYCHOTIC MEDICATIONS

The Evidence-Based Guide to
ANTIPSYCHOTIC MEDICATIONS

Edited by

Anthony J. Rothschild, M.D.

Irving S. and Betty Brudnick Endowed Chair and
Professor of Psychiatry, Department of Psychiatry
University of Massachusetts Medical School
UMass Memorial Healthcare
Worcester, Massachusetts

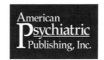

American Psychiatric Publishing, Inc.

Washington, DC
London, England

If you would like to buy between 25 and 99 copies of this or any other APPI title, you are eligible for a 20% discount; please contact APPI Customer Service at appi@psych.org or 800-368-5777. If you wish to buy 100 or more copies of the same title, please e-mail us at bulksales@psych.org for a price quote.

Copyright © 2010 American Psychiatric Publishing, Inc.
ALL RIGHTS RESERVED

Manufactured in the United States of America on acid-free paper
13 12 11 10 09   5 4 3 2 1
First Edition

Typeset in Adobe's Cushing and Optima

American Psychiatric Publishing, Inc.
1000 Wilson Boulevard
Arlington, VA 22209–3901
www.appi.org

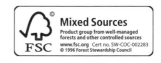

Library of Congress Cataloging-in-Publication Data
The evidence-based guide to antipsychotic medications / edited by Anthony J. Rothschild. — 1st ed.
    p. ; cm.
    Includes bibliographical references and index.
    ISBN 978-1-58562-366-2 (pbk. : alk. paper)
    1. Antipsychotic drugs. 2. Evidence-based psychiatry. I. Rothschild, Anthony J.
    [DNLM: 1. Mental Disorders—drug therapy. 2. Antipsychotic Agents—therapeutic use. 3. Evidence-Based Medicine. WM 402 E945 2010]
    RM333.5.E95 2010
    615′.7882–dc22
                                                                2009040345

British Library Cataloguing in Publication Data
A CIP record is available from the British Library.

To Judy, Rachel, and Amanda; my mother, Edith Rothschild, and the memory of my father, Ernest Rothschild; and the memory of my in-laws, Maye and Arnold Shindul.

The book is also dedicated to Betty Brudnick and in memory of Irving Brudnick, without whose generous support this book would not have been possible.

Contents

Contributors xiii

Acknowledgments xvii

Disclaimer xix

1 Introduction 1
Anthony J. Rothschild, M.D.

2 Schizophrenia and Schizoaffective Disorder . . 5
Jayendra K. Patel, M.D.
Kristina M. Deligiannidis, M.D.

TREATMENT GOALS 6

CLINICIAN-PATIENT RELATIONSHIP 7

ANTIPSYCHOTIC MEDICATIONS 8

TREATMENT OF SCHIZOPHRENIA 20

TREATMENT OF SCHIZOAFFECTIVE DISORDER . . . 37

TREATMENT ADHERENCE 39

KEY CLINICAL POINTS 39

REFERENCES 40

3 Mood and Anxiety Disorders 45
Kristina M. Deligiannidis, M.D.
Anthony J. Rothschild, M.D.

BIPOLAR DISORDER. 45
KEY CLINICAL POINTS: BIPOLAR DISORDER 53
PSYCHOTIC DEPRESSION. 54
KEY CLINICAL POINTS: PSYCHOTIC DEPRESSION. . 58
TREATMENT-RESISTANT DEPRESSION. 59
KEY CLINICAL POINTS: TREATMENT-RESISTANT
DEPRESSION 61
NONPSYCHOTIC DEPRESSION. 61
KEY CLINICAL POINTS: NONPSYCHOTIC
DEPRESSION 63
OBSESSIVE-COMPULSIVE DISORDER. 63
KEY CLINICAL POINTS: OBSESSIVE-COMPULSIVE
DISORDER 71
GENERALIZED ANXIETY DISORDER. 72
KEY CLINICAL POINTS: GENERALIZED ANXIETY
DISORDER 80
POSTTRAUMATIC STRESS DISORDER 81
KEY CLINICAL POINTS: POSTTRAUMATIC STRESS
DISORDER 90
SAFETY AND TOLERABILITY OF ANTIPSYCHOTICS
IN MOOD AND ANXIETY DISORDERS:
FUNDAMENTAL CONCEPTS 90
REFERENCES 92

4 Personality Disorders **101**
Kenneth R. Silk, M.D.
Michael D. Jibson, M.D., Ph.D.

HOW PSYCHOSIS IS VIEWED
IN PERSONALITY DISORDER. 102
HISTORICAL CONSIDERATIONS. 103
MECHANISM OF ACTION 104
INDICATIONS AND EFFICACY. 105
CLINICAL USE 106
GUIDELINES FOR SELECTION AND USE 108
SIDE EFFECTS AND THEIR MANAGEMENT 110
BORDERLINE PERSONALITY DISORDER 110
SCHIZOTYPAL PERSONALITY DISORDER 116
OTHER PERSONALITY DISORDERS 121
KEY CLINICAL POINTS 122
REFERENCES 123

5 Substance Abuse Disorders. **125**
Gerardo Gonzalez, M.D.
Ruben Miozzo, M.D., M.P.H.
Douglas Ziedonis, M.D., M.P.H.

SUBSTANCE-RELATED PSYCHOMOTOR
AGITATION 126
SUBSTANCE-ASSOCIATED
PSYCHOTIC SYMPTOMS AND DISORDERS. 133
CO-OCCURRING DISORDERS 136
SUBSTANCE USE DISORDERS. 141
KEY CLINICAL POINTS 142
REFERENCES 143

6 Use of Antipsychotics in Children and Adolescents 145

Bruce Meltzer, M.D.

INDICATIONS AND EFFICACY. 146
SECOND-GENERATION ANTIPSYCHOTICS 163
FIRST-GENERATION ANTIPSYCHOTICS 172
ANTIPSYCHOTIC TREATMENT OF
PEDIATRIC PSYCHIATRIC DISORDERS 180
DISCONTINUING ANTIPSYCHOTIC TREATMENT . . 185
KEY CLINICAL POINTS 185
REFERENCES 186

7 Use of Antipsychotics in Geriatric Patients . . 191

Ellen M. Whyte, M.D.
Charles Madeira

GENERAL PRINCIPLES OF MEDICATION
MANAGEMENT. 192
AGE-SPECIFIC ISSUES RELATED
TO SIDE EFFECTS 193
RISKS UNIQUE TO PATIENTS WITH DEMENTIA . . . 200
USE OF ANTIPSYCHOTIC MEDICATIONS
IN LONG-TERM-CARE FACILITIES. 202
MEDICATION MANAGEMENT FOR PATIENTS
WITH PSYCHIATRIC AND NEUROPSYCHIATRIC
DISORDERS 203
KEY CLINICAL POINTS 212
REFERENCES 213

8 Use of Antipsychotics in Medically Ill
Patients 215
  Marcus W. Tjia, M.D.
  David F. Gitlin, M.D.

    MEDICAL CONSIDERATIONS IN THE USE OF
    ANTIPSYCHOTICS 216
    GENERAL CONDITIONS.................... 218
    MEDICAL DISORDERS 222
    KEY CLINICAL POINTS.................... 238
    REFERENCES 238

Appendix 1
Names, Strengths, and Formulations of
First- and Second-Generation
Antipsychotics............................241

Appendix 2
Pharmacokinetics of First- and Second-
Generation Antipsychotics 249

Appendix 3
Dosing and Administration of First- and
Second-Generation Antipsychotics
in Schizophrenia..........................261

Appendix 4
Medical Workup When Initiating and
Continuing First- and Second-Generation
Antipsychotics............................275

Appendix 5
Medical Workup When Initiating and
Continuing Clozapine 279

Appendix 6

Use of First- and Second-Generation
Antipsychotics for Agitation Due to
Psychosis 283

Appendix 7

Side Effects of Commonly Used
Antipsychotics. 289

Appendix 8

Management of Treatment-Emergent
Side Effects of Antipsychotic Medications. . . .291

Appendix 9

Use of First- and Second-Generation
Antipsychotics in Pregnancy and Lactation . . .297

Index. 331

Contributors

Kristina M. Deligiannidis, M.D.
Director, Depression Specialty Clinic, and Assistant Professor of Psychiatry, Department of Psychiatry, University of Massachusetts Medical School, Worcester, Massachusetts

David F. Gitlin, M.D.
Assistant Professor of Psychiatry, Harvard Medical School; and Director, Division of Medical Psychiatry, Brigham and Women's Hospital, Boston, Massachusetts

Gerardo Gonzalez, M.D.
Associate Professor, Department of Psychiatry, University of Massachusetts Medical School, Worcester, Massachusetts

Michael D. Jibson, M.D., Ph.D.
Professor of Psychiatry and Director of Residency Education, University of Michigan Health System, Ann Arbor, Michigan

Charles Madeira
University of Pittsburgh School of Medicine, Pittsburgh, Pennsylvania

Bruce Meltzer, M.D.
Assistant Professor of Pediatrics and Child Psychiatry, University of Massachusetts Medical School, Worcester, Massachusetts; and Executive Medical Director, UMASS/DMH Continuing Care Programs, Worcester and Westborough State Hospital, Westborough, Massachusetts

Ruben Miozzo, M.D., M.P.H.
Assistant Professor, Department of Psychiatry, University of Massachusetts Medical School, Worcester, Massachusetts

Jayendra K. Patel, M.D.
Director, Schizophrenia Research; Director, Bipolar Disorder Program, Center for Psychopharmacologic Research and Treatment; and Associate Professor, Department of Psychiatry, University of Massachusetts Medical School, Worcester, Massachusetts

Anthony J. Rothschild, M.D.
Irving S. and Betty Brudnick Endowed Chair and Professor of Psychiatry, Department of Psychiatry, University of Massachusetts Medical School and UMass Memorial Healthcare, Worcester, Massachusetts

Kenneth R. Silk, M.D.
Professor of Psychiatry, Department of Psychiatry, University of Michigan Health System, Ann Arbor, Michigan

Marcus W. Tjia, M.D.
Instructor in Psychiatry, Harvard Medical School; and Assistant Director, Division of Medical Psychiatry, Brigham and Women's Hospital, Boston, Massachusetts

Ellen M. Whyte, M.D.
Assistant Professor of Psychiatry and Physical Medicine and Rehabilitation, University of Pittsburgh School of Medicine, Pittsburgh, Pennsylvania

Douglas Ziedonis, M.D., M.P.H.
Professor and Chair, Department of Psychiatry, University of Massachusetts Medical School, Worcester, Massachusetts

Disclosure of Competing Interests

The following contributors to this book have indicated a financial interest in or other affiliation with a commercial supporter, a manufacturer of a commercial product, a provider of a commercial service, a nongovernmental organization, and/or a government agency, as listed below:

Gerardo Gonzalez, M.D.: *Research support:* Bristol-Myers Squibb, UCB; *Honoraria as speaker:* Reckitt Benckiser

Michael D. Jibson, M.D., Ph.D.: *Speaker's bureau:* AstraZeneca; "Up-to-Date" author

Jayendra K. Patel, M.D.: *Research support:* Bristol-Myers Squibb, Foundation for National Institutes of Health, Forest, Johnson & Johnson, National Institute of Mental Health

Anthony J. Rothschild, M.D.: *Grants/Research support:* Cyberonics, National Institute of Mental Health, Takeda, Wyeth; *Consultant:* Forest, GlaxoSmithKline, Lilly, Pfizer; *Royalties:* Rothschild Scale for Antidepressant Tachyphylaxis (RSAT)™

Kenneth R. Silk, M.D.: *Royalties:* American Psychiatric Press, Cambridge University Press

Ellen M. Whyte, M.D.: *Grant funding:* National Institute of Mental Health, NICHD/NCMRR; *Investigator-initiated grants:* Forest, Lilly, Ortho-McNeil, Pfizer

The following authors have no competing interests to report:

Kristina M. Deligiannidis, M.D.
David F. Gitlin, M.D.
Charles Madeira
Bruce Meltzer, M.D.
Marcus W. Tjia, M.D.

Acknowledgments

I have many people to thank for their encouragement, advice, and support in preparing this book. My family has been patient and understanding of my need to spend time on this project. Irving and Betty Brudnick were instrumental by their endowment of the Irving S. and Betty Brudnick Endowed Chair at the University of Massachusetts Medical School, a position that allowed me the time to focus on projects such as this evidence-based guide. I am eternally grateful to Irving Brudnick's wisdom and support, and I miss his guidance greatly.

At American Psychiatric Publishing, Inc., Robert Hales, Editor-in-Chief; John McDuffie, Editorial Director; and Greg Kuny, Managing Editor, Books, deserve a great deal of credit for their unwavering confidence in me as an author and for their support throughout the development and production of this evidence-based guide.

A special thank-you goes to Dr. Kristina Deligiannidis of the University of Massachusetts Medical School for creating the informative tables in the Appendix of this book. My assistant Karen Lambert provided invaluable help in the typing of the manuscript, figures, and tables. I am also appreciative of the support and encouragement of colleagues and trainees at the University of Massachusetts Medical School and UMass Memorial Healthcare. Finally, this book could not have been written without the many patients and families with whom I have had the privilege of working.

Disclaimer

Specific treatment regimens for a particular patient remain the responsibility of the treating clinician, who has access to all of the patient's relevant clinical information, can make a complete assessment of the patient with the information in this textbook as appropriate, and can provide the most informed medical advice. The information provided in this textbook is educational in nature and for general use only and should not be seen as medical advice for a specific patient or as the rendering of professional services. The latest manufacturer's package information for any medications or devices discussed in this book should be reviewed before prescribing for use. Information provided may include a description of the uses of therapeutic and biological products that have not been approved by the U.S. Food and Drug Administration. Medical practice, research, and pharmacological advances will occur, and, therefore, changes in the information and therapies in this book are expected to occur.

CHAPTER 1

Introduction

Anthony J. Rothschild, M.D.

ANTIPSYCHOTIC MEDICATIONS revolutionized the practice of psychiatry after the discovery of chlorpromazine in 1952. Patients who would have otherwise been chronically psychotic and institutionalized began to receive treatment that alleviated many of their symptoms and permitted treatment as an outpatient. In the ensuing years, more than 20 antipsychotic compounds were identified that had pharmacological properties similar to those of chlorpromazine; namely, dopamine antagonism (Lehmann and Ban 1997). The antipsychotic medications in this first wave are referred to as *conventional antipsychotic medications, "typical" antipsychotics,* or *first-generation antipsychotics*. A second revolution occurred with the introduction of the first *"atypical,"* or *second-generation, antipsychotic*—clozapine—in the United States in 1990. Although clozapine was first discovered in 1959, it received little attention because clinicians doubted its efficacy, since clozapine did not produce the typical neuromotor effects in the animal model expected of a dopamine antagonist (Lehmann and Ban 1997). In addition, clozapine's side-effect profile of agranulocytosis, decreased seizure threshold, and hypotension limited its use. The perception of clozapine changed with a study by Kane and colleagues (1988), who reported that clozapine had greater efficacy in treatment-resistant schizophrenia than did chlorpromazine. This finding led to the second wave of antipsychotic medication development.

Although most of the antipsychotic medications were initially approved by regulatory bodies for the treatment of schizophrenia, over the years they have received additional regulatory approval for use in bipolar disorder and as adjunctive therapy for treatment-resistant unipolar depression. In addition, the use of antipsychotic medication by clinicians for non–U.S. Food and Drug Administration (FDA)–approved illnesses, so-called off-label use, has been growing. Hence the need arose for this evidence-based guide to antipsychotic medications. Each chapter in this guide will include the FDA-approved and off-label uses of the antipsychotic medications (both first- and second-generation antipsychotics) and the evidence base that supports (or does not support) each of their uses. All of the chapter authors have synthesized a large amount of medical literature to create a comprehensive yet understandable, concise, reader-friendly guide for the practicing clinician.

In Chapter 2, Drs. Patel and Deligiannidis discuss the use of antipsychotic medications in schizophrenia and schizoaffective disorder. They review the history and background of first- and second-generation antipsychotic medications and the goals of treatment. For each antipsychotic medication, they provide a brief description of its pharmacology. The initial medical workup for initiating antipsychotic medication treatment and the tests that should be done during treatment are clearly illustrated in informative tables that are included in the appendixes. Drs. Patel and Deligiannidis sort through the vast and complex literature on the use of antipsychotic medications in schizophrenia and schizoaffective disorder and distill the information for the practicing clinician with helpful, practical advice for the management of acute and long-term antipsychotic medication treatment.

In Chapter 3, the use of antipsychotic medications for the treatment of mood and anxiety disorders is reviewed by Drs. Deligiannidis and Rothschild. Some antipsychotic medications have received FDA indications for the treatment of bipolar disorder and as an adjunctive therapy for treatment-resistant unipolar depression, but the chapter also includes discussion of the evidence base for off-label uses of antipsychotic medications for several conditions, including major depression with psychotic features, obsessive-compulsive disorder, generalized anxiety disorder, and posttraumatic stress disorder.

In Chapter 4, the use of antipsychotic medications for borderline personality disorder, schizotypal personality disorder, and other personality disorders in general is discussed by Drs. Silk and Jibson. Although none of the antipsychotic medications have FDA indications for the treatment of personality disorders, they are often used by clinicians to treat psychosis and peripsychotic experiences in patients with personality disorders. Drs. Silk and Jibson discuss how the use of antipsychotics in this patient population differs in significant ways from their use in other illnesses.

In Chapter 5, Drs. Gonzalez, Miozzo, and Ziedonis discuss the use of antipsychotic medications in patients with substance abuse and co-occurring disorders. Substance abuse is a common co-occurring disorder in patients with schizophrenia, bipolar disorder, and major depression. Although none of the antipsychotic medications have an FDA indication for the treatment of substance abuse, symptoms of psychosis and agitation often are observed in patients either withdrawing from or intoxicated with various drugs of abuse. The authors focus on the off-label use of antipsychotic medications to treat these symptoms.

In Chapter 6, Dr. Meltzer reviews the use of antipsychotic medications in children and adolescents. He delineates the medications with FDA approval and those that are prescribed off label. The author discusses the use of antipsychotic medications in children and adolescents with psychosis (including schizophrenia), early-onset bipolar disorder, anorexia nervosa, pediatric autism spectrum disorder, pervasive developmental delay, and Tourette syndrome.

In Chapter 7, Dr. Whyte and Charles Madeira review the use of antipsychotic medications in the geriatric patient. After discussing the general principles of medication management in the older patient, they review age-specific side effects of antipsychotic medications with an emphasis on how these side effects can differ in older patients compared with younger patients. A review of the federal Omnibus Budget Reconciliation Act (OBRA) guidelines for the use of antipsychotic medications in long-term-care facilities is included. The chapter contains a detailed description of the use of antipsychotic medications in specific diseases, including schizophrenia, major depressive disorder, bipolar disorder, Alzheimer's disease, Parkinson's disease, dementia with Lewy bodies, and frontotemporal dementia. The authors also discuss the use of antipsychotic medications in the management of acutely dangerous agitation and aggression in geriatric patients with dementia.

In Chapter 8, Drs. Tjia and Gitlin review the use of antipsychotic medications in medically ill patients. They begin by discussing the unique issues that need to be addressed when using antipsychotic medications in this patient population, including drug-drug interactions, pharmacokinetics, routes of administration of the antipsychotic, sedation, and extrapyramidal side effects. They then discuss the use of antipsychotic medications for various medical conditions, including delirium, agitation or aggressive behavior, cardiovascular disease, renal disease, hepatic insufficiency, pulmonary disease, dementia, Parkinson's disease, traumatic brain injury, HIV infection, epilepsy, rheumatologic disorders, steroid-induced psychiatric disorders, burns, trauma, and pain. The use of antipsychotic medications during pregnancy and breast-feeding is also discussed.

This book is a condensed yet comprehensive overview of the current knowledge and evidence base regarding the use of antipsychotic medications. Chapters typically contain several useful tables pertaining to the topic being discussed. In addition, at the end of the book, the appendixes include clinically useful tables containing information on names, strengths, formulations, pharmacokinetics, and dosing of the antipsychotic medications; the medical workup when initiating and continuing antipsychotic medications; the use of antipsychotic medications for agitation due to psychosis; the common side effects and their management; and the use of antipsychotic medications in pregnancy and during breast-feeding. Finally, at the end of each chapter (and each individual section in Chapter 3), the important clinical pearls of information are summarized in the Key Clinical Points.

This book is designed for the busy clinician, and I hope it will prove useful to psychiatrists, family and general practitioners, internists, neurologists, nurses, psychologists, social workers, and advanced students.

References

Kane JM, Honigfeld G, Singer J, et al: Clozapine for the treatment resistant schizophrenic: a double-blind comparison versus chlorpromazine/benztropine. Arch Gen Psychiatry 45:789–796, 1988

Lehmann HE, Ban TA: The history of the psychopharmacology of schizophrenia. Can J Psychiatry 42:152–162, 1997

CHAPTER 2

Schizophrenia and Schizoaffective Disorder

Jayendra K. Patel, M.D.
Kristina M. Deligiannidis, M.D.

IN 1911, EUGEN BLEULER, a Swiss psychiatrist, coined the term *schizophreniegruppe*, or *schizophrenia*, to describe a heterogeneous group of illnesses with distinguishing characteristics and clinical courses. Schizophrenia is a chronic, severe, and debilitating mental illness that usually starts early in life and has a chronic downhill course with an associated mortality rate about twice that in the general population.

Several factors important to the observed increased mortality rates in schizophrenia patients include an increased incidence of accidents, more frequent association with medical illnesses (e.g., cardiovascular diseases, diabetes mellitus), comorbid substance abuse, general neglect of health, an increased rate of damaging behaviors (e.g., smoking cigarettes, poor diet), decreased access to health services, depression, and suicide (Harris and Barraclough 1998). Additionally, mortality rates were found to be 10 times higher in patients who were not taking medications compared with those who were (Tiihonen et al. 2006). Severe mental illness increases risk of death from coronary heart disease and stroke independent of antipsychotic medication, smoking, or social deprivation.

Approximately 10% of the increased mortality rate in schizophrenia is attributable to suicide. Several risk factors for suicide in schizophrenia include being young and male (especially during the early stages of their illness, when these patients are most likely to complete suicide), frequent relapses and rehospitalizations, social isolation, agitation, depression, hopelessness, recent losses, and a history of suicide attempts (Lester 2006).

Successful treatment of schizophrenia requires an appreciation of the chronicity of the illness, a greater level of clinical knowledge, and professional dexterity that starts with the formation of a therapeutic clinician-patient relationship. The treatment plan involves close coordination with patient, family members (when available), and other disciplines and combines the latest developments in pharmacological therapeutics and psychosocial interventions.

Treatment Goals

Successful pharmacological intervention in schizophrenia demands formulating specific treatment targets with realistic outcome expectations. Clinicians can expect significant pharmacological efficacy in positive symptoms, mood symptoms, abnormal behavior, and agitative and assaultive behavior. Moderate to significant efficacy can be expected for suicidal behavior, and modest efficacy can be expected for the negative symptoms. The cognitive symptoms of schizophrenia are less responsive to the pharmacological strategies currently available. The management of medication side effects remains a challenge because side effects can contribute to medical illness (e.g., diabetes, hyperlipidemia, weight gain), which increases total disease morbidity.

The overall treatment plan should cover the acute and maintenance phases and have short-term, intermediate-term, and long-term goals. The following stage- or state-specific issues are important to consider:

- Treatment outcomes during the first break and early stages of the illness are significantly better and rapidly achieved compared with the later stages of the illness.
- Duration of untreated psychosis appears to predict long-term outcome, with shorter duration having better prognosis.
- Frequent relapses may negatively affect the long-term course.
- Noncompliance is more common in the earlier stages of the illness and with lack of insight.

- It can be expected that 30%–40% of patients will have very good long-term response to medications, with another 30%–40% showing moderate response and the rest fair to poor response.

Achieving significant efficacy while maintaining a minimal side-effect burden may require juggling the antipsychotic medications, managing side effects, and preventing noncompliance. It is important to recognize that remission does not occur in most patients; only 20% may go on to have meaningful employment. However, this cannot be viewed pessimistically; current medications still significantly affect the symptoms and the course of illness and remarkably improve the overall quality of life. Thus, the clinician constantly measures the progress made with the interventions used against the predetermined targets, measures the time frame within which such progress is made, identifies and overcomes the obstacles in achieving these goals, and makes necessary and pragmatic changes in treatment as appropriate.

Clinician-Patient Relationship

The clinician-patient relationship is the key foundation for effectively treating schizophrenia, but several clinical manifestations of the illness render the formation of such a relationship difficult. For example, paranoid delusions may lead to mistrust of the clinician; conceptual disorganization and cognitive impairment make it difficult for patients to attend to what the clinician is saying or sometimes even to follow simple directions. The negative symptoms may result in lack of emotional expression and social withdrawal, which can be demoralizing for the clinician who is attempting to connect with the patient; command auditory hallucinations may further interfere with establishing an effective rapport with the patient. Thus, the clinician needs to understand the ways in which the psychopathology of the illness affects the therapeutic relationship.

Several strategies can aid the clinician in promoting the therapeutic relationship in patients with schizophrenia. For example, providing constancy to the patient may help anchor the patient in his or her turbulent world. Moreover, consistency, acceptance, and appropriate levels of warmth that respect the patient's need for titrating emotional intensity, nonintrusiveness, and caring are equally important in strengthening the therapeutic alliance.

With increasing medical morbidity secondary to lifestyle issues and side effects of medications in patients with schizophrenia, the clinician also assumes more responsibilities of coordinating care across various disciplines, integrating discussions about "wellness" with illness management, and heavily relying on this relationship to effect positive changes.

Antipsychotic Medications

Background

It was mere serendipity that the antipsychotic chlorpromazine's unusual tranquilizing properties were recognized during its use as a preoperative anesthetic medication in France. Subsequently, chlorpromazine was successfully used in the treatment of psychosis by Delay and Deniker in 1952 such that it forever changed the face of schizophrenia. With chlorpromazine treatment, chronically institutionalized patients were then able to achieve enough recovery to receive outpatient treatment and live in the community. Thus, chlorpromazine paved the way for the deinstitutionalization movement. The word *neuroleptic* (which means "nerve cutting") was used to describe the tranquilizing effects of these medications; 13 different classes of antipsychotics are currently available in the United States (see Appendix 1).

Antipsychotics developed subsequent to chlorpromazine, such as haloperidol and thiothixene, were modeled on the (misguided) belief that induction of extrapyramidal symptoms (EPS) was an integral part of achieving antipsychotic efficacy. Over the years, another myth developed that all antipsychotics were similar in their efficacy and varied only in their side effects. However, the antipsychotic clozapine challenged these beliefs because it was significantly superior in efficacy to the existing antipsychotics and had minimal to no EPS. This started the era of antipsychotic agents being referred to as either *typical* (conventional, first-generation, or traditional) or *atypical* (novel, second-generation, or serotonin-dopamine antagonists). *Atypicality* generally refers to the ability of an antipsychotic to be efficacious without causing significant neurological side effects (see Patel et al. 2008 for more details).

Chlorpromazine started the first revolution in the psychopharmacological treatment of schizophrenia, whereas clozapine ushered in the second, and more profound, revolution, whose effect has been felt beyond schizophrenia. Clozapine invigorated the psychopharmacology of schizophrenia and rekindled one of the most ambitious searches for new antipsychotic compounds. Perhaps the most pragmatic way to classify antipsychotics would be to call traditional, typical, or conventional antipsychotics *first-generation antipsychotics* (FGAs) and atypical, novel, or serotonin-dopamine antagonists *second-generation antipsychotics* (SGAs).

FGAs were the only treatments available for schizophrenia in the United States until 1990. Although prescriptions for SGAs have increased dramatically, FGAs are still an important and sometimes the only choice for some patients. Most—but not all—clinicians, educators, and researchers firmly believed that the nonclozapine SGAs were *markedly* superior to the FGAs. The psychiatry community was so enamored with SGAs that annual spending on antipsychotic medications increased dramatically from $1.4 billion in 1994 to more than $10 billion by 2006. SGAs are the most widely prescribed on-patent psychotropic drugs and as much as 100 times the cost of some FGAs. Each year saw SGAs eroding the market share of FGAs such that many believed it was only a matter of time before FGAs would be out of use.

However, meta-analyses have failed to find substantial differences between FGAs and the nonclozapine SGAs (Leucht et al. 2009). Furthermore, data from practical "real-world" clinical trials surprised the clinical and research community by failing to show meaningful differences in effectiveness, quality of life, and other important outcome measures between FGAs and SGAs (excluding clozapine) in patients with nonrefractory symptoms (Jones et al. 2006; Lieberman 2006; Lieberman et al. 2005; Rosenheck 2006). These data were further supported when studies failed to show substantial differences in efficacy and retention measures between SGAs and FGAs during the treatment of early and perhaps the most malleable stage of schizophrenia (Lieberman 2006).

These results have led prominent researchers to conclude that the nonclozapine SGAs are not as great a breakthrough as once thought but rather represent an incremental advance over FGAs. However, others believe that the differences between SGAs and FGAs are sufficiently important to justify the preferential use of SGAs. The debate rages on. For now, it appears that both SGAs and FGAs have a place in the treatment of schizophrenia until we find dramatically better alternatives. Increasingly, the opinions are converging on *individualizing* treatments for the patients that provide the most efficacy and the least number of side effects regardless of medication class used.

The names, strengths, and formulations of FGAs and SGAs are listed in Appendix 1. The pharmacokinetics and chlorpromazine equivalents of the FGAs and SGAs are illustrated in Appendix 2.

First-Generation Antipsychotics

Six major classes of FGAs, discussed below in order of appearance, are currently available in the United States (see Appendixes 1 and 2).

- The *phenothiazines* were the first antipsychotics used in the treatment of schizophrenia. These tricyclic compounds can be further classified into three subgroups:
  - *Aliphatic* phenothiazines are low-potency antipsychotics, such as chlorpromazine and triflupromazine, which are quite sedating and have substantial hypotensive and anticholinergic side effects.

- *Piperidine* phenothiazines include thioridazine, which also causes sedation, hypotension, and anticholinergic side effects. Moreover, this medication is likely to prolong QTc interval substantially such that it now carries a "black-box" warning requiring mandatory electrocardiogram (ECG) monitoring.
- *Piperazine* phenothiazines are more likely to produce EPS but less likely to produce drowsiness, anticholinergic side effects, and hypotension. These are also the most popular FGA phenothiazines and include compounds such as fluphenazine, perphenazine, and prochlorperazine.

- The *butyrophenones* include haloperidol, one of the most commonly used FGAs. Haloperidol is a potent dopamine D_2 receptor antagonist and thus more likely to cause acute dystonic reactions, EPS, and tardive dyskinesia (TD), but it does not cause anticholinergic and autonomic side effects. Droperidol, another member of this group, was commonly used in the emergency department to control agitation until it was reported to prolong QTc interval and cause torsades de pointes and sudden deaths.
- The *diphenylbutylpiperidines* have similarities with the butyrophenones. Pimozide is the only compound available from this group in the United States. Prolongation of QTc interval has emerged as a major concern limiting its use. It is often used in treatment of delusional disorders.
- The *thioxanthenes* include thiothixene, which has side effects similar to those of the phenothiazines.
- The *dibenzoxazepines* include loxapine, which is the only one of these compound available in the United States.
- The *dihydroindoles* include molindone, which was, before the advent of SGAs, widely used in individuals who gained weight while taking other FGAs. In a new trial in children and adolescents, molindone was reported to be an effective antipsychotic agent without the associated weight gain and metabolic side effects. This may cause a resurgence of its use in those patients who are struggling with metabolic issues (Sikich et al. 2008).

Second-Generation Antipsychotics

Seven major classes of SGAs are currently available in the United States.

Clozapine

Clozapine, a dibenzodiazepine compound, was approved for use in the United States in 1990. In a landmark double-blind, controlled study, clozapine showed superior clinical efficacy when compared with an FGA, without the associated EPS (Kane et al. 1988). It is superior to SGAs for treatment of psychosis.

Studies of patients with chronic and treatment-resistant schizophrenia suggest that approximately 50% of patients derive a better response from clozapine than from FGAs (Iqbal et al. 2003). It is very effective in treating negative symptoms; however, there is controversy as to whether the efficacy is with primary or secondary negative symptoms or both.

Substantial evidence indicates that clozapine decreases relapses, improves stability in the community, and diminishes suicidal behavior. It is the only antipsychotic that has received U.S. Food and Drug Administration (FDA) approval for treating suicidal patients. Clozapine may cause a gradual reduction in preexisting TD, improve tardive dystonia, decrease substance use, improve psychogenic polydipsia, decrease aggression, and decrease cigarette smoking among patients with schizophrenia.

Unfortunately, because clozapine is associated with agranulocytosis, frequent white blood cell (WBC) testing is required. Approximately 0.8% of the patients taking clozapine with regular WBC monitoring develop agranulocytosis. There are several groups at higher risk for agranulocytosis with clozapine treatment: women, the elderly, Ashkenazi Jews, and African Americans (they can have lower WBC counts at baseline compared with other races). The risk is greater at the start of treatment and during the first 6 months. Thus, weekly blood draws are mandatory in the first 6 months. After the first 6 months, the monitoring is every other week if a person has a history of WBC counts within normal range in the preceding 6 months. After 1 year of WBC counts being in normal range, the monitoring frequency decreases to once a month. If the WBC count is less than $3,500/mm^3$ or absolute neutrophil count (ANC) is less than $2,000/mm^3$, it is recommended to repeat the counts twice weekly until the WBC count is $3,500/mm^3$ or greater. Whenever the WBC count declines substantially, clinicians should repeat the WBC count. Current guidelines state that the medication must be held if the total WBC count is $3,000/mm^3$ or less *or* the ANC is $1,500/mm^3$ or less. The WBC count should be repeated daily until the WBC count is greater than $3,000/mm^3$ and the ANC is greater than $1,500/mm.^3$ However, if the WBC is less than $2,000/mm^3$ or the ANC is less than $1,000/mm^3$, clozapine should be discontinued and the patient should be placed in reverse isolation and daily blood counts taken. This patient *cannot* be rechallenged with clozapine. Patients who discontinue clozapine treatment for any reason require blood monitoring for at least 4 weeks after the last dose.

Sudden death from myocarditis and cardiomyopathy in physically healthy young adults with schizophrenia receiving clozapine therapy led to a black-box warning from the FDA in 2002. These cardiac events usually occur within the first 2 months of initiating treatment; thus, gradual titration of the medication is important. An ECG at baseline and within the first few weeks, or if the patient develops symptoms, is important.

Other significant side effects of clozapine include orthostatic hypotension, tachycardia, sialorrhea, sedation, elevated temperature, dysphagia, weight gain, hyperglycemia, and hyperlipidemia (Baldessarini and Frankenburg 1991). Furthermore, clozapine can lower the seizure threshold in a dose-dependent fashion, with a higher risk of seizures seen particularly at doses greater than 600 mg/day. Most patients can choose to continue clozapine with an antiepileptic medication if they develop seizures during treatment.

Clozapine has an affinity for dopamine receptors (D_1, D_2, D_3, D_4, and D_5), serotonin (5-hydroxytryptamine [5-HT]) receptors (5-HT_{2A}, 5-HT_{2C}, 5-HT_6, and 5-HT_7), α_1- and α_2-adrenergic receptors, nicotinic and muscarinic cholinergic receptors, and histamine (H_1) receptors. Because clozapine has a relatively short half-life, it is usually administered twice a day. Clozapine is not associated with hyperprolactinemia. Binding studies have shown it to be a relatively weak D_1 and D_2 antagonist, compared with the FGAs. Clozapine shares the property of a higher ratio of 5-HT_{2A} to D_2 blockade, which has been reported to impart atypicality. The noradrenergic system also may have a role in the mechanism of action of clozapine. Clozapine, but not FGAs, causes up to a fivefold increase in plasma norepinephrine levels. Moreover, this increase in norepinephrine has been found to correlate with clinical response. Clozapine is available in tablet form only and is available in a generic formulation.

Benzisoxazoles

The benzisoxazole group includes risperidone, the second SGA to be approved by the FDA (in 1994). Risperidone has a high affinity for 5-HT_{2A} and D_2 receptors and a high serotonin-to-dopamine receptor antagonism ratio. It also has a high affinity for α_1-adrenergic and H_1 histaminergic receptors and moderate affinity for α_2-adrenergic receptors. Risperidone is devoid of significant activity against the cholinergic system and dopamine D_1 receptors. Its efficacy is equal to that of other first-line SGAs, and it is well tolerated and can be given once or twice a day. The most common side effects reported are drowsiness, orthostatic hypotension, lightheadedness, anxiety, akathisia, constipation, nausea, nasal congestion, prolactin elevation, and weight gain. At dosages greater than 6 mg/day, EPS can become a significant issue. The risk of TD at regular therapeutic doses is low. Risperidone is also available in a liquid form, as rapidly disintegrating tablets (M-Tab), and as a long-acting intramuscular preparation (Risperdal Consta), which is given every 2 weeks. Risperidone (but not Risperdal Consta) is now available in a generic form.

Paliperidone, or 9-hydroxy-risperidone (an active metabolite of risperidone) was approved by the FDA in 2006 for treatment of schizophrenia. Paliperidone, like its parent compound risperidone, blocks dopamine D_2 receptors along with serotonin receptors. It was significantly efficacious in double-blind, placebo-controlled studies (Meltzer et al. 2008); however, prolactin levels were significantly increased in both men and women at any dosage. EPS, including dystonia and hyperkinesis, were more prevalent at 12 mg/day (10%) than at 6 mg/day (5%). Tachycardia was also more common than with placebo. Paliperidone does not undergo hepatic metabolism, thereby minimizing drug-drug interactions. An extended-release form of paliperidone is available through an osmotic-controlled release oral delivery system (OROS), in which there is an osmotic trilayer core, consisting of two distinct drug layers and an osmotic push layer. The extended-release formulation is reported to be well tolerated at dosages of 6, 9, and 12 mg/day.

Paliperidone palmitate extended-release injectable suspension (Invega Sustenna) was approved by the FDA in 2009 for the acute and maintenance treatment of schizophrenia. Therapeutic activity is mediated through central D_2 dopamine and serotonin (5-HT_{2A}) receptor antagonism, but it also has α_1- and α_2-adrenergic and H_1-histaminergic antagonism activity. The drug utilizes NanoCrystal® technology, which increases the rate of dissolution and allows monthly maintenance administration. After intramuscular injection, paliperidone palmitate dissolves slowly and then is hydrolyzed to paliperidone and absorbed into the general circulation, reaching maximum plasma concentrations in approximately two weeks. Paliperidone palmitate is initially dosed at 234 mg IM on day 1, followed by 156 mg on day 8, in the deltoid muscle; monthly maintenance doses can be administered in either the deltoid or gluteal muscle, with similar tolerability between injection sites (Hough et al. 2009). The most common treatment-emergent side effects are injection site reactions (deltoid > gluteal), sedation, dizziness, akathisia, and extrapyramidal disorder. FDA approval was based on four acute treatment studies and one longer-term maintenance study. Paliperidone palmitate was found to significantly increase time to relapse compared with the oral atypical antipsychotic quetiapine in a 2-year open-label, active-controlled, comparative international study (Medori et al. 2008).

Iloperidone was also approved by the FDA in 2009 for the acute treatment of schizophrenia. Efficacy is mediated through a combination of central D_2 dopamine and serotonin (5-HT_{2A}) receptor antagonism; it also has high binding affinity toward D_3 dopamine and moderate binding affinity toward D_4 dopamine, serotonin 5-$HT_{6/7}$ and α_1-adrenergic receptors. Iloperidone is available in tablets only and is dosed 12–24 mg daily. It is recommended that iloperidone be titrated slowly to reduce the incidence of treatment-emergent orthostatic hypotension. The slow initial titration may delay the onset of efficacy associated with a therapeutic dose level. Compared with placebo, the most commonly reported adverse reactions reported at dosages between 20 and 24 mg/day were dizziness (number needed to harm (NNH)=8), dry mouth (NNH=12), fatigue (NNH=34), nasal congestion (NNH=17), orthostatic hypotension (NNH=25), somnolence (NNH=10), tachycardia (NNH=10), and weight gain (NNH=13) (Citrome 2009). Extrapyramidal symptoms, including akathisia, bradykinesia, dyskinesia, dystonia, parkinsonism, and tremor, are reported to be rare with iloperidone.

Three 6-week double-blind, placebo-controlled studies of acute or sub-acute exacerbations of schizophrenia or schizoaffective disorder were conducted. The first study compared iloperidone (4, 8, or 12 mg/day) with halo-peridol (15 mg/day), the second study compared iloperidone (4–8 mg/day or 10–16 mg/day) with risperidone (4–8 mg/day), and the third compared ilo-peridone (12–16 mg/day or 20–24 mg/day) with risperidone (6–8 mg/day) (Potkin et al. 2008). In the first study, Positive and Negative Syndrome Scale scores significantly improved from baseline vs. placebo with iloperidone 12 mg/day only. In the second study, Brief Psychiatric Rating Scale (BPRS) scores significantly improved from baseline versus placebo with iloperidone 4–8 mg and 10–16 mg/day. In the third study, BPRS scores significantly improved from baseline versus placebo with iloperidone 20–24 mg/day only. Of note, mean improvements in the BPRS were numerically larger for the active competitors risperidone and haloperidol, but P values were not reported (Potkin et al. 2008). Long-term efficacy and safety of iloperidone were demonstrated in a pooled analysis of three 1-year double-blind prospective studies in patients with schizophrenia. Patients were randomly assigned to iloperidone 4–16 mg/day or haloperidol 5–20 mg/day after a 6-week stabilization phase. Iloperidone was not inferior to haloperidol in preventing relapse. Iloperidone was well tolerated and associated with a low risk for discontinuation due to adverse events (Kane et al. 2008).

Thienobenzodiazepines

The thienobenzodiazepines include olanzapine, the third SGA approved by the FDA (in 1996). Olanzapine has antagonistic effects at dopamine D_1 through D_5 receptors and serotonin 5-HT_{2A}, 5-HT_{2C}, and 5-HT_6 receptors. The anti-serotonergic activity is more potent than the antidopaminergic activity. Olanzapine also has affinity for α_1-adrenergic, M_1 muscarinic acetylcholinergic, and H_1 histaminergic receptors. Olanzapine differs from clozapine by not having high affinity for 5-HT_7, α_2-adrenergic, and other cholinergic receptors. It has significant efficacy against positive symptoms. EPS are reported to be minimal when olanzapine is used in the therapeutic range, with the exception of mild akathisia. Because the compound has a long half-life, it is used once a day; because it is well tolerated, it can be started at a higher dose or rapidly titrated to the most effective dose. Olanzapine is available as a rapidly disintegrating wafer (Zyprexa Zydis), which dissolves immediately in the mouth. A short-acting intramuscular form also has been approved by FDA. The major side effects of olanzapine are weight gain, hyperglycemia, hyperlipidemia, sedation, dry mouth, nausea, lightheadedness, orthostatic hypotension, dizziness, constipation, headache, akathisia, and transient elevation of hepatic transaminases. The risk of TD and neuroleptic malignant syndrome (NMS) is low. The average dosage of olanzapine is 15–20 mg/day. However, dosages higher than 20 mg/day are often used clinically. In the National Institute of Mental Health (NIMH)–sponsored Clinical Antipsychotic Trials of Intervention Effectiveness (CATIE) study, patients received olanzapine at dosages of up to 30 mg/day (Lieberman et al. 2005).

Dibenzothiazepines

The dibenzothiazepines include quetiapine, which was approved by the FDA in 1997 for use in treating schizophrenia. Quetiapine has a greater affinity for serotonin 5-HT$_2$ receptors than for dopamine D$_2$ receptors; it has considerable activity at dopamine D$_1$, D$_3$, D$_4$, D$_5$; serotonin 5-HT$_{1A}$; and α_1- and α_2-adrenergic receptors. Unlike clozapine, it lacks affinity for the muscarinic cholinergic receptors. Quetiapine is reported to be as effective as FGAs. In controlled studies, quetiapine at all doses used did not have a rate of EPS greater than that seen with placebo. This is in contrast to olanzapine, risperidone, and ziprasidone, which have dose-related effects on EPS levels. In addition, the rate of treatment-emergent EPS was very low, even in high-risk populations such as adolescents, parkinsonian patients with psychosis, and geriatric patients. Quetiapine has not been associated with hyperprolactinemia. Major side effects that have been reported are somnolence, postural hypotension, dizziness, agitation, dry mouth, and weight gain. Akathisia may occur on rare occasions. The package insert warns about the development of lenticular opacity or cataracts and advises that the patient have an eye examination every 6 months, although clinical data suggest that the risk of these ophthalmological conditions may be extremely low.

Quetiapine is available as tablets and as an extended-release version. It is usually administered twice a day because of its short half-life; however, the extended-release formulation, which can be given once a day, significantly decreases the titration rate because it can be started at 200 mg and quickly titrated to 600 to 800 mg within a few days. It may have a lower frequency of side effects than does the immediate-release form, which improves tolerance and provides patients an opportunity to take higher dosages within the therapeutic range.

Benzisothiazolyls

The benzisothiazolyl group of SGAs includes ziprasidone, which was approved by the FDA in 2001. It has a very strong 5-HT$_{2A}$ receptor binding relative to D_2 binding among the SGA agents currently in use. Ziprasidone has $5\text{-}HT_{1A}$ agonist and $5\text{-}HT_{1D}$ antagonist properties and a high affinity for $5\text{-}HT_{1A}$, $5\text{-}HT_{2C}$, and $5\text{-}HT_{1D}$ receptors. It does not cause anticholinergic side effects and produces little orthostatic hypotension and relatively little sedation. Just like some antidepressants, ziprasidone blocks presynaptic reuptake of serotonin and norepinephrine. Ziprasidone has a relatively short half-life and thus should be administered twice a day; it is most effective at dosages between 80 and 160 mg/day for treating symptoms of schizophrenia. Ziprasidone should be taken with meals to obtain adequate blood levels. The major side effects reported with the use of ziprasidone are somnolence, nausea, insomnia, dyspepsia, and prolongation of the QTc interval. Dizziness, weakness, nasal discharge, orthostatic hypotension, and tachycardia occur less commonly. Ziprasidone should not be used in combination with other drugs that cause *significant* prolongation of the QTc interval. It is also contraindicated for patients with a known history of significant QTc prolongation, recent myocardial infarction, or symptomatic heart failure. Ziprasidone has low EPS potential, does not elevate prolactin levels, and causes approximately 1 pound (0.45 kg) of weight gain in short-term studies. Ziprasidone is available in pill form and as a short-acting intramuscular preparation.

Quinolinones

The quinolinone group of SGAs includes aripiprazole, which was approved by the FDA in 2002 for the treatment of schizophrenia. Aripiprazole has a different mechanism of action; as a partial agonist at the dopamine D_2 receptor, it behaves as a functional dopamine D_2 antagonist in hyperdopaminergic environments and as a functional dopamine agonist in hypodopaminergic environments. This mechanism of action is thought to "modulate" and "stabilize" the dopaminergic system. It is also a serotonin $5\text{-}HT_{2A}$ antagonist and partial agonist at $5\text{-}HT_{1A}$ receptors. It has moderate affinity for α_1-adrenergic and histamine H_1 receptors, with no significant effect at the anticholinergic receptors. Aripiprazole has a long half-life (75 hours). It is dosed once a day, is well absorbed orally, and is not affected by administration of food.

As an antipsychotic medication in nongeriatric adults, aripiprazole offers the following advantages: 1) it is perhaps the least sedating antipsychotic agent currently available; 2) it does not increase prolactin levels and may even decrease them from baseline; 3) it causes significantly less weight gain in adults (1 kg/year); 4) it does not significantly elevate mean serum glucose levels; 5) it does not significantly elevate mean serum lipid levels; 6) it does not prolong the QTc interval; and 7) it has a relatively low rate of EPS.

However, aripiprazole may cause nausea and akathisia during the early phase of the treatment. Because it is metabolized by cytochrome P450 (CYP)

3A4 and 2D6, the aripiprazole dose may need to be adjusted with 3A4 inducers such as carbamazepine and 3A4 and 2D6 inhibitors such as fluoxetine. It is available in oral tablets, as liquid, and as a short-acting intramuscular preparation (for details, see Patel et al. 2008).

Dibenzo-oxepino Pyrroles

Asenapine was approved by the FDA in 2009 for the treatment of schizophrenia. Belonging to the dibenzo-oxepino pyrrole class, treatment effects are mediated through a combination of antagonist activity at D_2 and 5-HT_{2A} receptors. Asenapine has high binding affinity for dopamine D_2, D_3, D_4, and D_1 receptors, serotonin 5-HT_{1A}, 5-HT_{1B}, 5-HT_{2A}, 5-HT_{2B}, 5-HT_{2C}, 5-HT_5, 5-HT_6, and 5-HT_7, α_1- and α_2-adrenergic receptors, and histamine H_1 receptors. As it does not have affinity for muscarinic cholinergic receptors, there is minimal risk of anticholinergic side effects compared with some other antipsychotics. Asenapine may be started and maintained at 5 mg sublingually twice daily. The tablet is placed under the tongue and left to dissolve; it should not be swallowed, and eating and drinking should be withheld for 10 minutes after administration. The most commonly reported side effects are akathisia, oral hypoesthesia, and somnolence. Short-term efficacy was demonstrated in a double-blind, three-arm fixed-dose, 6-week placebo- and risperidone-controlled trial (Potkin et al. 2007). Compared with placebo, mean improvements on PANSS total, negative subscale, and general psychopathology subscale scores were all statistically significantly greater with asenapine than with placebo from week 2 or 3 onward. There were no significant between-group (risperidone vs. asenapine) differences in medication adherence rates during the study, and there were no reports of QT interval prolongation >500 ms in any treatment group. There was a higher incidence of clinically significant weight gain in the risperidone group (17%) versus the asenapine (4.3%) or placebo (1.9%) groups. End-of-study prolactin levels 2 times the upper limit of normal were more prevalent in the risperidone (79%) than in the asenapine (9%) or placebo (2%) groups.

Mechanism of Action of Second-Generation Antipsychotics

Dopamine

Dopamine hyperactivity was proposed to underlie the pathophysiology of schizophrenia in 1973 and quickly became the dominant hypothesis for many years. This was not surprising because all commercially available antipsychotic agents at that time had antagonistic effects on the dopamine D_2 receptor in relation to their clinical potencies. Furthermore, dopamine agonists, such as amphetamine and methylphenidate, exacerbated psychotic symptoms in a subgroup of patients with schizophrenia. However, the dopamine hyperactivity hypothesis and the primacy of D_2 antagonism for antipsychotic drug action were seriously questioned largely because of clozapine, the most efficacious treatment for chronic schizophrenia despite having one of the lowest levels of D_2 occupancy of all antipsychotic drugs. In vivo brain imaging studies found that clozapine D_2 occupancy levels were as low as 20% more than 12 hours after the last dose of medication in patients deriving excellent antipsychotic efficacy (compared with more than 80% D_2 occupancy for haloperidol). This started an extensive search for explanations underlying the extraordinary efficacy of clozapine.

FGAs and SGAs are effective only when their D_2 receptor occupancy exceeds 50%–65%, reinforcing the importance of D_2 antagonism in producing antipsychotic effects. The five subtypes of dopamine receptors are D_1, D_2, D_3, D_4, and D_5. Dopamine agonists improve negative symptoms of schizophrenia. These and other data led to a revised model of dopamine dysfunction, which stated that deficits in dopamine, perhaps in the prefrontal cortex, may result in negative and cognitive symptoms and that concomitant dopamine dysregulation causing dopamine increases in the striatum, perhaps related to faulty presynaptic control of dopamine release, may be involved in positive symptoms. However, the dopaminergic system interacts with serotonergic, glutamatergic, and other systems such that changes in one system affect the balance of the other systems too.

Serotonin

Interest in serotonin as a pathophysiological candidate in schizophrenia arose in 1956 with the discovery that the hallucinogen lysergic acid diethylamide (LSD), which produces psychosis, with similarities to schizophrenia, had primary effects on serotonin neurotransmission. Clozapine has a relatively high affinity for specific serotonin receptors (5-HT_{2A} and 5-HT_{2C}), and risperidone has even greater serotonin antagonistic properties. Most SGAs have a greater ratio of serotonin 5-HT_{2A} to dopamine D_2 binding affinity. This led to the hypothesis that the balance between serotonin and dopamine may be altered in schizophrenia. Serotonin 5-HT_{2A} (and other serotonin) receptor occupancy by the antipsychotic drugs (depending on the areas of the brain involved), along with the synergistic effect of dopamine D_2 and 5-HT_{2A} antagonism, could be associated with improvement in cognition, depression, and D_2 receptor–mediated EPS.

Glutamate and NMDA

Glutamate is the primary brain excitatory amino acid neurotransmitter and is critically involved in learning, memory, and brain development. Approximately 60% of the neurons in the brain, including all cortical pyramidal neurons and thalamic relay neurons, use glutamate as their primary neurotransmitter. The glutamate receptors are divided into ionotropic and metabotropic receptors. The ionotropic receptors are linked directly to ion channels and include N-methyl-D-aspartate (NMDA), α-amino-3-hydroxy-5-methyl-4-isoxazole propionic acid (AMPA), and kainate; metabotropic receptors are linked to second-messenger systems and are divided into groups I, II, and III according to their functional activity. Interest in glutamate and the NMDA receptor in schizophrenia arose because of the similarity between phencyclidine (PCP) psychosis and the psychosis of schizophrenia. PCP is a noncompetitive antagonist of the NMDA receptor and produces a psychotic state that includes conceptual disorganization, auditory hallucinations, delusions, and negative symptoms. PCP produces more symptoms that are similar to those of schizophrenia than do most other pharmacological agents.

The glutamate hypothesis of schizophrenia is one of the most active areas of research currently. Thus, hypoglutamatergia in schizophrenia may have very important downstream modulatory effects on catecholaminergic neurotransmission and play a critical role during neurodevelopment. It also plays an important role in synaptic pruning and underlies important aspects of neurocognition.

Issues Underlying Mechanism of Actions of Antipsychotics

A higher ratio of the serotonin 5-HT_{2A} receptor to dopamine D_2 receptor blockade is reported to predict atypicality. This finding, along with other data, formed the basis of the *serotonin-dopamine hypothesis* that explains the possible mechanism of action underlying the efficacy of SGAs (Meltzer et al. 1989). However, studies that used positron emission tomography (PET) failed to detect differences in the serotonin receptor affinities between FGAs and SGAs. Moreover, SGAs produce high 5-HT_{2A} receptor occupancy at doses that are not sufficient to produce antipsychotic effects. Although FGAs, compared with SGAs, show a much higher affinity for the D_2 receptors, both are effective only when their D_2 receptor occupancy exceeds 50%–65%, suggesting that D_2 antagonism is important in producing antipsychotic effects.

A major difference between FGAs and SGAs may lie in their affinity for the D_2 receptor. *Affinity* is the ratio of the rate at which the drug moves off of and on to the receptor. PET studies suggest that all antipsychotics (FGAs and SGAs) attach to the D_2 receptor with a similar rate constant but differ in how fast they come off of the receptor (K_{off}). Kapur and Seeman (2001) proposed that this relation between fast K_{off} and low receptor affinity of the antipsychotic drug for dopamine D_2 receptor may explain atypicality. Furthermore, antipsychotic agents modulate dopaminergic transmission and compete with endogenous dopamine. Thus, drugs with fast K_{off} (e.g., clozapine, quetiapine) modulate dopamine transmission differently from drugs with a slow K_{off} (e.g., haloperidol). Clinically, a significant difference between the FGA and the SGA medications is the extent to which EPS occur during treatment with therapeutic doses of antipsychotic drugs. PET studies suggest that the threshold for clinical antipsychotic response is lower than that for developing EPS and can be separated on the basis of D_2 receptor occupancy.

Specifically, D_2 occupancy of 65% or more significantly predicted clinical response, whereas D_2 occupancy of 78% or higher significantly predicted EPS. Similarly, D_2 occupancy of 72% or higher resulted in prolactin elevation. Risperidone and olanzapine achieve strong antipsychotic activity only at doses that occupy 65% or more D_2 receptors, which is similar to haloperidol. On the contrary, although clozapine and quetiapine show less than 60% D_2 occupancy 12 hours after drug administration, these differences partly reflect a fast decline in D_2 occupancy. Antipsychotic agents, both FGAs and SGAs, give rise to EPS only when they exceed 78%–80% D_2 occupancy. Because clozapine and quetiapine never exceed this threshold of D_2 occupancy, they do not give rise to EPS. Because olanzapine and risperidone exceed this threshold in a dose-dependent fashion, they give rise to EPS also in a dose-dependent fashion.

Partial Agonism of D_2 Receptors

Partial dopamine agonists such as aripiprazole bind to the D_2 receptor and block the effects of extracellular physiologically active dopamine but also have intrinsic agonistic effects at this receptor. Aripiprazole, in therapeutic doses, occupies about 95% of the striatal D_2 receptors but does not rapidly dissociate because it has one of the highest D_2 receptor affinities. Yet in clinical situations, it has a low risk for EPS. This is probably a result of approximately 30% intrinsic agonistic activity at the D_2 receptor. The delayed onset of action of antipsychotic drugs is thought to be due to remodeling of neuronal structures and circuits rather than exclusively receptor blockade or changes in neurotransmitter levels.

Treatment of Schizophrenia

Medical Workup When Initiating and Continuing Antipsychotics

The recommended medical workup when antipsychotic medications are being initiated is shown in Appendix 4. Also shown there are the recommended medical tests when antipsychotic medications are being continued. The recommended medical tests for initiation and continued treatment with clozapine are shown in Appendix 5.

Randomized controlled trials suggest that, on average, an antipsychotic agent is associated with at least 20% improvement in symptoms. Recent pragmatic real-world studies and meta-analyses give olanzapine an edge over the other SGAs, except clozapine, for clinical efficacy. However, excessive weight gain and lipid elevations with olanzapine and clozapine have been reported. Clozapine is the only antipsychotic agent that is more effective than most currently available antipsychotics in managing treatment-resistant schizophrenia (Kane et al. 1988, 2001; McEvoy et al. 2006). Unfortunately, its potential for treatment-emergent agranulocytosis, seizures, and myocarditis precludes its use as a first-line agent for schizophrenia.

Dosing and Administration

The dosing and administration of FGAs and SGAs, including dosing in patients with hepatic impairment, renal impairment, and special populations, are summarized in Appendix 3.

Acute Treatment

Acute symptoms or relapses are heralded by positive symptoms, including delusions, hallucinations, disorganized speech or behavior, severe negative symptoms, or catatonia. Frequently, a relapse is a result of antipsychotic discontinuation, and resumption of antipsychotic treatment aids in the resolution of symptoms. A high degree of variability in response rates is seen among individuals. Improvement in clinical symptoms can be seen over hours, days, or weeks of treatment. The primary goal of acute treatment is the amelioration of any behavioral disturbances that would put the patient or others at risk for harm. Although FGAs are effective, no convincing evidence indicates that one FGA is more efficacious as an antipsychotic than any other; however, a given individual may respond better to a specific drug.

With so many antipsychotics available, making an informed choice between using an FGA or an SGA by the patient and the clinician should be based on efficacy, side-effect profile, history of prior response (or nonresponse) to a specific agent, or history of response of a family member to a certain antipsychotic agent. Among FGAs, low-potency and sedating agents such as chlorpromazine are as effective as the high-potency agents such as haloperidol in the treatment of agitated patients. The low-potency antipsychotics, however, are frequently associated with orthostatic hypotension and lowered seizure threshold and are often not as well tolerated at higher doses. Higher-potency antipsychotics, such as haloperidol and fluphenazine, are safely used at higher doses and are effective in reducing agitation and psychosis. However, they are more likely to cause EPS than are the low-potency agents and SGAs.

The significantly low potential to cause EPS or dystonic reactions, and thus the decreased long-term consequences of TD, has made SGAs more acceptable in acute treatment of schizophrenia. Other significant advantages adding to the popularity of some SGAs include the beneficial effect on mood symptoms. They are easy to use, have rapid action depending on the type of preparation used (e.g., liquid, rapidly disintegrating forms, or intramuscular), and may have a better side-effect profile for acute treatment (depending on the SGA used), promoting individualized treatment.

Thus, the selection of the antipsychotic will depend on the circumstances under which the medications are started; for example, extremely agitated or incompetent patients who are refusing court-mandated treatments or catatonic patients would require an intramuscular preparation, rapidly disintegrating oral tablets, or a liquid preparation of antipsychotics. Available data suggest that SGA intramuscular preparations such as ziprasidone, olanzapine, and aripiprazole may hold significant advantages over the intramuscular FGAs such as haloperidol. However, they are also significantly more expensive).

Except for clozapine, which is not considered first-line treatment because of substantial and potentially life-threatening side effects, no convincing data support the preference of one FGA or SGA over another.

However, if the patient's symptoms do not respond to one antipsychotic, a trial with another antipsychotic is reasonable and may produce response. Once the decision is made to use an antipsychotic agent, an appropriate dose must be selected. Initially, higher doses or repeated dosing may be helpful in preventing grossly psychotic and agitated patients from doing harm. In general, doses of high-potency antipsychotics such as haloperidol can be maintained up to 10 mg/day in an acute setting. Early adjuvant anticholinergic medications may facilitate compliance by decreasing side effects. Extremely agitated or aggressive patients may benefit from concomitant administration of high-potency benzodiazepines such as lorazepam, at 1–2 mg, until they are stable. Benzodiazepines rapidly decrease anxiety, calm the person, and help with sedation to break the cycle of agitation. They also help decrease agitation due to akathisia. The use of these medications should be limited to the acute stages of the illness to prevent tachyphylaxis and dependency.

Maintenance Treatment

Long-term follow-up studies suggest that patients have a higher risk of relapse and exacerbations if adequate antipsychotic regimens are not maintained (Hogarty et al. 1986). Noncompliance with medication, possibly because of intolerable antipsychotic side effects or other factors, may contribute to increased relapse rates. Approximately two-thirds of patients relapse after 9–12 months without antipsychotic medication, compared with 10%–30% who relapse when FGAs are maintained. Long-term studies suggest that patients with persistent symptoms that do not respond to FGA therapy have a greater risk of rehospitalization. Nonpharmacological interventions may help decrease relapse rates. The CATIE study and others have shown that almost 75% of subjects will switch or discontinue antipsychotic medications within the first 18 months (Lieberman et al. 2005). This occurs even with antipsychotics that have low potential for EPS. Unfortunately, even with SGAs, treatment compliance rates are not substantially better (Keith 2006).

Long-term medication treatment of schizophrenia is inherently complex because most of these patients require maintenance antipsychotic medication. A small group of patients may do well while taking stable doses of antipsychotics for years without any exacerbations, whereas another group of patients who are receiving maintenance therapy with a stable antipsychotic dose have episodic breakthroughs of their psychotic symptoms. Unfortunately, side effects often contribute to medication noncompliance. It is prudent to assess patients for medication compliance when signs of relapse are suspected, especially if prodromal cues are present such as recent change in sleep pattern, changes in activities of daily living, or disorganization.

In a landmark study comparing risperidone with haloperidol for effects on maintenance treatment, at the end of 1 year, patients taking risperidone were significantly better clinically, were more compliant, had fewer relapses (34% for the risperidone group and 60% for the haloperidol group), and had fewer EPS than those in the haloperidol group (Csernansky et al. 2002). These findings led to an FDA indication for the use of risperidone for the maintenance treatment of schizophrenia.

Long-term use of olanzapine, quetiapine, aripiprazole, and ziprasidone also was reported to have significant beneficial effects in comparison to either placebo or an FGA such as haloperidol. Although reviewing all the data would be beyond the scope of this chapter, some of the important studies are reviewed in the next section. Clozapine enjoys superiority compared with other treatments, especially for treatment-refractory symptoms; long-term randomized trials have found significant reduction in rehospitalization (Essock et al. 1996; for more details, see Patel et al. 2008) and suicide rates (Meltzer and Okayli 1995).

For patients for whom compliance is a problem, long-acting preparations of antipsychotics are available in the United States for fluphenazine, haloperidol, paliperidone, and risperidone. Fluphenazine or haloperidol is esterified in an oily solution that is injected every 1–6 weeks to circumvent the need for daily oral antipsychotic medications and daily monitoring. This alternative should be considered if noncompliance has led to relapses and re-hospitalization. With these patients, maintenance treatment with long-acting preparations should begin as early as possible.

Depot antipsychotic medications are effective maintenance therapy for patients with schizophrenia. Unlike the decanoate compounds of FGAs, Risperdal Consta has risperidone, an SGA, which is encapsulated into microspheres made of biodegradable polymer suspended in an aqueous diluent. After injection, very little active moiety is released for up to 3 weeks, and thus oral therapy should be continued during this period. With repeated administration every 2 weeks, steady-state plasma levels are reached after the fourth injection and are maintained for 4–6 weeks after the last injection. Another SGA, paliperidone palmitate injection, which is administered every 4 weeks, utilizes NanoCrystal® technology for monthly maintenance treatment.

Compared with the daily immediate-release oral therapy, treatment with Risperdal Consta is associated with reductions in peak blood levels of approximately 30% and also decreased plasma peak-to-trough ratios by 32%–42% and may cause fewer adverse effects. Long-term data report significant decreases in hospitalization rates with a better tolerability profile than with FGAs. Effective maintenance treatment is defined as that which prevents or minimizes the risks of symptom exacerbation, relapse, and subsequent morbidity.

In dose-finding studies to determine the minimal dosage required to prevent relapse and to reduce the risk of EPS and TD, the relapse rate (56%) for patients taking lower doses of fluphenazine decanoate (1.25–5 mg every 2 weeks) was significantly greater than the relapse rate (14%) for patients receiving standard doses (12.5–50 mg every 2 weeks). Low dosage range may appear to prevent relapse for a certain period but fails to do so if patients are followed up for more than 1 year. Unfortunately, no specific dosage reliably prevents relapse, and there is no way to predict future relapse. This is true for SGAs as well.

Plasma drug levels and their correlation with clinical response remain controversial. At this time, plasma drug levels are not recommended for dosage determination. They are clinically useful, however, for confirming compliance with medication and may provide information about toxicity or altered metabolism.

Second-Generation (Except Clozapine) Versus First-Generation Antipsychotics in Management of Schizophrenia

Clozapine is superior to all other antipsychotics in treating patients who are

- Treatment refractory
- Hostile and aggressive

- Suicidal
- Concurrently using drugs and alcohol
- Having polydipsia and water intoxication
- Intolerant to neurological side effects of other antipsychotic agents

SGAs and FGAs are reported to have generally equivalent efficacy against positive symptoms. Among the antipsychotics available in the United States, clozapine is clearly more effective than FGAs. Risperidone, paliperidone, and olanzapine belong to the group of antipsychotics that are considered more effective than FGAs. Aripiprazole, quetiapine, and ziprasidone are viewed as not superior to FGAs. These results were not likely a result of higher and unfavorable doses of FGAs. According to data from meta-analyses, it appears that SGAs may be better than FGAs in the maintenance treatment of schizophrenia because restoration of social functions and better efficacy against negative symptoms, depression, and thought disorder may favor their use (Davis and Chen 2005). However, data from a recent meta-analysis do not support this (except for clozapine) (Leucht et al. 2009). Since asenapine and iloperidone were just introduced to the market, we will have to wait and see how they work in "real world" patients.

Data from clinical trials often provide confusing and inconsistent results. When 42 head-to-head studies of SGAs were analyzed, there appeared to be a bias in industry-sponsored studies because in 90% of the studies supported by pharmaceutical companies, the outcome favored the sponsoring company. To address such shortcomings, including study design issues, the NIMH embarked on its most ambitious and expensive project, called CATIE. With the increase in number of antipsychotic agents and lingering questions about FGA use in light of perceived superiority of SGAs, CATIE investigators compared the effectiveness of olanzapine, quetiapine, risperidone, ziprasidone, and perphenazine on the primary outcome measure of *discontinuation of treatment for any cause,* a discrete outcome selected because stopping or changing medication is a frequent occurrence and a major problem in the treatment of schizophrenia. This measure also integrates patients' and clinicians' judgments of efficacy, safety, and tolerability into a global measure of effectiveness that reflects their evaluation of therapeutic benefits in relation to undesirable effects. This all-cause treatment discontinuation measure is a proxy for the decision process in the real world and reflects the ongoing joint evaluation by clinicians and patients as to whether a particular treatment is acceptable or needs to be changed. Perphenazine was chosen as a representative FGA on the basis of its intermediate potency among the FGAs and lower likelihood of EPS. The study was done in a real-world setting and with a representative patient sample to inform clinical practice directly.

The study had three phases. In Phase 1, the study enrolled 1,460 subjects, and this made it the largest study of its kind. Patients with any comorbid condition, active substance abuse, and medical issues that were stable were allowed to participate, whereas first-episode subjects and subjects with treatment-refractory symptoms were excluded. Patients were randomly assigned to double-blind treatment and followed up for 18 months. Aripiprazole, asenapine, iloperidone, and paliperidone were not included because they were approved after the study started. The 231 patients who had TD at study entry were randomly assigned to only SGAs rather than to perphenazine. The most prominent finding of the CATIE study was the 74% all-cause discontinuation rate for all antipsychotic drugs studied. The time to discontinuation was significantly longer for olanzapine than for risperidone and quetiapine. The differences between olanzapine and either perphenazine or ziprasidone were no longer significant after adjustment for multiple comparisons, possibly because of lower sample sizes for the latter two agents.

Although olanzapine was associated with a longer duration of treatment than were the other antipsychotic drugs, it was associated with the highest frequency of metabolic side effects, including increases in weight, blood glucose, cholesterol, triglycerides, and glycosylated hemoglobin. In contrast, patients receiving ziprasidone had the best overall metabolic profile. More patients (8%) discontinued the FGA perphenazine because of neurological side effects compared with those taking SGAs (2%–4%). Overall, most of the patients in each group discontinued their assigned treatment because of inefficacy or intolerable side effects or for other reasons. These and other data from the CATIE study exposed the significant limitations of both FGAs and SGAs. Moreover, the cost-effectiveness data suggested that there were no significant differences between perphenazine and SGAs on quality-of-life improvements, and the average total monthly costs were 20%–30% lower for perphenazine than for SGAs mainly because of lower drug costs.

The Phase 2 trial in the CATIE study consisted of two pathways. Those in Phase 1 who discontinued the medication because of lack of efficacy before 18 months could be randomly assigned to the efficacy arm, called the "clozapine arm." The other pathway was called the "tolerability arm" or "ziprasidone arm"; patients who had problems with tolerability and/or refused clozapine were assigned to this arm. Clozapine was given open label, but other medications were administered in a double-blind manner. The time to treatment discontinuation was significantly longer for clozapine at 10.5 months compared with quetiapine at 3.3 months, risperidone at 2.8 months, and olanzapine at 2.7 months. In the ziprasidone arm, the median time to treatment discontinuation was longest for risperidone (7 months) and olanzapine (6.3 months) compared with both quetiapine (4 months) and ziprasidone (2.8 months). Relatively small sample sizes and the fact that clozapine was administered open label prevented definitive conclusions; however, these data are directionally consistent with previous studies (Lieberman et al. 2005; McEvoy et al. 2006).

Cost Utility of the Latest Antipsychotic Drugs in Schizophrenia Study (CUtLASS 1), a pragmatic multicenter, rater-blinded, randomized controlled study funded by the U.K. National Health Service, was designed to test the effectiveness of antipsychotics in routine clinical practice. Using broad inclusion criteria, the study followed up on 287 patients for 1 year at 14 community psychiatric services while the patients were receiving either FGAs or SGAs. The main outcome measures were quality-of-life scale scores, symptoms, adverse effects, participant satisfaction, and costs of care. The main results of the study were that participants in the FGA arm showed a trend toward greater improvements in quality-of-life scale and symptom scores. Participants did not report preference for either drug group, and the costs were comparable. Only 59% of the subjects continued taking their originally assigned medication for the full year (Jones et al. 2006).

Thus, the important message from these studies is that current antipsychotic medications are imperfect drugs, with no one group of drugs being preferred over the other. The positive effect of olanzapine was modest and offset by serious metabolic side effects. These studies strongly made the case for individualizing treatments for schizophrenic patients.

Depression and Schizophrenia

Symptoms of depression occur in a substantial percentage of patients with schizophrenia (up to 75%) and are associated with poor outcome, impaired functioning, suffering, higher rates of relapse or rehospitalization, and suicide. It is important to distinguish depression as a symptom or as a syndrome when it occurs because there is an important overlap of symptoms of depression with the negative symptoms. Differentiating these states can sometimes be difficult, especially in patients who lack the interpersonal communication skills to articulate their internal subjective states well. A link between FGA use and depression has been suggested, with some considering depression to be a form of medication-induced akinesia. Many patients have a reaction of disappointment, a sense of loss or powerlessness, or awareness of psychotic symptoms or psychological deficits that contributes to depression (Lysaker et al. 1995).

Depression in schizophrenia is heterogeneous and requires careful diagnostic clarification. DSM-IV-TR (American Psychiatric Association 2000) suggests that the term *postpsychotic depression* be used to describe depression that occurs at any time after a psychotic episode of schizophrenia, even after a prolonged interval. However, many patients still end up with a depression that will require treatment with an antidepressant. Finally, it is also important to differentiate "postpsychotic depression" in schizophrenia from major depression, with psychotic features (see Chapter 3, "Mood and Anxiety Disorders," in this volume).

Risks and Side Effects

The side effects of commonly used antipsychotics are shown in Appendix 7. The recommendations for management of various side effects of antipsychotic medications are summarized in Appendix 8.

Extrapyramidal Symptoms and Neurological Side Effects

Neurological side effects more commonly associated with FGA medications are dystonias, oculogyric crisis, pseudoparkinsonism, akinesia, and akathisia. They are referred to collectively as *extrapyramidal symptoms,* or EPS, because they are mediated at least in part by dopaminergic transmission in the extrapyramidal system. Prevalence rates vary among the different types of EPS. When present, they can be uncomfortable for the patient and a reason for noncompliance.

Dystonias are involuntary muscular spasms that can be brief or sustained, involving any muscle group. They can occur with even a single dose of medication. When they develop suddenly, these spasms can be quite frightening to the patient and potentially dangerous, as in the case of laryngeal dystonias. They are more likely to be seen in young patients. Prevalence rates for dystonias secondary to FGA exposure range from 2% to 20%. Dystonias occur less commonly with SGAs.

Pseudoparkinsonism and akinesia are characterized by muscular rigidity, tremor, and bradykinesia. Patients typically have masked facies, cogwheel rigidity, slowing, and decreased arm swing with a shuffling gait. These symptoms occur in 15%–35% of patients taking FGAs and significantly less commonly with SGAs. Akathisia affects more than 20% of patients taking FGA medications. Patients report motor restlessness accompanied by an internal sense of restlessness. Often patients experiencing akathisia are unable to sit still during an interview. It is very important, but often difficult, to differentiate akathisia from agitation. Use of increased doses of antipsychotics may exacerbate akathisia; similarly, psychotic agitation would worsen if the dose of antipsychotic were decreased, making treatment decisions challenging.

Treatment of EPS can be difficult but usually involves administration of anticholinergic medications. Some advocate the use of prophylactic anticholinergic agents when beginning FGA treatment to decrease the incidence of EPS. This option may be appropriate, but it should be used with caution, considering the side effects associated with anticholinergic agents and their potential for abuse.

Treatment of acute dystonic reactions usually involves acute intramuscular administration of either an anticholinergic medication or diphenhydramine. Akathisia may not respond to anticholinergic medications. Both antipsychotic dosage reduction and the use of β-blocking agents such as propranolol have been found to be efficacious in the treatment of akathisia.

A major risk of antipsychotic treatment, especially with FGAs, is that of tardive dyskinesia, a potentially irreversible syndrome of involuntary choreoathetoid movements and chronic dystonias associated with long-term antipsychotic exposure. These buccal, orofacial, truncal, or limb movements can be exacerbated by anxiety and disappear during sleep. They can present with a range of severity, from subtle tongue movements to truncal twisting and pelvic thrusting movements and even possible respiratory dyskinesias. The prevalence rates for this syndrome range from less than 10% to more than 50%, but it is generally accepted that the risk increases 3%–5% per year for each year the patient takes FGAs (Kane et al. 1988).

- Older age is a considerable risk factor for TD.
- Some evidence suggests that women are at increased risk for the development of TD.
- A withdrawal dyskinesia that resembles TD may appear on cessation of the antipsychotic.
- The specific mechanism involved in TD remains unclear, although supersensitivity of dopaminergic receptors has been implicated.

All patients receiving antipsychotic treatment should be monitored regularly for any signs of a movement disorder. If TD is suspected, the benefits of antipsychotic treatment must be carefully weighed against the risk of TD. This should be discussed with the patient, and the antipsychotic should be removed if it is clinically feasible to do so or at least maintained at the lowest possible dose that provides antipsychotic effect. This would also be an indication to switch to an antipsychotic agent with reduced risk of TD or, in the case of clozapine, no risk of TD. In many instances, clozapine (and possibly quetiapine or olanzapine) may be the best treatment that can be offered for the TD itself. Unfortunately, there is no specific treatment for TD, and adrenergic agents such as clonidine, calcium channel blockers, vitamin E, benzodiazepines, valproic acid, or reserpine to reduce the spontaneous movements have been suggested as possible treatment options.

Neuroleptic Malignant Syndrome

Neuroleptic malignant syndrome is a rare but potentially serious phenomenon seen in approximately 1% of patients taking FGAs. It can be fatal in 15% of cases if not properly recognized and treated. To address the difficulties in making the diagnosis of NMS, Levenson (1985) proposed three major or two major and four minor manifestations as indicative of a high probability of NMS. Major manifestations of NMS are fever, rigidity, and increased creatine kinase levels, and minor manifestations include tachycardia, abnormal blood pressure, tachypnea, altered consciousness, diaphoresis, and leukocytosis. (It should be noted that not everyone subscribes to the major–minor manifestation distinctions.) In general, NMS is considered to be a constellation of symptoms that usually develops during 1–3 days. Although its pathogenesis is poorly understood, it has been associated with all antidopaminergic antipsychotic agents and can present at any time during treatment. It must be distinguished from other clinical entities, including catatonia, malignant hyperthermia, and serotonin syndrome.

The mainstay of treatment of NMS is cessation of antipsychotic therapy and supportive care, including intravenous hydration, reversal of fever with antipyretics and cooling blankets, and careful monitoring of vital signs because of the risk of cardiac and respiratory disturbance. Rhabdomyolysis, one of the most serious sequelae of NMS, can lead to renal failure unless patients are well hydrated (Levenson 1985). In some cases, dantrolene and bromocriptine have been reported to be effective pharmacological treatments.

Although quite rare, NMS has been reported even with the use of SGAs. The decision to rechallenge the patient with antipsychotics after an episode of NMS must be made with caution. Given the potential risk involved, informed consent related to a rechallenge is important and should be obtained unless there is a valid clinical or legal basis that it would not be required.

Sudden Death

Sudden death in psychiatric patients taking FGA drugs has been reported for a long time. Sudden cardiac deaths probably occur from prolongation of the ventricular action potential duration, represented as the QT interval (or QTc when corrected for heart rate) on the ECG, resulting in a polymorphic ventricular tachycardia termed *torsades de pointes* that can degenerate into ventricular fibrillation. The incidence of torsades de pointes is unknown, and the specific duration of the QTc interval at which the risk of an adverse cardiac event is greatest has not been established. QTc prolongation alone does not appear to explain torsades de pointes; several other risk factors must be present simultaneously with QT prolongation before torsades de pointes occurs. These risk factors may include hypokalemia, hypomagnesemia, hypocalcemia, bradycardia, preexisting cardiac diseases (life-threatening arrhythmias, cardiac hypertrophy, heart failure, and congenital long QT syndrome), female gender, advancing age, baseline QTc interval of more than 460 msec, and medications that prolong QTc interval (Tamargo 2000). In some instances, torsades de pointes may be associated with an increase in drug plasma concentrations (e.g., combination with drugs that inhibit the CYP systems). The frequency of ECG abnormalities in patients taking antipsychotic drugs is unclear. QTc prolongation has been reported with virtually all antipsychotic drugs. QTc prolongation by more than 2 standard deviations was reported in 8% of psychiatric patients taking antipsychotics and especially in those receiving thioridazine (Zarate and Patel 2001). Cardiac consultation should be considered in any patient with a QTc interval greater than 450 msec because a QTc interval greater than 500 msec significantly increases the risk for cardiac arrhythmias.

Of the FGA drugs, haloperidol, chlorpromazine, trifluoperazine, mesoridazine, prochlorperazine, droperidol, and fluphenazine all have been reported to cause QTc prolongation and torsades de pointes, but thioridazine may be the worst offender. Pimozide also has been associated with QTc prolongation, torsades de pointes, and deaths. A reevaluation by the FDA of the cardiac safety parameters of thioridazine, mesoridazine, and droperidol resulted in a black-box warning because of significant QTc prolongation. New data from a large Medicaid sample suggest that commonly used FGAs and SGAs such as haloperidol, thioridazine, clozapine, olanzapine, quetiapine, and risperidone are associated with a similar and dose-related increased risk of sudden cardiac death (Ray et al. 2001, 2009). Thus, it is important to monitor QTc interval frequently, especially in the high-risk population, to prevent this rare but potentially fatal side effect.

Weight and Metabolic Side Effects

Treatment-emergent substantial weight gain and changes in metabolic measures and their long-term health consequences undermine the significant neurological advantages offered by the SGAs. Moreover, metabolic issues are a frequent and important reason for noncompliance with medication. Accumulated data clearly imply that among the SGAs, clozapine and olanzapine are associated with the most weight gain; ziprasidone and aripiprazole are associated with the lowest weight gain; and risperidone, paliperidone, and quetiapine are associated with intermediate weight gain. Based on limited data, recently approved iloperidone may belong to the intermediate group, while asenapine may belong to the lowest weight gain group. Molindone, an FGA, is not associated with weight gain. However, it is important to recognize that patients with schizophrenia, independent of the use of antipsychotic agents, are already at higher risk for developing diabetes mellitus relative to the general population (Thakore et al. 2002). Diabetes mellitus and obesity among patients with major mental illness were substantially higher even before the advent of SGAs, especially in women and the nonwhite population (Dixon et al. 2000). Thus, patients with schizophrenia are at a higher risk to develop major medical problems such as central obesity even *before* they are exposed to antipsychotic medications. Higher rates of diabetes have been associated with several SGAs, including clozapine, olanzapine, risperidone, and quetiapine.

In 2003, an FDA warning for hyperglycemia and diabetes mellitus was added to the package insert of all SGAs. It stated that

> hyperglycemia, in some cases extreme and associated with ketoacidosis or hyperosmolar coma or death, has been reported in patients treated with atypical antipsychotics. Assessment of the relationship between atypical antipsychotic use and glucose abnormalities is complicated by the possibility of an increased background risk of diabetes mellitus in patients with schizophrenia and the increasing incidence of diabetes in the general population. Given these confounders, the relationship between atypical antipsychotic use and hyperglycemia-related adverse events is not completely understood. Epidemiological studies suggest an increased risk of treatment-emergent hyperglycemia-related adverse events in patients treated with the atypical antipsychotics. Precise estimates for hyperglycemia-related adverse events in patients treated with atypical antipsychotics are not available.

This risk is substantially exacerbated when patients with schizophrenia are given some of the SGAs that result in significant weight gain, hyperlipidemia, and hyperglycemia (see, e.g., Haupt 2006; Newcomer 2007), including diabetic ketoacidosis and deaths occurring during the first 6 months of treatment. Diabetic ketoacidosis–related deaths have not been reported with all SGAs. The risk of antipsychotic-induced weight gain, associated diabetes (type 2 diabetes mellitus), and metabolic syndrome may result from changes in glucose metabolism and insulin resistance. In approximately 25%–40% of the cases of hyperglycemia, insulin resistance appears to occur even in the absence of significant weight gain, raising some interesting questions about how these medications may interact with the insulin–glycemic control. Even though some patients were prediabetic or undiagnosed with diabetes prior to SGA administration, it fails to explain the higher rates seen with SGAs. Unfortunately, in the case of clozapine, the risk of developing abnormal glucose levels and diabetes mellitus appears to be cumulative over the years.

Effective countermeasures available to help with weight gain and hyperglycemia are limited. The substantial increased risk to the health of patients with schizophrenia as a result of these effects is worrisome and an important shortcoming of these efficacious and important medications. Hyperlipidemia is a common problem with SGAs, especially in women; significant elevations of serum triglycerides are reported following SGA treatment. Baseline data from the CATIE study suggest that the rate of diabetes mellitus was 12.5%, hyperlipidemia was 53%, and hypertension was 37%, but a significant number of these individuals were not receiving medical treatment for the same. At CATIE baseline, significantly large groups of subjects were already obese or

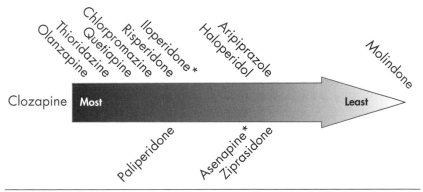

FIGURE 2–1. Antipsychotic medications associated with weight gain, by frequency.
[a]Based on limited data; may change in the future.

overweight. In a subgroup of the CATIE study, 41% of the subjects met criteria for metabolic syndrome at baseline. Olanzapine was associated with the highest mean weight gain (0.9 kg/month) among all the antipsychotics studied; about 30% of the subjects receiving olanzapine gained 7% or more weight from baseline compared with 7%–16% in other treatment groups (Lieberman et al. 2005). Olanzapine also was associated with greater increases in glycosylated hemoglobin, total cholesterol, and triglycerides compared with other study drugs. Ziprasidone was associated with improvement in each metabolic variable. Schizophrenia is already associated with a high mortality rate, and the dramatic increase in obesity and metabolic syndrome in this group further increases risk for medical morbidity and mortality. Moreover, heavy smoking rates and unhealthy lifestyle only compound the grim picture. Finally, there have been reports of acute pancreatitis associated with SGA use.

Metabolic issues are also evident during treatment of first episodes with SGAs. These concerns led to a conference of experts in psychiatry and medicine at Mount Sinai Medical Center in 2002 at which specific recommendations were made regarding obesity, diabetes, hyperlipidemia, and other health-related concerns in persons with schizophrenia (Marder et al. 2004). Similarly, the American Diabetes Association, American Psychiatric Association, American Association of Clinical Endocrinologists, and North American Association for the Study of Obesity provided consensus guidelines (modified version as in Appendixes 4 and 5). The Mount Sinai group also recommended interventions for management of weight gain and metabolic syndrome as early as when the body mass index changes by 1 unit. Many studies suggest that the gain in weight is reversible when the patient is switched to another antipsychotic. Mean weight reductions of approximately 10 kg with a switch from olanzapine and 7 kg with a switch from risperidone have been reported. Figure 2–1 illustrates, in descending order, the frequency by which antipsychotic medications are associated with weight gain so that clinicians may consider possible switching of antipsychotics to decrease weight. However, switching medications is not always easy because it may result in relapse.

Prolactin

Among the SGAs, risperidone (and paliperidone), because of its potent dopamine D_2 blockade, results in a significant increase in prolactin levels. High-potency FGAs also result in elevated prolactin levels. The increase in prolactin with risperidone and paliperidone is significantly more than that usually seen with FGAs. Clozapine and quetiapine are less potent at the D_2 receptors and do not cause elevations in prolactin levels. Ziprasidone and olanzapine, within the therapeutic dose range, also do not cause significant increases in prolactin levels. Iloperidone was associated with modest prolactin level elevation in short-term trials. Aripiprazole, because of its unique effects on dopamine receptors, does not increase prolactin levels and may in fact decrease them from baseline. Long-term asenapine studies show a decline or minimal changes in prolactijn levels. In some individuals, prolactin elevations lead to amenorrhea, galactorrhea, and gynecomastia and may decrease bone mineral density. Figure 2–2 illustrates, in descending order, the frequency by which antipsychotic medications may increase prolactin levels so that clinicians may consider possible switching of antipsychotics to decrease prolactin levels. However, as discussed earlier, switching medications is not always easy because it may result in relapse.

Other Side Effects

Other side effects, which are more commonly seen with the low-potency antipsychotics, include sedation, tachycardia, and anticholinergic side effects such as urinary hesitancy or retention, blurred vision, or constipation. Other nonextrapyramidal side effects include cardiac conduction disturbances, retinal changes, sexual dysfunction, lowered seizure threshold, and a risk of agranulocytosis.

Treatment Resistance and Negative Symptoms

Treatment resistance was originally defined for research purposes (as a threshold to start clozapine) as a failure to respond to or an inability to tolerate adequate trials of three FGAs from different biochemical classes (Kane et al. 1988). However, this concept has undergone significant modification. The current definition states that the patient should fail to respond to at least one

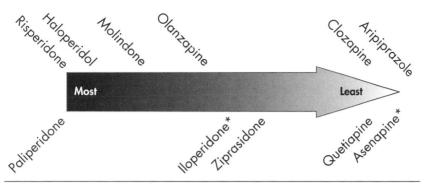

FIGURE 2–2. Antipsychotic medications associated with increase in prolactin levels, by frequency.

[a]Based on limited data; may change in the future.

SGA agent before a trial of clozapine is initiated (mainly to avoid the side effects of clozapine). The definition of the duration of a drug trial also has evolved over the years so that 4–6 weeks of an antipsychotic treatment at therapeutic doses can be considered an adequate trial. The recommended dosing also has undergone changes. The original recommendation considered a trial of 1,000 mg equivalent of chlorpromazine as a necessary minimum requirement, but this threshold has been reduced to 400–600 mg equivalent. The recommendation for a lower threshold is based on the knowledge that these doses block sufficient dopamine D_2 receptors, and higher doses provide no additional benefit. In those patients whose symptoms are considered treatment refractory, subsequent FGA use results in a lower than 5% response rate (Kane et al. 1988). Clozapine is the only antipsychotic drug proven more efficacious in rigorously defined treatment-refractory groups. Patients with treatment-resistant schizophrenia had more favorable outcomes when receiving clozapine than when receiving an FGA agent. However, monitoring of blood counts and fear of its side effects make it one of the most underused effective treatments for schizophrenia.

Risperidone may be superior to FGAs in treatment-refractory schizophrenia but does not appear to be as efficacious as clozapine. Olanzapine has been reported to lead to a better outcome than haloperidol in the treatment-resistant schizophrenia group. However, in a double-blind study, when olanzapine was compared with chlorpromazine in a treatment-refractory group, the outcome with olanzapine was not comparable to what is typically seen with the use of clozapine. When patients with symptoms refractory to olanzapine in this trial were subsequently given clozapine, the response rate was similar to what is seen with the use of clozapine in a treatment-refractory group. Thus, although olanzapine appears to have had better efficacy than

FGAs, it was not as efficacious as clozapine for treatment-refractory schizophrenia. Higher dosages of olanzapine (up to 50 mg/day) appear to be better
and lead to efficacy comparable to that of clozapine (Volavka et al. 2002),
suggesting that patients with treatment-refractory symptoms may need
higher doses of olanzapine for a meaningful outcome to occur.

Negative symptoms, such as apathy, amotivational syndrome, flattened
affect, and alogia, are often the most problematic for patients and account for
much of the morbidity associated with this illness. These symptoms are often
very difficult to treat. Clozapine has been used extensively in treatment of
negative symptoms with significant effect on general negative symptoms, but
its effect on primary negative symptoms is disputed. Data about risperidone
and olanzapine use are mixed. Selective serotonin reuptake inhibitors (SSRIs)
in combination with antipsychotic medications have shown mixed but encouraging results (see Murphy et al. 2006).

Switching Antipsychotics

Switching antipsychotics occurs as a result of problems with efficacy or un-
manageable side effects or a combination of both. It is extremely important to
establish that the side effect is indeed related to the antipsychotic and not
something else. Other strategies such as lowering the dose or adding another
medication to overcome the side effect should be tried before changing antipsychotics. Switching antipsychotics may have the potential to lead to a loss
of efficacy.

Antipsychotic Polypharmacy

Antipsychotic polypharmacy beyond the short-term stage of switching from
one antipsychotic to another, although practiced frequently, is viewed as unnecessary by some and as a necessary evil by others. However, when a large
segment of patients with chronic schizophrenia respond poorly or have significant side effects or both, clinicians are forced to individualize treatment by
seeking solutions outside the realm of evidence-based practice. Polypharmacy
is expensive and increases the burden of side effects, including mortality, but
few data have systematically evaluated the risk-benefit ratio and cost-effectiveness.

To logically approach the issue of polypharmacy, one should reevaluate
the case to

- Clarify the primary diagnosis.
- Diagnose comorbid conditions and their contribution to treatment resistance.

- Consider treatment of comorbid conditions such as obsessive-compulsive disorder with an SSRI.
- Determine compliance with past treatments.
- Evaluate the adequacy of previous clinical trials.
- Consider a trial with clozapine before starting polypharmacy.
- Consider nonpharmacological interventions.

Combination treatments worth considering from a pharmacokinetic or pharmacodynamic perspective would be based on the goals of such treatments. Sometimes these treatments are directed to improve efficacy, and other times they are combined to decrease side effects. High-potency with low-potency antipsychotics (e.g., clozapine or quetiapine with aripiprazole) may help decrease the side effects of sedation, metabolic effects, akathisia, insomnia, and so forth. Risperidone and haloperidol have been used with clozapine too. Combination of two high-potency antipsychotics, such as aripiprazole with loxapine, may improve efficacy without worsening the metabolic side effects.

Sometimes the issue of compliance forces clinicians to use a long-acting intramuscular antipsychotic with an oral form of antipsychotic. The long-acting antipsychotic ensures compliance, whereas the oral medication such as clozapine ensures improved efficacy. In some instances, this combination with lower doses also decreases the side-effect burden. Combination treatments should be used only after obtaining an adequate informed consent; complex treatments warrant close monitoring for side effects and ensuring that the therapeutic goals are achieved.

Pregnancy and Lactation

Pregnancy is not uncommon in women with schizophrenia and schizoaffective disorder. Discontinuation of antipsychotic medications in pregnant women with schizophrenia often leads to rapid relapse, which poses risks to the fetus and the mother. Most antipsychotics cross the placenta and are secreted in the breast milk to some extent (see Appendix 9). FGAs, especially high-potency ones, appear to be relatively safe for the fetus. A detailed discussion of the use of antipsychotic medication during pregnancy and breastfeeding can be found in Tjia and Gitlin, Chapter 8, in this volume.

Treatment of Schizoaffective Disorder

Kasanin (1933) coined the term *schizoaffective disorder*. The criteria for schizoaffective disorder have evolved over the years and have undergone major changes. According to DSM-IV-TR, a patient with schizoaffective disorder must have an uninterrupted period of illness during which, at some time, he or she meets the diagnostic criteria for a major depressive episode, manic episode, or a mixed episode concurrently with the diagnostic criteria for the active phase of schizophrenia. The DSM-IV-TR diagnosis of schizoaffective disorder can be further classified as schizoaffective disorder, bipolar type, or schizoaffective disorder, depressive type.

Regarding the prognosis of schizoaffective disorder, to the extent that this illness has symptoms from both a major mood disorder and schizophrenia, theoretically one can confer a relatively better prognosis than for schizophrenia and a relatively poorer prognosis than for bipolar disorder. Regardless of the subtype, the following variables are harbingers of a poor prognosis:

- Poor premorbid history
- Insidious onset
- Absence of precipitating factors
- Predominance of psychotic symptoms
- Deficit or negative symptoms
- Early age at onset
- Unremitting course
- Family history of schizophrenia

As in schizophrenia, the risk of relapse is diminished by antipsychotic maintenance treatment. Mood stabilizers, antidepressants, and antipsychotic medications clearly have a role in management of these symptoms. The presenting symptoms, their duration and intensity, and patient choices need to be incorporated into deciding what treatment(s) to choose.

SGAs appear more effective than FGAs in the treatment of schizoaffective disorder. SGAs appear to have more broad-spectrum effects than do FGAs. Optimizing antipsychotic treatment, especially with SGAs, is more likely to be effective than the routine use of adjunctive antidepressants or mood stabilizers. However, when indicated, the use of antidepressants is well supported in schizoaffective patients who present with a full depressive syndrome after stabilization of psychosis.

All currently available SGAs are reported to be effective treatments either alone or in combination with mood stabilizers. SGAs are better tolerated than FGAs. Recent data from paliperidone may result in an FDA indication for the same if accepted and approved. Persistent and enduring improvements with clozapine lasting 1–2 years have been reported. Clozapine also helps decrease suicidality. Clozapine use may be beneficial in treatment-refractory schizoaffective disorder because it has both mood-stabilizing and antipsychotic properties, a substantial advantage.

Treatment Adherence

To achieve short- and long-term goals of a treatment plan successfully in a patient with schizophrenia and schizoaffective disorder, adherence to pharmacological and nonpharmacological interventions is crucial. Most data evaluating the risks across a continuum of adherence behaviors report a direct correlation between adherence and hospitalization. When patients were 100% compliant with treatment, significantly less hospitalization occurred. In one study, poor adherence to antipsychotic treatment increased risk for suicide attempts up to fourfold.

The quality of a patient's relationship with clinicians during an acute admission is critical in forming his or her attitude toward medication and adherence. Psychosocial interventions, especially psychoeducation for patients and family, are effective avenues to improve adherence and reduce relapse and readmission rates. However, despite the effectiveness of psychoeducation, the number of family members and patients exploiting this approach is quite low. When patients are at high risk for noncompliance or partial compliance, long-acting injectable antipsychotics can help improve adherence and reduce relapse and hospitalization rates. This mode of medication administration can detect noncompliance early and reliably and provide an opportunity to intervene when the medication is still in the person's system (Kane 2006). VNA (Visiting Nurse Association) services can provide at-home psychoeducation as well as supervision of treatment compliance in patients who are living independently or reluctant to have family members provide the medication supervision.

If schizophrenia is progressive and has neurodegenerative components and treatments for schizophrenia have neuroprotective effects (by arresting gray matter loss in important areas of the brain) either as a primary effect or secondary to prevention of relapses, then treatment adherence provides perhaps the most important opportunity to optimize these imperfect treatments. Otherwise, these losses may not be reversible.

KEY CLINICAL POINTS

- Schizophrenia is a progressive, severe, chronic mental illness associated with such significant morbidity and mortality that it obliges the psychiatrist to coordinate care among medical and psychosocial service providers to maximize positive clinical outcomes.

- Because studies have not shown clinically meaningful differences between FGAs and SGAs (excluding clozapine), the goal is to provide individualized patient treatment that is maximally efficacious and associated with the fewest side effects, regardless of medication class used.

- Clozapine is superior to SGAs for the treatment of psychosis, and its use decreases relapses, improves stability in the community, and diminishes suicidal behavior. Clozapine is the only antipsychotic that has received an FDA indication for the treatment of recurring suicidal behavior in patients with schizophrenia or schizoaffective disorder.

- Most patients switch or discontinue their antipsychotic medications because of inefficacy or intolerable side effects.

- For patients for whom adherence is a problem, long-acting preparations of fluphenazine, haloperidol, and risperidone are available in the United States.

- All currently available SGAs are reported to be effective treatments for schizoaffective disorder either alone or in combination with mood stabilizers; SGAs are associated with better tolerability and efficacy than are FGAs in this patient population.

References

Adams CE, Fenton MK, Quraishi S, et al: Systematic meta-review of depot antipsychotic drugs for people with schizophrenia. Br J Psychiatry 179:290–299, 2001

American Psychiatric Association: Diagnostic and Statistical Manual of Mental Disorders, 4th Edition, Text Revision. Washington, DC, American Psychiatric Association, 2000

Asenapine [package insert], Kenilworth, NJ, Schering-Plough, 2009

Baldessarini RJ, Frankenburg FR: Clozapine: a novel antipsychotic agent. N Engl J Med 324:746–754, 1991

Citrome L: Iloperidone for schizophrenia: a review of the efficacy and safely profile for this newly commercialized second-generation antipsychotic. Int J Clin Prac 63:1237–1248, 2009

Csernansky JG, Mahmoud R, Brenner R, et al: A comparison of risperidone and haloperidol for the prevention of relapse in patients with schizophrenia. N Engl J Med 346:16–22, 2002

Davis JM, Chen N: Old versus new: weighing the evidence between the first and second-generation antipsychotics. Eur Psychiatry 20:7–14, 2005

Dixon L, Weiden P, Delahanty J, et al: Prevalence and correlates of diabetes in national schizophrenia samples. Schizophr Bull 26:903–912, 2000

Essock SM, Hargreaves WA, Covell NH, et al: Clozapine's effectiveness for patients in state hospitals: results from a randomized trial. Psychopharmacol Bull 32:683–697, 1996

Harris EC, Barraclough B: Excess mortality of mental disorder. Br J Psychiatry 173:11–33, 1998

Haupt DW: Differential metabolic effects of antipsychotic treatments. Eur Neuropsychopharmacol Suppl 3:S149–S155, 2006

Hogarty GE, Anderson CM, Reiss DJ, et al: Family psychoeducation, social skills training, and maintenance chemotherapy in the aftercare treatment of schizophrenia, I: one-year effects of a controlled study on relapse and expressed emotion. Arch Gen Psychiatry 43:633–642, 1986

Hough D, Lindenmayer JP, Gopal S, et al: Safety and tolerability of deltoid and gluteal injections of paliperidone palmitate in schizophrenia. Prog Neuropsychopharmacol Biol Psychiatry 33:1022–1031, 2009

Iloperidone [package insert], Rockville, MD, Vanda, 2009

Iqbal MM, Rahman A, Husain Z, et al: Clozapine: a clinical review of adverse effects and management. Ann Clin Psychiatry 15:33–48, 2003

Jones PB, Barnes TRE, Davies L, et al: Randomized controlled trial of the effect on quality of life of second- vs first-generation antipsychotic drugs in schizophrenia: Cost Utility of the Latest Antipsychotic Drugs in Schizophrenia Study (CUtLASS 1). Arch Gen Psychiatry 63:1079–1087, 2006

Kane JM: Review of treatments that can ameliorate nonadherence in patients with schizophrenia. J Clin Psychiatry 67 (suppl 5):9–14, 2006

Kane JM, Honigfeld G, Singer J, et al: Clozapine for the treatment resistant schizophrenic: a double-blind comparison versus chlorpromazine/benztropine. Arch Gen Psychiatry 45:789–796, 1988

Kane JM, Marder SR, Schooler NR, et al: Clozapine and haloperidol in moderately refractory schizophrenia: a 6-month randomized and double-blind comparison. Arch Gen Psychiatry 58:965–972, 2001

Kane JM, Lauriello J, Laska E, et al: Long-term efficacy and safety of iloperidone: results from 3 clinical trials for the treatment of schizophrenia. J Clin Psychopharmacol 28(2 Suppl. 1):S29–35, 2008

Kapur S, Seeman P: Does fast dissociation from the dopamine D2 receptor explain the action of atypical antipsychotics? A new hypothesis. Am J Psychiatry 158:360–369, 2001

Kasanin J: The acute schizoaffective psychoses. Am J Psychiatry 13:97–126, 1933

Keith S: Advances in psychotropic formulations. Prog Neuropsychopharmacol Biol Psychiatry 30:996–1008, 2006

Lester D: Sex differences in completed suicide by schizophrenic patients: a meta-analysis. Suicide Life Threat Behav 36:50–56, 2006

Leucht S, Corves C, Arbter D, et al: Second-generation antipsychotic drugs versus first-generation antipsychotic drugs for schizophrenia: meta-analysis. Lancet 373:31–41, 2009

Levenson JC: Neuroleptic malignant syndrome. Am J Psychiatry 142:1137–1145, 1985

Lieberman JA: Comparative effectiveness of antipsychotic drugs: a commentary on Cost Utility of the Latest Antipsychotic Drugs in Schizophrenia Study (CUtLASS 1) and Clinical Antipsychotic Trials of Intervention Effectiveness (CATIE). Arch Gen Psychiatry 63:1069–1072, 2006

Lieberman JA, Stroup TS, McEvoy JP, et al: Effectiveness of antipsychotic drugs in patients with chronic schizophrenia. N Engl J Med 353:1209–1223, 2005

Lysaker PH, Bell MD, Bioty SM, et al: The frequency of associations between positive and negative symptoms and dysphoria in schizophrenia. Compr Psychiatry 36:113–117, 1995

Marder SR, Essock SM, Miller AL, et al: Physical health monitoring of patients with schizophrenia. Am J Psychiatry 161:1334–1349, 2004

McEvoy JP, Lieberman JA, Stroup TS, et al: Effectiveness of clozapine versus olanzapine, quetiapine, and risperidone in patients with chronic schizophrenia who did not respond to prior atypical antipsychotic treatment. Am J Psychiatry 163:600–610, 2006

Medori R, Wapenaar R, de Arce R, et al: Relapse prevention and effectiveness in schizophrenia with risperidone long-acting injectable (RLAI) versus quetiapine. Poster presented at the 161st annual meeting of the American Psychiatric Association, Washington, DC, May 2008

Meltzer HY, Okayli G: The reduction of suicidality during clozapine treatment in neuroleptic-resistant schizophrenia: impact on risk-benefit assessment. Am J Psychiatry 152:183–190, 1995

Meltzer HY, Matsubara S, Lee JC: The ratios of serotonin-2 and dopamine-2 affinities differentiate atypical and typical antipsychotic drugs. Psychopharmacol Bull 25:390–392, 1989

Meltzer HY, Bobo WV, Naamah IF, et al: Efficacy and tolerability of oral paliperidone extended-release tablets in the treatment of acute schizophrenia: pooled data from three 6-week placebo-controlled studies. J Clin Psychiatry 69:817–829, 2008

Murphy BP, Chung YC, Park TW, et al: Pharmacological treatment of primary negative symptoms in schizophrenia: a systematic review. Schizophr Res 88:5–25, 2006

Newcomer JW: Metabolic considerations in the use of antipsychotic medications: a review of recent evidence. J Clin Psychiatry 68 (suppl 1):20–27, 2007

Paliperidone palmitate [package insert]. Titusville, NJ, Janssen, 2009

Patel JK, Pinals DA, Breier A: Schizophrenia and other psychosis, in Psychiatry, 3rd Edition. Edited by Tasman A, Kay J, Leiberman J, et al. Chichester, UK, Wiley, 2008, pp 1201–1282

Potkin SG, Cohen M, Panagides J: Efficacy and tolerability of asenapine in acute schizophrenia. J Clin Psychiatry 68:1492–1500, 2007

Potkin SG, Litman RE, Torres R, et al: Efficacy of iloperidone in the treatment of schizophrenia: initial phase 3 studies. J Clin Psychopharmacol 28 (2, suppl 1):S4–S11, 2008

Ray WA, Meredith S, Thapa PB, et al: Antipsychotics and the risk of sudden cardiac death. Arch Gen Psychiatry 58:1161–1167, 2001

Ray WA, Chung CP, Murray KT, et al: Atypical antipsychotic drugs and the risk of sudden cardiac death. N Engl J Med 360:225–235, 2009

Rosenheck RA: Outcomes, costs, and policy caution: a commentary on the Cost Utility of the Latest Antipsychotic Drugs in Schizophrenia Study (CUtLASS I). Arch Gen Psychiatry 63:1074–1076, 2006

Sikich L, Frazier JA, McClellan J, et al: Double-blind comparison of first- and second-generation antipsychotics in early onset schizophrenia and schizoaffective disorder: findings from the Treatment of Early Onset Schizophrenia Spectrum Disorders (TEOSS) study. Am J Psychiatry 165:1420–1431, 2008

Tamargo J: Drug-induced torsades de pointes: from molecular biology to bedside. Jpn J Pharmacol 83:1–19, 2000

Thakore JH, Mann JN, Vlahos I, et al: Increased visceral fat distribution in drug-naïve and drug-free patients with schizophrenia. Int J Obes Relat Metab Disord 26:137–141, 2002

Tiihonen J, Wahlbeck K, Lönnqvist J, et al: Effectiveness of antipsychotic treatments in a nationwide cohort of patients in community care after first hospitalisation due to schizophrenia and schizoaffective disorder: observational follow-up study. BMJ 333:224, 2006

Volavka J, Czobar P, Sheitman B, et al: Clozapine, olanzapine, risperidone, and haloperidol in the treatment of patients with chronic schizophrenia and schizoaffective disorder. Am J Psychiatry 159:255–262, 2002

Zarate CA Jr, Patel JK: Sudden cardiac death and antipsychotic drugs: do we know enough? (commentary). Arch Gen Psychiatry 58:1168–1171, 2001

CHAPTER 3

Mood and Anxiety Disorders

Kristina M. Deligiannidis, M.D.
Anthony J. Rothschild, M.D.

IN RECENT YEARS, the use of antipsychotic medications has expanded beyond the treatment of schizophrenia to mood and anxiety disorders, with some antipsychotic medications receiving U.S. Food and Drug Administration (FDA) indications for the treatment of these conditions. In this chapter, we review the evidence base for the use of antipsychotic medications in the treatment of bipolar disorder, psychotic depression, treatment-resistant depression (TRD), nonpsychotic depression, obsessive-compulsive disorder (OCD), generalized anxiety disorder (GAD), and posttraumatic stress disorder (PTSD).

Bipolar Disorder

Bipolar disorder is a severe, long-term illness characterized by cyclical episodes of mania and depression. About 5.7 million American adults, or about 2.6% of the population age 18 and older, in any given year have bipolar disorder (Kessler et al. 2005). The classic form of the illness, which involves recurrent episodes of mania and depression, is called *bipolar I disorder*. Some people, however, never develop severe mania but instead experience milder episodes of hypomania that alternate with depression; this form of the illness is called *bipolar II disorder*. When four or more episodes of illness occur within a 12-month period, a person is said to have *rapid-cycling* bipolar disorder. Some people experience multiple episodes within a single week, or even within a single day. Rapid cycling tends to develop later in the course of illness and is more common among women than among men.

The first episode of bipolar disorder may occur at any age from childhood to old age. The average age at onset is 21. More than 90% of the individuals who have a single manic episode go on to have future episodes. Untreated patients with bipolar I disorder typically have 8–10 episodes of mania and depression in their lifetime. Often, 5 years or more may elapse between the first and second episode, but thereafter the episodes become more frequent and more severe.

Several antipsychotic medications have FDA approval for the treatment of bipolar disorder. The various FDA indications of antipsychotic medications for the treatment of bipolar disorder are shown in Table 3–1.

Acute Mania and Mixed States

Almost all conventional and atypical antipsychotic medications have been studied in bipolar patients in manic or mixed states and have been shown to be effective either as monotherapy or in combination with another antimanic agent such as lithium or valproate. The American Psychiatric Association's "Practice Guideline for the Treatment of Patients With Bipolar Disorder (Revision)" (Hirschfield et al. 2002) and the Texas Consensus Conference Panel on Medication Treatment of Bipolar Disorder (Suppes et al. 2002) include the atypical antipsychotic medications, along with lithium, valproate, and conventional antipsychotic medications, as first-line treatments for bipolar mania. Little to no differences have been observed among the atypical antipsychotic medications in their efficacy for the treatment of bipolar mania, whether these medications are used as monotherapy or as add-on therapy (Perlis et al. 2006).

Patients with acute mania often require medication doses at the higher end of the therapeutic ranges listed in Appendix 3. For example, aripiprazole can be started at 10–15 mg/day, and then the dosage can be increased, if necessary, to 30 mg/day, although it is unclear if additional efficacy occurs at dosages greater than 15 mg/day. Olanzapine can be started at 15 mg/day. Quetiapine can be started at 100 mg/day, and then the dosage can be increased by 100 mg/day to a target of 400–600 mg/day. Risperidone can be started at

TABLE 3–1. U.S. Food and Drug Administration indications of antipsychotic medications for bipolar disorder

MEDICATION	BIPOLAR MANIA		BIPOLAR MIXED STATE		BIPOLAR DEPRESSION	BIPOLAR MAINTENANCE	
	MONOTHERAPY	ADJUNCTIVE[a]	MONOTHERAPY	ADJUNCTIVE[a]	MONOTHERAPY	MONOTHERAPY	ADJUNCTIVE[a]
Aripiprazole	√	√	√	√		√	
Asenapine	√		√				
Chlorpromazine	√						
Olanzapine	√	√	√	√		√	
Quetiapine	√	√		√	√		√
Risperdal Consta						√	√
Risperidone	√	√	√				
Ziprasidone	√		√				√

[a]As adjunct to lithium or valproate.

2 mg/day, and then the dosage can be rapidly increased to 4–6 mg/day as needed over the next couple of days. Long-acting injectable risperidone is the only long-acting injectable antipsychotic approved as both monotherapy and adjunctive therapy to lithium or valproate in the maintenance treatment of bipolar I disorder. Long-acting injectable risperidone may be initiated at 25 mg IM every 2 weeks as either adjunctive or monotherapy, though some patients may benefit from a higher dose (37.5 mg or 50 mg IM every two weeks). Asenapine, a newly approved antipsychotic for the treatment of acute bipolar I manic and mixed states, can be initiated and maintained at 10 mg sublingually twice daily—twice the initial dose recommended for its indication in the treatment of schizophrenia. Finally, ziprasidone can be started at 80 mg/day, and then the dosage can be increased to 160 mg/day on day 2.

Evidence suggests that the combination of an atypical antipsychotic medication and either lithium or valproate may lead to a faster response. As one would expect, combining medications leads to the potential for more side effects than with either medication alone. The current evidence base would deem it appropriate to treat patients with acute bipolar mania with either one medication, the addition of a second medication during treatment, or two medications. Which treatment is initiated will depend on the individual clinical situation and patient factors such as severity of symptoms or sensitivity to side effects.

Acute Bipolar Depression

Bipolar I Depression

Most experts agree that the depressive phase of bipolar disorder is more disabling and difficult to treat than the manic or hypomanic phase. Quetiapine as a monotherapy and olanzapine (in combination with fluoxetine) are approved by the FDA for the treatment of bipolar depression.

Quetiapine monotherapy

Evidence for the acute efficacy of quetiapine monotherapy in patients with bipolar I or bipolar II depression comes from two large, 8-week randomized, double-blind studies that evaluated quetiapine monotherapy (300 and 600 mg/day) (Calabrese et al. 2005; Thase et al. 2006). In the first study, involving 360 patients with bipolar I depression (Calabrese et al. 2005), quetiapine monotherapy at both dosages significantly improved depression (as measured by the Montgomery-Åsberg Depression Rating Scale [MADRS]) in patients with bipolar I depression compared with placebo at week 8 ($P<0.001$). The effect of quetiapine was observed as early as week 1. These findings were confirmed in the second study, involving 338 patients with bipolar I depression (Thase et al. 2006), at 300 mg/day ($P<0.001$) and 600 mg/day ($P<0.01$).

The efficacy of quetiapine monotherapy was further evaluated in a double-blind, placebo-controlled study in bipolar I and bipolar II depression (Young et al. 2008). The primary end point of the acute phase of the study was the change from baseline to week 8 in MADRS total score. In the bipolar I subgroup of patients ($n=487$), the mean change in MADRS total score at week 8 was -14.8 with quetiapine 300 mg/day ($P<0.05$ vs. placebo) and -16.5 with quetiapine 600 mg/day ($P<0.05$ vs. placebo) compared with -11.2 for placebo.

Another study with a similar design (McElroy et al. 2008) that evaluated the efficacy of quetiapine (300 and 600 mg/day) and paroxetine (20 mg/day) as monotherapy in patients with bipolar I and bipolar II depression found that in the bipolar I subgroup ($n=448$), both dosages of quetiapine (300 and 600 mg/day) significantly ($P<0.05$) reduced the MADRS total score from baseline to week 8 compared with placebo.

Olanzapine-fluoxetine combination

In an 8-week double-blind, randomized controlled study (Tohen et al. 2003) of 833 patients with bipolar I depression randomly assigned to receive placebo ($n=377$); olanzapine, 5–20 mg/day ($n=370$); or an olanzapine-fluoxetine combination, 6 and 25, 6 and 50, or 12 and 50 mg/day ($n=86$), the olanzapine and olanzapine-fluoxetine groups showed statistically significant improvement in depressive symptoms compared with the placebo group ($P<0.001$ for all). The olanzapine-fluoxetine combination group also showed statistically greater improvement than the olanzapine group at weeks 4 through 8. At week 8, MADRS total scores were lower than at baseline by 11.9, 15.0, and 18.5 points in the placebo, olanzapine, and olanzapine-fluoxetine combination groups, respectively. Remission criteria were met by 24.5% (87 of 355) of the placebo group, 32.8% (115 of 351) of the olanzapine group, and 48.8% (40 of 82) of the olanzapine-fluoxetine combination group. Treatment-emergent mania (Young Mania Rating Scale [YMRS] score <15 at baseline and ≥15 subsequently) did not differ among groups (placebo, 6.7% [23 of 345]; olanzapine, 5.7% [19 of 335]; and olanzapine-fluoxetine combination, 6.4% [5 of 78]). Adverse events for olanzapine-fluoxetine therapy were similar to those for olanzapine therapy but also included higher rates of nausea and diarrhea.

Bipolar II Depression

Unfortunately, less attention has been paid to the treatment of bipolar II depression than to the treatment of bipolar I depression. Consequently, even though patients with bipolar II depression spend considerably more time with depression than do patients with bipolar I depression, less is known about the treatment of bipolar II depression.

Quetiapine was studied as a monotherapy for bipolar II depression in the two studies discussed earlier (Calabrese et al. 2005; Thase et al. 2006). Calabrese and colleagues (2005) found that in the subgroup of 182 patients with bipolar II disorder, the mean change in MADRS total score from baseline to last assessment was smaller than that observed in the bipolar I patients. Although the change in MADRS total score from baseline in the patients with bipolar II disorder taking quetiapine was statistically superior to that in the placebo group at most assessments, it did not reach statistical significance at the final assessment: −14.06 in the group taking 600 mg/day of quetiapine and −14.78 in the group taking 300 mg/day compared with −12.35 in the placebo group.

In the study by Thase and colleagues (2006), of the 152 patients with bipolar II depression, the mean change in MADRS total score from baseline was significantly greater ($P<0.05$) at week 1 in the 300-mg/day group compared with the placebo group. This improvement was sustained through the last assessment (−17.61 vs. −12.86 for placebo; $P<0.05$). In the 600-mg/day group, the change in MADRS total score from baseline in the patients with bipolar II disorder was statistically superior to that seen with placebo from week 3 onward (mean change in MADRS total score at final assessment=−18.27; $P<0.01$).

Relapse Prevention

Because bipolar disorder is a recurrent or chronic condition that requires extended therapy, identifying medications that prevent relapses is important. At present, the only antipsychotic medications that are FDA approved for relapse prevention are olanzapine, aripiprazole, and long-acting risperidone as monotherapy and quetiapine and long-acting risperidone as an adjunct therapy to lithium or valproate (other FDA-approved medications for relapse prevention of bipolar disorder include lithium and lamotrigine). Conventional antipsychotics have not been shown to be effective maintenance treatments (Keck et al. 2000) and have long-term side-effect risks such as tardive dyskinesia and hyperprolactinemia. Consequently, they have a limited role in the long-term maintenance treatment of bipolar disorder.

Olanzapine

Olanzapine has an FDA indication for relapse prevention in bipolar disorder. In a double-blind, placebo-controlled study, Tohen and colleagues (2006) investigated the efficacy and safety of olanzapine as monotherapy in relapse prevention in bipolar I disorder. Patients achieving symptomatic remission from a manic or mixed episode of bipolar I disorder (YMRS total score≤12 and 21-item Hamilton Rating Scale for Depression [Ham-D] score≤8) at two consecutive weekly visits following 6–12 weeks of open-label acute treatment with 5–20 mg/day of olanzapine were randomly assigned to double-blind maintenance treatment with olanzapine ($n=225$) or placebo ($n=136$) for up to 48 weeks. The primary measure of efficacy was time to symptomatic relapse into any mood episode (YMRS score≥15, Ham-D score≥15, or hospitalization). Time to symptomatic relapse into any mood episode was statistically significantly longer among patients receiving olanzapine (a median of 174 days, compared with a median of 22 days in patients receiving placebo). Times to symptomatic relapse into manic, depressive, and mixed episodes were all statistically significantly longer among patients receiving olanzapine than among patients receiving placebo. The relapse rate was significantly lower in the olanzapine group (46.7%) than in the placebo group (80.1%). During olanzapine treatment, the most common treatment-emergent adverse event was weight gain; during the open-label phase, patients who received olanzapine gained a mean of 3.1 kg (standard deviation [SD]=3.4). In double-blind treatment, placebo patients lost a mean of 2.0 kg (SD=4.4), and patients who continued to take olanzapine gained an additional 1.0 kg (SD=5.2).

Aripiprazole

Aripiprazole has an FDA indication for the prevention of relapse in bipolar disorder. Two important studies evaluated the efficacy and safety of aripiprazole for the maintenance therapy of bipolar disorder. In a randomized, double-blind, parallel-group, placebo-controlled multicenter study (Keck et al. 2006), 161 patients with bipolar I disorder who had recently been hospitalized and treated for a manic or mixed episode entered an open-label stabilization phase (aripiprazole monotherapy=15 or 30 mg/day for 6–18 weeks). After meeting stabilization criteria (YMRS score≤10 and MADRS score≤13 for 6 consecutive weeks), the patients were randomly assigned to aripiprazole or placebo for the 26-week double-blind phase. Sixty-seven patients completed the 26-week double-blind phase. The primary end point was time to relapse for a manic, mixed, or depressive episode (defined by discontinuation caused by lack of efficacy). The authors reported that aripiprazole was superior to placebo in delaying the time to relapse ($P=0.020$). Aripiprazole-treated patients had significantly fewer relapses (25%) compared with the patients receiving placebo (43%; $P=0.013$). Aripiprazole was superior to placebo in delaying the time to manic relapse ($P=0.01$); however, no significant differences were observed in time to depressive relapse ($P=0.68$). Weight gain (≥7% increase) occurred in 7 (13%) aripiprazole-treated and 0 placebo-treated patients. Adverse events (≥5% incidence and twice that of placebo) reported by aripiprazole-treated patients were akathisia, pain in the extremities, tremor, and vaginitis.

Patients who completed this 26-week study without a relapse were offered the option to continue in a second study: a 74-week double-blind, placebo-controlled extension phase for a total of 100 weeks of double-blind treatment (Keck et al. 2007), allowing for further evaluation of the efficacy and tolerability of aripiprazole for relapse prevention in bipolar I disorder. Sixty-six patients entered this 74-week double-blind extension phase of the study. At 100 weeks, time to relapse was significantly longer with aripiprazole ($n = 7$) than with placebo ($n = 5$; hazard ratio$= 0.53$; $P = 0.011$; 95% confidence interval [CI]$= 0.32$–0.87); however, a further 24 patients had discontinued the medication as a result of study closure. Aripiprazole was superior to placebo in delaying time to manic relapse ($P = 0.005$; hazard ratio$= 0.35$; 95% CI$= 0.16$–0.75); however, no significant differences were observed in time to depressive relapse ($P = 0.602$; hazard ratio$= 0.81$; 95% CI$= 0.36$–1.81). The adverse events reported during 100 weeks of treatment with aripiprazole versus placebo ($\geq 5\%$ incidence and twice placebo rate) were tremor, akathisia, dry mouth, hypertension, weight gain, vaginitis, abnormal thinking, pharyngitis, and flu syndrome. Mean weight change from baseline to 100 weeks (last observation carried forward) was $+0.4 \pm 0.8$ kg with aripiprazole and -1.9 ± 0.8 kg with placebo.

Quetiapine

For quetiapine, in both the study by Young and colleagues (2008) and the study by McElroy and colleagues (2008) discussed earlier, patients who achieved remission after treatment with quetiapine 300 mg/day or 600 mg/day after 8 weeks were then randomly assigned to either continued treatment with quetiapine 300 mg/day or placebo for an additional 26–52 weeks. Quetiapine significantly increased the time to recurrence of depression compared with placebo in both studies in patients with bipolar I and II depression. Other studies have found that over a 2-year period, the addition of quetiapine to either lithium or valproate was more effective than the addition of placebo in preventing the recurrence of both any mood event ($P < 0.001$) and a depression event ($P < 0.001$) in patients with bipolar I depression (Suppes et al. 2007; Vieta et al. 2007).

Olanzapine-Fluoxetine Combination

The olanzapine-fluoxetine combination has not been evaluated in placebo-controlled trials. One study (Brown et al. 2006) compared the olanzapine-fluoxetine combination at various dosages (6 and 25, 6 and 50, 12 and 25, or 12 and 50 mg/day; $n = 205$) with lamotrigine (maximum dosage$= 200$ mg/day, $n = 205$) in a 25-week double-blind, randomized study of patients with bipolar I depression. The olanzapine-fluoxetine combination was associated with significantly greater improvements in Clinical Global Impressions (CGI) Scale and MADRS total scores than was lamotrigine from baseline to week 25 ($P < 0.01$).

Long-Acting Injectable Risperidone

Studies demonstrating the efficacy of long-acting injectable risperidone for relapse prevention have begun to emerge. In a small 2007 study by Han and colleagues, patients with bipolar I disorder whose condition was stable were switched from their existing oral antipsychotic medications to open-label long-acting injectable risperidone (25–37.5 mg IM every 2 weeks) for 12 months. Patients in this study had had stable YMRS scores of 12 for at least 4 continuous weeks, were taking oral atypical antipsychotics, and were not prescribed concomitant mood-stabilizing drugs. YMRS scores were stable over the 12-month study as were Ham-D and Brief Psychiatric Rating Scale (BPRS) scores, and this was indicative of efficacy in relapse prevention. Clinical Global Improvement–Severity scale (CGI-S) scores showed a statistically significant decrease from baseline (3.10±0.57) to post–12 month treatment (1.70±0.48). A separate study found that open-label continuation of oral atypical antipsychotic augmentation therapy over 6 months was as effective in preventing relapse of bipolar disorder as switching to long-acting injectable risperidone augmentation therapy (Yatham et al. 2007). In this study, patients were maintained on stable doses of lithium, valproate, or lamotrigine and, if applicable, one antidepressant. There were no significant between-group differences on any of the efficacy measures—CGI-S, YMRS, MADRS, or Hamilton Rating Scale for Anxiety (Ham-A). Study weaknesses included the lack of a double-blind and the fact that changes in dosage with oral atypical antipsychotics were allowed throughout the study, but changes in dosages of long-acting injectable risperidone were made only under stringent improvement criteria.

Asenapine

Efficacy of asenapine in bipolar disorder was demonstrated in two 3-week trials in which asenapine performed better than placebo in both (Traynor 2009). Asenapine has high binding affinity for dopamine D_2, D_3, D_4, and D_1 receptors; serotonin 5-HT$_{1A}$, 5-HT$_{1B}$, 5-HT$_{2A}$, 5-HT$_{2B}$, 5-HT$_{2C}$, 5-HT$_5$, 5-HT$_6$, and 5HT 7; α_1- and α_2-adrenergic receptors, and histamine H_1 receptors (Asenapine [package insert] 2009). The most frequently reported side effects in clinical trials including bipolar patients were drowsiness, dizziness, movement disorders, and weight gain.

KEY CLINICAL POINTS: BIPOLAR DISORDER

- Almost all conventional and atypical antipsychotic medications have been shown to be effective as monotherapy or in combination with an antimanic agent such as lithium or valproate for the acute treatment of manic or mixed states.

- Quetiapine as a monotherapy and olanzapine (in combination with fluoxetine) are approved by the FDA for the treatment of bipolar I depression.

- Aripiprazole, olanzapine, and long-acting injectable risperidone (as monotherapy) and quetiapine and long-acting injectable risperidone (as an adjunct to lithium or valproate) are FDA approved for relapse prevention in bipolar disorder.

- Conventional antipsychotic medications have a limited role in the long-term maintenance treatment of bipolar disorder.

Psychotic Depression

Psychotic depression (major depression with psychotic features, delusional depression) is a serious illness during which a person experiences the dangerous combination of depressed mood and psychosis, with the psychosis commonly manifesting itself as nihilistic, "bad things are about to happen"–type delusions (Rothschild 2009). In samples of patients with major depression, a European study found that 18.5% of them also fulfilled criteria for major depressive episode with psychotic features (Ohayon and Schatzberg 2002), and in a study in the United States (Johnson et al. 1991), 14.7% of the patients who met criteria for major depression had a history of psychotic features. In outpatient studies of adolescents with major depression, the prevalence of psychotic symptoms has been reported to be 18% (Ryan et al. 1987). In people older than 60, the prevalence of psychotic depression in the community is even higher at between 14 and 30 per 1,000 (Baldwin and Jolley 1986; Blazer 1994). In a Finnish community sample of people older than 60, the rate of psychotic depression was found to be 12 per 1,000 in women and 6 per 1,000 in men (Kivela and Pahkala 1989).

Currently, no drugs, devices, or treatments, including any antipsychotic medication, are approved by the FDA specifically for the treatment of major depression with psychotic features. The American Psychiatric Association's (2000) "Practice Guideline for the Treatment of Patients With Major Depressive Disorder (Revision)" recommends, with substantial clinical confidence, the use of a combination of an antipsychotic and an antidepressant or electroconvulsive therapy (ECT) for the pharmacological treatment of psychotic depression. However, despite these recommendations, recent data have shown that only 5% of patients with psychotic depression receive an adequate combination of an antidepressant and an antipsychotic (Andreescu et al. 2007). These findings show a persisting low rate of adequate dose and duration of treatment (particularly the use of an antipsychotic medication) of psychotic depression and little change from a study published a decade earlier that also reported inadequate dose and duration of medication treatment prescribed to patients with psychotic depression (Mulsant et al. 1997).

Use of an Antipsychotic With an Antidepressant

Five randomized clinical trials have compared antipsychotic monotherapy with the combination of an antipsychotic and an antidepressant medication for the treatment of psychotic depression (Meyers et al. 2009; Muller-Siecheneder et al. 1998; Rothschild et al. 2004 [two studies]; Spiker et al. 1985). All five studies found a significantly greater efficacy of the combination treatment. A meta-analysis (Wijkstra et al. 2006) of three of the studies (Rothschild et al. 2004; Spiker et al. 1985) showed a statistically significant difference favoring the combination compared with antipsychotic monotherapy (relative risk [RR]=1.92; 95% CI=1.32–2.80; $P=0.0007$).

In two large randomized controlled trials (Rothschild et al. 2004), a combination of the selective serotonin reuptake inhibitor (SSRI) fluoxetine plus the second-generation antipsychotic olanzapine was compared with olanzapine monotherapy or placebo in 249 hospitalized patients with psychotic depression. In both studies, patients were randomly assigned to receive placebo, olanzapine (mean dosages=11.9 and 14.0 mg/day) plus placebo, or olanzapine (mean dosages=12.4 and 13.9 mg/day) plus fluoxetine (mean dosages=23.5 and 22.6 mg/day) and followed up for 8 weeks. The first trial showed a reduction in Ham-D score that was statistically greater in the combination group than in the olanzapine monotherapy group or the placebo group throughout the 8 weeks. The second trial did not detect any statistically significant differences among the three treatment groups except for the Ham-D score in the combination group, which was statistically lower than that in the placebo group at the end of week 1. However, several aspects of the study design were biased against the combination of fluoxetine and olanzapine. First, the study was powered to show a difference between olanzapine monotherapy and placebo and not the combination therapy, resulting in a small sample size in the combination group, which limited statistical power. Additionally, the study design limited fluoxetine dosing according to olanzapine dosing, such that most subjects received only a starting dose of fluoxetine (20 mg/day). It is plausible that if higher doses of fluoxetine had been used, greater reductions in depressive symptoms or higher response or remission rates could have been achieved.

Wijkstra and colleagues (2009) reported on a double-blind, randomized controlled study of 122 hospitalized patients (ages 18–65 years) with psychotic depression at eight sites in the Netherlands. The patients were treated for 7 weeks with either imipramine ($n=42$), venlafaxine ($n=39$), or the combination of venlafaxine and quetiapine (n=41). The dosage of imipramine was adjusted to adequate plasma levels of 200–300 ng/mL. The maximum dosage was 375 mg/day for venlafaxine and 375/600 mg/day for venlafaxine-quetiapine. The primary outcome measure was a response on the Ham-D ($\geq$50% decrease and final score $\leq$14). Remission was defined as a final Ham-D score of 7 or less. Response rates for imipramine, venlafaxine, and venlafaxine-quetiapine were 22 of 42 (52.4%), 13 of 39 (33.3%), and 27 of 41 (65.9%), respectively. For the primary outcome measure of response, the venlafaxine-quetiapine combination was statistically significantly more effective than venlafaxine; there were no statistically significant differences in the response rates between venlafaxine-quetiapine and imipramine or between imipramine and venlafaxine. Remission rates for the venlafaxine-quetiapine combination (17 of 41, or 41.5%) were statistically significantly higher than those for imipramine (9 of 42, or 21.4%), with no statistically significant difference compared with venlafaxine (11 of 39, or 28.2%) and no significant difference between imipramine and venlafaxine. The authors concluded that the combination of venlafaxine and quetiapine was more effective than venlafaxine alone on the primary outcome measure (response) and was well tolerated (Wijkstra et al. 2009).

The recently completed National Institute of Mental Health (NIMH) Study of Pharmacotherapy of Psychotic Depression (STOP-PD) reported results that indicated that the combination of an antidepressant and an atypical antipsychotic medication was more efficacious than monotherapy with the atypical antipsychotic (Meyers et al. 2009). The study included 259 subjects with psychotic depression, 142 subjects 60 years or older, and 117 subjects younger than 60 years. The investigators randomly assigned 129 subjects to combination treatment and 130 to olanzapine plus placebo. Remission was defined as a Ham-D score of 10 or lower at two consecutive assessments without delusions, as classified by a Schedule for Affective Disorders and Schizophrenia delusion severity score of 1 at the second assessment when the 2-week Ham-D depression remission criterion was met. Subjects who achieved a Ham-D score of 10 or lower for the first time at week 12 were assessed again at week 13 to determine whether the 2-week duration criterion for remission was met.

The dosing regimen in the STOP-PD was as follows: 1) administer initial doses of 50 mg of sertraline or placebo and 5 mg of olanzapine as tolerated (frail elderly subjects initially received 25 mg of sertraline or placebo and 2.5 mg of olanzapine); 2) increase the dosage of sertraline or placebo by 50 mg/day and of olanzapine by 5 mg/day every 3 days as tolerated; 3) attempt to reach minimum dosage of 100 mg/day of sertraline or placebo and 10 mg/day of olanzapine before the end of week 1; 4) increase dosage to 150 mg/day of sertraline or placebo and 15 mg/day of olanzapine during week 2; 5) allow use of sertraline or placebo at 200 mg/day and olanzapine at 20 mg/day for residual symptoms beginning in week 3; 6) allow slower titration or temporary dose reductions of one or both medications if side effects are suspected; however, subsequent dose increases were required to attempt to achieve minimum target dosage of 150 mg/day of sertraline or placebo and 15 mg/day of olanzapine.

Meyers et al. (2009), in the STOP-PD, reported that 67% of the study completers who received the olanzapine-sertraline combination achieved remission by week 12, compared with only 49% of the study completers who received olanzapine monotherapy ($\chi^2 = 10.42$; $P=0.04$). An analysis of all randomly assigned subjects found that the combination of olanzapine and sertraline was associated with a greater frequency of remission (42% of 129 subjects) than was olanzapine monotherapy (24% of 130 subjects) ($\chi^2 = 9.53$; $P=0.002$). The superior efficacy of olanzapine plus sertraline increased over time (odds ratio [OR]=1.28; 95% CI=1.12–1.47; $P<0.001$). Separation began at week 8 and continued through week 12. Remission rates in young adult and geriatric samples were comparable; however, geriatric patients also were more likely to discontinue study medication because of a lack of efficacy than were younger adults. The rates and severity of adverse events were similar in older and younger patients, and older subjects did not have poorer overall tolerability. With the exception of a greater frequency of pedal edema, older subjects were not more likely to experience falls, sedation or somnolence, or greater extrapyramidal symptoms. Both age groups experienced significant increases in weight, triglycerides, and cholesterol levels. However, older age was associated with less weight gain, which may be partially explained by the lower cumulative olanzapine dose (Smith et al. 2008). Fasting glucose levels increased significantly only in younger adults.

In the Muller-Siecheneder et al. (1998) study, risperidone monotherapy was compared with the combination of amitriptyline plus haloperidol in a 6-week double-blind study in 123 patients with psychotic depression ($n=38$) but also with schizoaffective disorder ($n=66$) and schizophrenia spectrum disorder with major depressive symptoms ($n=19$). A significantly greater decrease in scores on the Bech-Rafaelson Scale (70% vs. 51%) and the Positive and Negative Syndrome Scale (PANSS) derived from the BPRS (51% vs. 37%) occurred with combination therapy. However, given the mixed sample, it is not clear to what extent these results apply specifically to patients with psychotic depression.

Taken together, these five studies provide little support for using antipsychotic monotherapy rather than the combination of an antidepressant and an antipsychotic.

Selecting a Combination of Antidepressant and Antipsychotic

Four combinations of antidepressant plus antipsychotic medications have been studied in randomized controlled clinical trials of patients with psychotic depression and have been shown to be effective: 1) sertraline plus olanzapine (Meyers et al. 2009; 259 subjects); 2) fluoxetine plus olanzapine (Rothschild et al. 2004; 249 subjects); 3) venlafaxine plus quetiapine (Wijkstra et al. 2009; 122 subjects); and 4) amitriptyline plus perphenazine (Spiker et al. 1985; 51 subjects) (see Table 3–2).

Other combinations of antidepressants and antipsychotics have not been studied within a randomized, double-blind study design. We would recommend using one of the combinations described above until evidence indicates that other combinations are effective. If a patient does not respond to trials of one or two of these combinations, ECT should be seriously considered.

TABLE 3–2. Combinations of antidepressant and antipsychotic medications with demonstrated efficacy in psychotic depression in randomized controlled clinical trials

STUDY	SAMPLE SIZE	ANTIDEPRESSANT	ANTIPSYCHOTIC
Meyers et al. 2009	259	Sertraline	Olanzapine
Rothschild et al. 2004[a]	249	Fluoxetine	Olanzapine
Wijkstra et al. 2009	122	Venlafaxine	Quetiapine
Spiker et al. 1985	51	Amitriptyline	Perphenazine

[a]Only study with a placebo control group.

KEY CLINICAL POINTS: PSYCHOTIC DEPRESSION

- The most effective somatic treatments for psychotic depression are ECT and the combination of an antidepressant and an antipsychotic.

- No medication treatments have an FDA indication for the treatment of psychotic depression.

- Four combinations of antidepressant plus antipsychotic medications have been studied in randomized controlled clinical trials of patients with psychotic depression and have been shown to be effective: sertraline plus olanzapine, fluoxetine plus olanzapine, venlafaxine plus quetiapine, and amitriptyline plus perphenazine.

Treatment-Resistant Depression

A significant proportion of patients with major depressive disorder fail to achieve remission with standard antidepressant therapies and are classified as having TRD. TRD occurs along a continuum, with degrees of resistance ranging from failure to respond to one class of antidepressants to failure to respond to several different classes of antidepressants and ECT. At present, only one antipsychotic medication, olanzapine, has an FDA indication for the acute treatment of TRD, when combined with fluoxetine. For this FDA indication, TRD is defined as two failed attempts of adequate dose and duration with other antidepressants in the current episode.

Olanzapine-Fluoxetine Combination

The use of olanzapine for the treatment of TRD was first investigated in a small study that compared the effects of olanzapine alone (i.e., olanzapine plus placebo), olanzapine plus fluoxetine, and fluoxetine alone in patients who had previously failed adequate trials of an SSRI and a non-SSRI antidepressant, as well as a prospective treatment period with fluoxetine alone (up to 60 mg/day) (Shelton et al. 2001). The average maximum dosages in the double-blind period were as follows: 12.5 mg/day for olanzapine alone; 52 mg/day for fluoxetine alone; and 13.5 and 52 mg/day, respectively, for the olanzapine-fluoxetine combination. The continuation of fluoxetine for this period yielded essentially no further improvement.

Olanzapine administered alone achieved a modest benefit over fluoxetine, whereas the olanzapine-fluoxetine combination resulted in consistent and significantly greater improvement in depressive symptoms than with either monotherapy. Remission, defined as a 17-item Ham-D score of 7 or less, was achieved in 60% of the patients receiving the combination, 25% receiving olanzapine alone, and 20% receiving fluoxetine alone (Shelton et al. 2001).

Following the initial study of Shelton and colleagues (2001), two large-scale clinical trials testing the effects of the olanzapine-fluoxetine combination were undertaken (Corya et al. 2006; Shelton et al. 2005). Both trials failed to show significant, positive effects of the olanzapine-fluoxetine combination at end point compared with antidepressant monotherapies. Possible explanations for the results (Papakostas and Shelton 2008) include the fact that patients had only one failed adequate trial of an SSRI before entry and that the doses of olanzapine and fluoxetine were lower than in the pilot study of Shelton and colleagues (2001).

In two additional trials, each with the same design (Thase et al. 2007), 1,313 patients with a single drug failure were given fluoxetine. Those who did not respond ($n=605$) were randomly assigned to continuation fluoxetine (plus placebo), olanzapine (plus placebo), or olanzapine-fluoxetine combination. After 8 weeks of double-blind treatment, Study 1 reported no statistically significant therapy differences in MADRS mean change (–11.0, olanzapine-fluoxetine combination; –9.4, fluoxetine; –10.5, olanzapine). In Study 2, the olanzapine-fluoxetine combination resulted in significantly greater MADRS improvement (–14.5) compared with fluoxetine (–8.6; $P<0.001$) and olanzapine (–7.0; $P<0.001$). Pooled study results indicated significant differences for olanzapine-fluoxetine combination (–12.7) versus fluoxetine (–9.0; $P<0.001$) and olanzapine (–8.8; $P<0.001$). Pooled remission rates were 27% for olanzapine-fluoxetine combination, 17% for fluoxetine, and 15% for olanzapine. There was statistically significantly more weight gain, increased appetite, dry mouth, somnolence, peripheral edema, and hypersomnia with the olanzapine-fluoxetine combination compared with fluoxetine monotherapy but not olanzapine monotherapy (Thase et al. 2007).

Aripiprazole, Quetiapine, Risperidone, and Ziprasidone

Several studies have suggested that other atypical antipsychotic medications, such as aripiprazole, quetiapine, risperidone, and ziprasidone, also may have efficacy for the treatment of TRD (Papakostas and Shelton 2008), although except for aripiprazole, none has the indication as yet from the FDA. Most of the studies involved the use of the atypical antipsychotic as an augmentation strategy of an antidepressant.

A recent meta-analysis of 16 acute-phase, placebo-controlled randomized trials of atypical antipsychotic augmentation of treatment-resistant nonpsychotic major depression demonstrated that augmentation with atypical antipsychotic agents was significantly more effective than placebo for response and remission. The fixed-effect meta-analytic trial included augmentation trials of olanzapine, risperidone, quetiapine, and aripiprazole: no acute-phase double-blind trials of adjunctive ziprasidone or paliperidone were located to include in the analysis. Of the 3,480 patients included in the meta-analysis, 2,014 were randomly assigned to receive adjunctive atypical antipsychotic treatment and 1,466 to receive placebo. The pooled response rates were 44.2% compared with 29.9% for atypical antipsychotic treatment or placebo, respectively. The pooled remission rates were 30.7% and 17.2% for atypical antipsychotic treatment and placebo, respectively. The odds ratio for remission was 2.0, and the number needed to treat with atypical antipsychotic augmentation to response or remission was 9. No between–antipsychotic agent differences in efficacy or discontinuation rates were observed, but discontinuation rates due to adverse events were significantly higher for the atypical agents, with a number needed to harm of 17.

In summary, augmenting antidepressants with an atypical antipsychotic medication can be effective for acute treatment in some patients with TRD. However, the long-term efficacy, tolerability, and safety of this treatment regimen remain to be determined. In particular, adverse events during treatment with these agents— the risk of metabolic (weight gain and hyperlipidemia or dyslipidemia), endocrine (hyperprolactinemia), cardiac (QTc prolongation and arrhythmogenesis), and central nervous system (akathisia, parkinsonism, tardive dyskinesia, neuroleptic malignant syndrome)—in major depressive disorder need to be better quantified (Papakostas and Shelton 2008). In addition, the efficacy and safety of atypical antipsychotic medications as augmentation strategies of antidepressants for the treatment of TRD need to be compared with the efficacy and safety of other treatments for TRD such as cognitive-behavioral psychotherapy; other classes of antidepressants, such as tricyclic antidepressants and monoamine oxidase inhibitors; ECT, and vagus nerve stimulation, transcranial magnetic stimulation, and deep brain stimulation (DBS).

KEY CLINICAL POINTS: TREATMENT-RESISTANT DEPRESSION

- Only olanzapine (when combined with fluoxetine) has an FDA indication for the acute treatment of TRD.
- Several studies have suggested that other atypical antipsychotic medications such as aripiprazole, quetiapine, risperidone, and ziprasidone also may have efficacy for the treatment of TRD when combined with an antidepressant.
- The long-term efficacy, tolerability, and safety of antipsychotic medication for TRD remain to be determined.

Nonpsychotic Depression

Over the past several years, there has been increasing off-label use of atypical antipsychotic medications for the treatment of nonpsychotic depression. At present, one atypical antipsychotic medication, aripiprazole, has an FDA indication as an addition to antidepressant treatment for the treatment of nonpsychotic major depressive disorder.[1] The decision to use an atypical antipsychotic medication for nonpsychotic depression needs to take into account the potential benefits of this class of medications and the risks (see discussion of risks in the section "Treatment-Resistant Depression" earlier in this chapter), as well as whether the patient has been given adequate treatment (both dose and duration) with medications from the various FDA-approved classes of antidepressants. In addition, the long-term efficacy, tolerability, and safety of atypical antipsychotic medications for the treatment of nonpsychotic major depressive disorder need to be determined.

Aripiprazole

The FDA approval of aripiprazole as an augmentation agent of antidepressants in nonpsychotic major depressive disorder was based on two large clinical trials. In the first study (Berman et al. 2007), patients with major depressive disorder who showed an incomplete response to one prospective and one to three historical courses of antidepressant treatment within the current episode were studied in an 8-week prospective treatment phase and a 6-week double-blind treatment phase. During prospective treatment, patients received escitalopram, fluoxetine, paroxetine controlled-release, sertraline, or venlafaxine extended-release, each with single-blind, adjunctive placebo. Those patients who had an incomplete response continued the antidepressant and were randomly assigned to double-blind, adjunctive placebo or adjunctive aripiprazole (2–15 mg/day with fluoxetine or paroxetine; 2–20 mg/day with all others). A total of 178 patients were randomly assigned to adjunctive placebo and 184 to adjunctive aripiprazole. Mean change in MADRS total score was significantly greater with adjunctive aripiprazole (−8.8) than with adjunctive placebo (−5.8; $P<0.001$). Adverse events that occurred in 10% or more of patients with adjunctive placebo or adjunctive aripiprazole were akathisia (4.5% vs. 23.1%), headache (10.8% vs. 6.0%), and restlessness (3.4% vs. 14.3%). Discontinuations because of adverse events were low with adjunctive placebo (1.7%) and adjunctive aripiprazole (2.2%); only one adjunctive aripiprazole-treated patient discontinued the antipsychotic because of akathisia.

The second study (Marcus et al. 2008) had the same design as the first study. Subjects with an inadequate response to either escitalopram, fluoxe-

---

[1]In April 2009, an FDA advisory committee recommended that quetiapine be approved as an add-on to antidepressant treatment but should not be used as a monotherapy and should be used only after the failure of other medications. A final decision of the FDA is expected in the future.

tine, paroxetine controlled-release, sertraline, or venlafaxine extended-release were randomly assigned to adjunctive placebo (n = 190) or adjunctive aripiprazole (n = 191) (starting dosage = 5 mg/day; dosage adjustments 2–20 mg/day; mean end-point dosage of 11 mg/day). The mean change in MADRS total score was significantly greater with adjunctive aripiprazole than with placebo (–8.5 vs. –5.7; P=0.001). Remission rates were significantly greater with adjunctive aripiprazole than with placebo (25.4% vs. 15.2%; P= 0.016) as were response rates (32.4% vs. 17.4%; P<0.001). Adverse events occurring in 10% or more of the patients with adjunctive placebo or aripiprazole were akathisia (4.2% vs. 25.9%), headache (10.5% vs. 9.0%), and fatigue (3.7% vs. 10.1%). Incidence of adverse events leading to discontinuation was low (adjunctive placebo: 1.1% vs. adjunctive aripiprazole: 3.7%).

KEY CLINICAL POINTS: NONPSYCHOTIC DEPRESSION

- At present, one atypical antipsychotic medication, aripiprazole, has an FDA indication as an addition to antidepressant treatment for the treatment of nonpsychotic major depressive disorder.

- In April 2009, an FDA advisory committee recommended that quetiapine be approved as an add-on to antidepressant treatment but should not be used as a monotherapy and should be used only after the failure of other medications.

- The long-term efficacy, tolerability, and safety of antipsychotic medications for the treatment of nonpsychotic major depressive disorder are not known.

Obsessive-Compulsive Disorder

Psychopharmacological Treatment Strategies: Initial Treatment Options

OCD affects 2%–3% of the U.S. population (Karno and Golding 1991) and is characterized by the presence of distressful, recurrent obsessions or compulsions that significantly interfere with the patient's social or occupational functioning. OCD can follow a long but variable course, with some patients experiencing a relapsing and remitting course and others experiencing a chronically disabling one. Patients with OCD commonly present with comorbid psychiatric illness—most notably, major depression (67%), social phobia (25%), and tic disorder (20%–30%).

The American Psychiatric Association (2007), in its "Practice Guideline for the Treatment of Patients With Obsessive-Compulsive Disorder," recommends behavior therapy consisting of exposure and response prevention as the first-line treatment for OCD. For patients who do not have an adequate response after 13–20 weekly sessions, additional treatment with an SSRI is recommended. Six serotonin reuptake inhibitors, including clomipramine, fluvoxamine, Luvox CR (fluvoxamine extended-release), fluoxetine, sertraline, and paroxetine, have been approved by the FDA for the treatment of OCD in adults. Current treatment recommendations (Bloch et al. 2006; Kaplan and Hollander 2003) include that the dose of the SSRI should be titrated to the maximum tolerated dose and that the treatment trial should last at least 12 weeks before changing the SSRI or augmenting it because continued response occurs through the twelfth week of SSRI treatment. An estimated 40%–60% of patients, however, do not respond to adequate treatment trials of SSRIs, when treatment response is defined as a reduction of the Yale-Brown Obsessive Compulsive Scale (Y-BOCS) total score by 35% or more (Erzegovesi et al. 2001). An even greater percentage of patients do not achieve symptom remission (Goodman et al. 1993). The literature defines partial response as reduction in Y-BOCS score of greater than 25% but less than 35%, nonresponse as reduction in Y-BOCS score of less than 25%, and refractory OCD as a failure to achieve any change in Y-BOCS score or a worsening of the score with all available therapies (Pallanti and Quercioli 2006).

When a patient achieves only a partial response or does not respond to serotonin reuptake inhibitors, clinicians have several treatment strategies to select from. Although the FDA has approved several initial serotonin reuptake inhibitor treatments, no pharmacological treatments have FDA approval for the adjunctive treatment of OCD. We discuss here off-label, non-FDA-approved antipsychotic augmentation strategies for partial and nonresponders; for an exceptional overview of other pharmacotherapeutic class adjunctive options, see the review by Kaplan and Hollander (2003). For patients who have exhausted these treatments, other biological approaches include ECT, repetitive transcranial magnetic stimulation, and neurosurgical approaches such as anterior capsulotomy, anterior cingulotomy, and DBS. For a recent and thorough review of DBS for treatment-resistant OCD, see the article by Lipsman et al. (2007).

Antipsychotic Augmentation Treatment Strategies in Treatment-Resistant OCD

Rationale

The use of augmentation agents in the treatment of OCD is based on the hypothesis that neurotransmitter circuits in addition to serotonin (i.e., 5-hydroxytryptamine; 5-HT) may be important in SSRI nonresponders or partial responders with OCD. Evidence from basic and clinical research indicates that the dopaminergic and serotonergic neural networks are intricately linked both anatomically and physiologically, especially in the basal ganglia (Goodman et al. 1990). The efficacy of atypical antipsychotics may be a result of a synergistic antagonism of the serotonin receptor subtypes (5-HT_{2A}, 5-HT_{2C}, 5-HT_{1A}, 5-HT_{1D}, and 5-HT_7) and/or antagonism of the dopamine receptors. Functional neuroimaging studies have implicated the dysfunction of the cortico-striatal-thalamic circuit during symptom provocation tasks in patients with OCD. The activity of the cortico-striatal-thalamic circuit is regulated by multiple neurotransmitters, including glutamate, serotonin, dopamine, and γ-aminobutyric acid (GABA). As evidence of a role for antipsychotics in the treatment of OCD, recent positron emission tomography (PET) studies have reported a downregulation of striatal dopamine D_1 receptors (Olver et al. 2009) in medication-free OCD patients compared with control subjects. Moresco et al. (2006) identified a link between the serotonergic and the dopaminergic circuits in OCD when they found that chronic fluvoxamine treatment induced the normalization of D_2 striatal receptor binding in previously medication-naïve OCD patients.

Acute Treatment

A growing literature and several recent meta-analyses show that antipsychotic augmentation is an effective treatment intervention for OCD patients who have not responded to a maximally dosed serotonin reuptake inhibitor after 12 weeks of treatment. In their systematic review of nine randomized, double-blind clinical trials (Bystritsky et al. 2004; Carey et al. 2005; Denys et al. 2004; Erzegovesi et al. 2005; Fineberg et al. 2005; Hollander et al. 2003; McDougle et al. 1994, 2000; Shapira et al. 2004), including 143 OCD patients receiving antipsychotic augmentation and 135 receiving placebo augmentation, Bloch et al. (2006) found that the rate of treatment response (defined as a 35% decline in Y-BOCS scores) in the antipsychotic augmentation group was 32% compared with 11% in the placebo group. The study authors calculated the number needed to treat (NNT; i.e., for one patient with treatment-resistant OCD to benefit from antipsychotic augmentation) as 4.5. This is a larger effect size than that typically reported for serotonin reuptake inhibitor treatment of major depression. The forest plot, comparing the absolute risk difference between the proportions of treatment responders in the antipsychotic augmentation and those in the placebo augmentation group, graphically demonstrated that all nine studies in the meta-analysis, individually and collectively, favored antipsychotic augmentation over augmentation with placebo. In addition, this group determined that all patients who would ultimately benefit from antipsychotic augmentation did so by 4 weeks of antipsychotic augmentation. Thus, clinically, patients who fail to respond to antipsychotic augmentation by the end of 4 weeks of treatment are unlikely to do so with continued augmentation.

Consistent with the results of earlier individual studies (those not included in this meta-analysis), Bloch et al. (2006) found that OCD patients with comorbid tic disorders had an even more favorable response to antipsychotic augmentation compared with placebo augmentation than did OCD patients without comorbid tic disorder. The NNT in this subpopulation of OCD patients was calculated as 2.3, compared with an NNT of 5.9 for OCD patients without comorbid tic disorder. Current evidence supports the use of risperidone or haloperidol in OCD treatment-resistant patients with comorbid tic disorders, given the dual evidence of efficacy of these agents in both Tourette syndrome and OCD (Scahill et al. 2003; Shapiro et al. 1989).

Four antipsychotics were represented among the nine studies included in Bloch et al.'s meta-analysis: haloperidol, risperidone, olanzapine, and quetiapine. Stratification by specific antipsychotic indicated strongest evidence of efficacy for risperidone or haloperidol augmentation compared with placebo augmentation but did not establish efficacy for olanzapine or quetiapine. The study authors noted that either haloperidol or risperidone is more efficacious than olanzapine or quetiapine as augmentation therapy or study heterogeneity invalidated the comparison among antipsychotics across different studies.

In a separate meta-analysis of antipsychotic augmentation of SSRIs in treatment-resistant OCD, Skapinakis et al. (2007) reviewed the nine studies in Bloch's meta-analysis and the Atmaca et al. (2002) single-blind, placebo-controlled study of quetiapine augmentation in treatment-resistant OCD. In this group's analysis, the use of standard and high doses of antipsychotic drugs was associated with better response rates (OR=5.51 for standard or high dose vs. 2.69 for low dose). Also, among the antipsychotics studied (haloperidol, risperidone, olanzapine, and quetiapine), the use of risperidone was associated with positive outcome and less heterogeneous results. Trials of antipsychotic augmentation lasting at least 8 weeks were associated with better outcomes. Contrary to the favorable response to antipsychotic augmentation in OCD patients with comorbid tic disorder reported in Bloch et al.'s meta-analysis, Skapinakis's group did not find a statistically significant response rate ratio in this subgroup. The authors noted that in the studies that included patients with OCD and comorbid tic disorder, compared with those that excluded comorbid tic disorder, the dose of antipsychotic was lower, and that may have contributed to the lower response rate ratio in this subgroup analysis.

Table 3–3 summarizes the key clinical features of the 10 studies included in these meta-analyses, including antipsychotic agent, mean dose, duration of study, and response rates. The mean baseline Y-BOCS score was similar across studies, ranging from 19.1 to 29.3, indicating moderate to severe symptomatology.

Four other studies that were not included in either of the above analyses deserve mention. Li et al. (2005) conducted a 9-week double-blind, placebo-controlled crossover study comparing the efficacy and tolerability of risperidone and a conventional antipsychotic, haloperidol, with that of placebo in patients with SSRI-refractory OCD and severe symptoms as assessed by Y-BOCS. In this study, patients were maintained on their current dose of SSRI and randomly assigned to receive 2 weeks of placebo, risperidone (1 mg/day), or haloperidol (2 mg/day) in a crossover design, with a 1-week placebo washout between each treatment. Li's group reported that risperidone (1 mg/day) and haloperidol (2 mg/day) augmentation in this patient population resulted in rapid improvement of obsessive symptoms but not compulsion symptoms. The percentage drop in total Y-BOCS score after 2 weeks of augmentation was 27% for placebo, 38% for risperidone, and 45% for haloperidol. Clinically, all patients began the study with severe symptoms (Y-BOCS score>24). After haloperidol or risperidone augmentation for 2 weeks, patients' symptoms were in the mild range (Y-BOCS score<15). In addition, augmentation with risperidone, but not haloperidol, was associated with significantly improved depressed mood as measured by the Ham-D-17. Overall, patients tolerated risperidone better than haloperidol: patients receiving haloperidol reported mild to moderate dystonia and lethargy. No abnormal movements were observed in the placebo or risperidone groups. In summary, the prominent clinical finding was that patients whose symptoms had not adequately responded to a 12-week trial of SSRIs were able to benefit from just 2 weeks of antipsychotic augmentation, with OCD symptoms decreasing from the severe to the mild range. This was a very brief augmentation trial, with substantial placebo effect still present at week 2 of analysis. It is unclear if there would be even further separation from placebo if the study were longer. Evidence from other studies indicates that patients who will ultimately respond to antipsychotic augmentation will start to do so by the end of 4 weeks, and for those patients who respond, additional evidence (Skapinakis et al. 2007) shows that an 8-week augmentation trial is associated with better outcomes.

Comparisons between pharmacological agents across different placebo-controlled trials, as with the meta-analyses, can lead to erroneous conclusions because of the heterogeneity of the studies. The Li et al. (2005) study is one of few head-to-head trials that were designed to make efficacy comparisons between antipsychotics (i.e., an atypical versus a typical antipsychotic).

TABLE 3–3. Randomized controlled antipsychotic augmentation trials in patients with treatment-resistant obsessive-compulsive disorder

STUDY	METHODS	N	DURATION OF STUDY (WEEKS)	ANTIPSYCHOTIC TREATMENT, MEAN DOSAGE (SD), MG/DAY	RESPONSE RATE (ANTIPSYCHOTIC ARM VS. PLACEBO ARM, %)
Atmaca et al. 2002	Single-blind, placebo-controlled study	27	8	Quetiapine 91.4 (41.1)	71.4 vs. 0
Bystritsky et al. 2004	Double-blind, placebo-controlled study	26	6	Olanzapine 11.2 (6.5)	46 vs. 0
Carey et al. 2005	Multicenter, double-blind, placebo-controlled study	41	6	Quetiapine 168.7 (120.8)	40 vs. 47.6
Denys et al. 2004	Double-blind, placebo-controlled study	40	8	Quetiapine 300	31 vs. 6
Erzegovesi et al. 2005	Double-blind, placebo-controlled study	20	6	Risperidone 0.5	50 vs. 20
Fineberg et al. 2005	Double-blind, placebo-controlled study	21	16	Quetiapine 215 (124)	27 vs. 10
Hollander et al. 2003	Double-blind, placebo-controlled study	16	8	Risperidone 2.2 (0.9)	50 vs. 0
McDougle et al. 1994	Double-blind, placebo-controlled study	34	4	Haloperidol 6.2 (3.0)	65 vs. 0
McDougle et al. 2000	Double-blind, placebo-controlled study	36	6	Risperidone 2.2 (0.7)	50 vs. 0
Shapira et al. 2004	Double-blind, placebo-controlled study	44	8	Olanzapine 6.1 (2.1)	41 vs. 41

The most recent head-to-head study (Maina et al. 2008) compared two atypical agents, risperidone and olanzapine, in 50 patients who did not have a 35% or greater decrease in Y-BOCS score after a 16-week SSRI trial. This trial, although not placebo controlled, found that risperidone (1–3 mg/day) and olanzapine (2.5–10 mg/day) were equally effective (response rates of 50% and 57%, respectively) in reducing total Y-BOCS score over 8 weeks. One challenge that arises with designing head-to-head studies is how to dose the medications so that they are comparable in terms of their potency and tolerability. In this study, the mean dosages of risperidone (2 mg/day) and olanzapine (5 mg/day) had differing D_2 and 5-HT_2 receptor occupancy rates, with risperidone having greater D_2 binding and olanzapine having greater serotonin binding. Future head-to-head studies should investigate fixed-dose comparisons so that the most effective dosing strategies may be determined.

The equivocality of the data regarding quetiapine prompted Kordon et al. (2008) to design a study that would overcome some of the weaknesses of prior quetiapine augmentation trials to assess efficacy and tolerability in patients with OCD who had not achieved a response to SSRI therapy (i.e., at least 25% reduction in Y-BOCS score) after 12 weeks. Despite using a larger sample size and a higher dose of quetiapine, 400–600 mg/day, no difference between placebo and quetiapine augmentation therapy was seen after 12 weeks of treatment. There were also no significant differences in any other variable measured, including Y-BOCS, CGI-S, or Ham-D-21.

The studies discussed thus far have ranged from 4 to 8 weeks' duration, with the exception of the 16-week Fineberg et al. (2005) study of quetiapine augmentation in SSRI-refractory OCD. Matsunaga and colleagues (2009) investigated the effectiveness and safety of long-term atypical antipsychotic augmentation to SSRI-refractory OCD. Subjects were initially treated with either paroxetine or fluvoxamine for 12 weeks, and those who achieved treatment response, defined in this study as a 25% reduction in Yale-Brown Obsessive Compulsive Scale (Y-BOCS) score, continued taking SSRI monotherapy and began receiving CBT, both for 1 year. Subjects who did not achieve at least 10% reduction in Y-BOCS at the end of 12 weeks of SSRI monotherapy continued taking SSRIs and were additionally randomly assigned to receive either olanzapine, quetiapine, or risperidone augmentation combined with CBT for 1 year. Augmentation with an atypical antipsychotic plus CBT resulted in a significant reduction in Y-BOCS total scores, from 29.3 ± 9.9 to 19.3 ± 6.8, as did SSRI continuation plus CBT (25.8 ± 11.4 to 13.7 ± 4.6) in the comparison group. The SSRI-refractory group had significantly higher YBOCS score at study entry compared with the SSRI-responder group, and continued to have higher YBOCS total scores at the end of 1 year of treatment. Interestingly, subjects in the SSRI-refractory group had a significantly higher prevalence of symmetry obsessions, repeating rituals, and hoarding symptoms than the SSRI-responder group. These symptoms have been associated with SSRI-refractoriness in other studies (Baer 1994; Mataix-Cols et al. 2005). Although the SSRI-refractory group had more severe symptoms at baseline, there was no between group difference in the rate of subjects who achieved >50% improvement in Y-BOCS total score after 1 year of treatment. There were, however, significant between-group differences in metabolic side effects. The SSRI + atypical antipsychotic group had a higher prevalence of subjects with BMI increases >10% (50% vs. 15.2%) and elevated fasting blood sugar (88.6±7.3 vs. 80.9±9.3) compared with the SSRI responder group. Thus, some patients with SSRI-refractory OCD may benefit from atypical antipsychotic augmentation, but the risks of body weight and metabolic side effects that may manifest with long-term treatment must be considered.

In summary, risperidone and haloperidol currently have the strongest evidence for antipsychotic augmentation in patients with OCD who have failed an adequate 12-week trial of SSRI therapy. There is growing evidence that olanzapine may be effective in this patient population, but limited evidence suggests that quetiapine is effective in reducing OCD symptoms when used as an augmentation agent. The American Psychiatric Association (2007), in its "Practice Guideline for the Treatment of Patients With Obsessive-Compulsive Disorder," recommends atypical antipsychotic augmentation when patients fail to respond fully to 4–6 weeks of adequate SSRI treatment plus 13–20 weekly sessions of behavior therapy (including ERP).

Dosing Strategies

Previous authors have recommended that dose ranges for antipsychotics used in the augmentation of OCD mirror those used for psychotic disorders (McDonough and Kennedy 2002). To determine whether the patient's symptoms will respond to antipsychotic augmentation, a minimum of a 4-week trial at the maximum tolerated dose is recommended, and some data (Skapinakis et al. 2007) suggest that an 8-week augmentation trial is associated with better outcomes.

Evidence for Maintenance Treatment

We were not able to locate any prospective studies that investigated maintenance treatment with antipsychotic augmentation in OCD. Two clinically important questions that still need to be addressed are 1) How long should patients who have responded to antipsychotic augmentation be maintained without precipitating relapse? and 2) When during maintenance therapy do the long-term side-effect risks of these agents outweigh benefit? In a retrospective chart review, Maina et al. (2003) reported that 83.3% of the patients who had responded to antipsychotic augmentation to an SSRI relapsed, where relapse was defined as a worsening of Y-BOCS total score by 35% or more with respect to last evaluation during maintenance therapy, or for patients with a Y-BOCS score lower than 16, a Y-BOCS score of 16 or greater anytime after discontinuation. Most patients who relapsed (13 of 15) did so by 8 weeks after discontinuation of the antipsychotic. Thus, the time of highest relapse risk is within 2 months of antipsychotic discontinuation. These statistics are striking, and the authors of this study recommended that patients with OCD whose symptoms are resistant to SSRIs but that respond to augmentation with low-dose antipsychotics should be maintained on this combination therapy, even for long periods, to prevent relapses.

Antipsychotic Monotherapy Treatment Strategies in Treatment-Resistant OCD

To our knowledge, there is no evidence that monotherapy with typical antipsychotics, and insufficient evidence that monotherapy with atypical antipsychotics, is efficacious in the treatment of OCD. McDougle et al. (1995) reported that clozapine monotherapy was not efficacious in treatment-resistant OCD. Ten years later, Connor et al. (2005) reported on the use of aripiprazole monotherapy in OCD. In this small pilot study, eight patients with OCD with varied prior SSRI responses were drug-free at baseline and had a mean baseline total Y-BOCS score of 23.9. All of the patients received 10–30 mg of aripiprazole as monotherapy. Five patients completed the trial, and three patients achieved a 30% or greater reduction in total Y-BOCS score. The study had no placebo arm given its small size. At this time, larger placebo-controlled trials need to be undertaken before any recommendations about the use of aripiprazole in the treatment of OCD can be made. Finally, case reports indicated that clozapine, risperidone, and olanzapine may induce or worsen obsessive-compulsive symptoms in patients with schizophrenia (Baker et al. 1992; Lykouras et al. 2000). Generally, the addition of an SSRI to the antipsychotic improves the obsessive-compulsive symptoms in schizophrenia (Poyurovsky et al. 1996).

KEY CLINICAL POINTS: OBSESSIVE-COMPULSIVE DISORDER

- OCD is a common disorder, and an estimated 40%–60% of patients do not respond to adequate treatment trials of SSRIs.
- A growing literature shows that antipsychotic augmentation is an effective treatment intervention for OCD that has not responded to a maximally dosed SSRI after 12 weeks of treatment.

- Risperidone and haloperidol have the strongest evidence for antipsychotic augmentation in patients with OCD who have failed an adequate 12-week trial of SSRI therapy.

- Growing evidence indicates that olanzapine may be effective in this patient population, but there is limited evidence that quetiapine is effective in reducing OCD symptoms when used as an augmentation agent.

- Antipsychotic augmentation trials should last a minimum of 4 weeks at the maximum tolerated dose.

- Discontinuation of a successful antipsychotic augmentation trial is associated with high rates of relapse, especially within 2 months of antipsychotic discontinuation.

- There is no evidence that monotherapy with typical antipsychotics, and insufficient evidence that monotherapy with atypical antipsychotics, is efficacious in the treatment of OCD.

- Generally, the combination of an SSRI and an antipsychotic is well tolerated, but important cytochrome P450 antidepressant-antipsychotic interactions must be considered.

Generalized Anxiety Disorder

Psychopharmacological Treatment Strategies: Initial Treatment Options

GAD affects approximately 5% of the U.S. population (Wittchen et al. 1994) and is characterized by the presence of excessive anxiety and worry about several events or activities for most days during at least a 6-month period. Patients find the worry distressful, difficult to control, and accompanied by somatic complaints, including irritability, muscle tension, autonomic hyperactivity, restlessness, and sleep disturbance, which ultimately affects social or occupational functioning. Patients with GAD commonly present with co-morbid psychiatric illness—most notably, social phobia, specific phobia, panic disorder, or a depressive disorder.

Initial treatment strategies include cognitive-behavioral therapy, SSRIs, benzodiazepines, and buspirone. Four antidepressants, including duloxetine (Cymbalta), venlafaxine extended-release (Effexor XR), escitalopram (Lexapro), and paroxetine (Paxil), have been approved by the FDA for the treatment of GAD in adults. In addition, several benzodiazepines, doxepin, buspirone, meprobamate, and hydroxyzine have FDA indications for anxiety. Short-term studies report response rates with SSRIs and benzodiazepines ranging from 40% to 70% in GAD (Gelenberg et al. 2000; Pollack et al. 2001). One analysis of data from a longitudinal study found that, despite the efficacy of initial pharmacotherapies, symptoms did not remit with treatment in 87% of patients at 1 year and 63% of patients at 5 years, and half of the patients remained symptomatic at 8-year follow-up (Yonkers et al. 2003). In addition, relapses are increasingly common as the patient is further from the initial GAD episode. Given that remission rates for GAD are low and that relapse is common, long-term treatment strategies include, for more than half of patients, two or more pharmacotherapies (Yonkers et al. 1996). Although the FDA has approved several first-line treatments for GAD, no pharmacological adjunctive treatments have FDA approval. For patients who have failed to remit after initial antidepressant and benzodiazepine trials, augmentation with anticonvulsants or antipsychotics may be considered as an off-label treatment strategy. We discuss the FDA-approved typical antipsychotic trifluoperazine in the short-term treatment of GAD and non-FDA-approved antipsychotic augmentation strategies for partial and nonresponders to the first-line GAD therapies mentioned earlier.

Antipsychotic Augmentation Treatment Strategies in GAD

Rationale

The use of antipsychotic augmentation in the treatment of refractory GAD is based on the understanding of the neurobiological etiology of GAD and the pharmacology of serotonergic and dopaminergic drugs known to be effective in its treatment.

Serotonergic neurons that arise from the rostral dorsal raphe nuclei along the brain stem project to several areas of the brain involved in anxiety, including the hypothalamus and other limbic system structures. The effects of serotonin in the brain, essential to anxiety responses, are mediated through the interaction of presynaptic $5\text{-}HT_1$ autoreceptors and postsynaptic $5\text{-}HT_2$ receptors (Salzman et al. 1993). For this reason, SSRIs are the foundation of GAD treatment.

Dopaminergic circuits hypothesized to be relevant in anxiety include the mesolimbic pathway, which runs from the ventral tegmental area of the midbrain and connects to the limbic system via the nucleus accumbens; the amygdala; the hippocampus; and the medial prefrontal cortex. Preclinical studies of the fear response in animals have identified alterations in dopamine transmission in key anxiety regions, including the amygdala, the medial prefrontal cortex, and the nucleus accumbens (Pezze and Feldon 2004). Thus, dopaminergic agents may prove effective in the treatment of anxiety disorders.

Early studies with typical antipsychotics, which have a very high relative affinity to D_2 receptors, compared with their relative affinity to 5-HT_2 receptors, indicated efficacy in the treatment of neurosis and anxiety disorders. With the development of the atypical antipsychotics, which have a greater relative affinity to 5-HT_2 receptors as compared with D_2 receptors, an interest in their use has ensued.

Acute Treatment

Several small studies published in the 1970s and 1980s investigated the treatment of tension, anxiety, and neurosis with typical antipsychotics in comparison to a benzodiazepine and placebo (Doongagi et al. 1976; Rickels et al. 1974; Yamamoto et al. 1973). Among the studies, trial design varied widely, as did inclusion and exclusion criteria and outcome measurement scales. Several randomized, double-blind studies in GAD (Kragh-Sørensen et al. 1990; Lehmann 1989; Pöldinger 1984) have identified anxiolytic properties of chlorprothixene, fluspirilene, and melperone, respectively. Overall, the evidence indicated that typical antipsychotics were as effective as benzodiazepines, and superior to placebo, in the treatment of a variety of anxiety symptoms.

The largest randomized clinical trial conducted with a typical antipsychotic, trifluoperazine, was completed by Mendels and colleagues (1986). In this multicenter, placebo-controlled study, 415 outpatients with GAD were given trifluoperazine, 2–6 mg/day, or placebo over 4 weeks. Trifluoperazine was superior ($P<0.001$) to placebo on the basis of the Hamilton Anxiety Scale (Ham-A) total score and subscore outcome measures. Trifluoperazine was well tolerated. These findings led to FDA approval of trifluoperazine for the short-term treatment of GAD. As long-term therapy is often indicated in GAD, typical antipsychotic use has not been embraced by clinicians because of the potential for irreversible neurological side effects (e.g., tardive dyskinesia) that can manifest over time.

More recently, studies have investigated the efficacy and safety of the atypical antipsychotics in treatment-resistant GAD. In 2006, Pollack and colleagues reported the efficacy of olanzapine (mean dosage=8.7 ± 7.1 mg/day) augmentation over a 6-week trial in patients with GAD who failed to achieve more than 50% reduction in Ham-A scores after a 6-week trial of fluoxetine, 20 mg/day. Patients who received olanzapine were more likely to have a greater than 50% reduction in Ham-A score than were those who received placebo ($P=0.046$). Weight gain and sedation were more common with olanzapine.

Two recent studies have found that risperidone is efficacious as augmentation treatment in refractory GAD. Brawman-Mintzer and colleagues (2005) reported that risperidone, 0.5–1.5 mg, added to patients' current anxiolytic, resulted in greater reductions in Ham-A total scores ($P=0.034$) and Ham-A psychic anxiety factor scores ($P=0.047$) than did placebo, although response rates did not reach statistical significance. The most commonly reported adverse effects associated with a mean dose of 1.1 ± 0.4 mg of risperidone were somnolence, dizziness, and blurred vision.

An open-label study by Simon and colleagues (2006) evaluated the efficacy of risperidone augmentation in patients with GAD, panic disorder, or social phobia that was refractory to initial pharmacotherapy with an adequate antidepressant and/or benzodiazepine trial of at least 8 weeks' duration. Patients with GAD experienced a mean 6.8-point decrease in Ham-A total score ($P=0.0055$) by the end of the 8-week augmentation trial. The mean dosage, 1.12 ± 0.68 mg/day, and side-effect profile of risperidone were similar to those in the Brawman-Mintzer study. GAD patients in both studies had similar baseline Ham-A scores, although because the CGI-S scores in the Simon study were reported collectively for GAD, panic disorder, and social phobia, it is unclear if patients had similar scores on this global severity measure as well. Of interest, the risperidone-associated reduction in Ham-A score for the Brawman-Mintzer and colleagues (2005) controlled study was more robust than that reported in the Simon and colleagues (2006) study. However, strict comparison of the studies is difficult given their construct differences, including treatment duration, inclusion or exclusion of comorbid illness, and definition of refractoriness.

The same research group that earlier investigated olanzapine and risperidone augmentation in GAD recently examined quetiapine (Simon et al. 2008) and aripiprazole (Hoge et al. 2008) augmentation of anxiolytic therapy. The quetiapine phase of the study failed to detect a statistical difference between quetiapine 25–400 mg/day and placebo over 8 weeks on the study's primary (Ham-A) and secondary measures (rate of remission and response). The first phase included open-label treatment with paroxetine controlled-release (mean dosage=47.3 ± 16.2 mg/day) over 10 weeks, which resulted in a 40% remission rate. Patients whose symptoms did not remit (defined as ≤7 Ham-A total score) were then randomly assigned to the quetiapine versus placebo phase. It is noteworthy that patients who, after completing 10 weeks of paroxetine controlled-release open-label treatment, were randomly assigned to placebo augmentation did not show further improvement over the subsequent 8 weeks of study. The authors recommended that to determine whether a patient's symptoms will respond to the initial SSRI trial, a 10-week trial, at the maximum tolerated dose, be undertaken prior to initiation of augmentation therapy. This is comparable to the recommendation in treatment-resistant OCD; a 12-week SSRI treatment trial is recommended prior to initiation of augmentation.

As mentioned earlier, Hoge and colleagues (2008) recently evaluated the efficacy of aripiprazole as augmentation therapy in a small open-label study in patients with GAD and panic disorder. Patients received an 8-week open-label trial of aripiprazole (mean dosage = 10.5 ± 4.95 mg/day) augmentation to their current anxiolytic treatment, which was held stable throughout the study. In the GAD subgroup, patients experienced a significant decrease in Ham-A (23.5 ± 3.5 to 16.8 ± 6.3; $P<0.01$) and CGI-S scores (4.8 ± 0.44 to 3.6 ± 1.2; $P<0.01$). Side effects reported in more than 10% of the patients included sedation, insomnia, jitteriness, dyspepsia, nausea, constipation, dry mouth, weight gain, and irritability.

In summary, trifluoperazine has the most evidence of efficacy and is approved by the FDA for the short-term treatment of refractory GAD. Further controlled clinical trials with the atypical antipsychotics are needed to increase the currently limited evidence for adjunctive atypical antipsychotic efficacy in GAD. In addition, controlled head-to-head studies between antipsychotics are needed to determine whether specific antipsychotics are more efficacious or better tolerated than others. Table 3–4 summarizes the key clinical features from the randomized controlled antipsychotic augmentation trials in patients with refractory GAD discussed earlier.

Dosing Strategies

According to the reviewed evidence, clinicians can consider using lower doses in augmentation than those used in primary psychotic disorders. For example, trifluoperazine's usual effective dosage range in the treatment of schizophrenia is 15–20 mg/day, with a maximum of 40 mg/day, but its efficacy in GAD augmentation studies was shown at dosages of 2–6 mg/day. The ideal length of an antipsychotic augmentation trial has not yet been established.

We were not able to locate any prospective studies that evaluated the issue of maintenance treatment with antipsychotic augmentation in GAD. It is not known how long to maintain patients who have responded to antipsychotic augmentation without precipitating relapse on antipsychotic discontinuation. Because long-term pharmacotherapy is often needed in chronic, refractory GAD, the risks and benefits of potential long-term use of antipsychotics should be evaluated in every patient prior to initiation of augmentation treatment.

TABLE 3–4. Randomized controlled antipsychotic augmentation trials in patients with treatment-resistant generalized anxiety disorder

STUDY	METHODS	DURATION OF STUDY (WEEKS)	TREATMENT ARM: DOSE (SD OR DOSE RANGE), N	OUTCOME
Yamamoto et al. 1973	Randomized double-blind	4	Chlordiazepoxide 25 mg/day (25 mg–200 mg/day), N=40 vs. Chlorpromazine 25 mg/day (12.5 mg–200 mg), N=41	No statistically significant difference in measured anxiety between groups.
Rickels et al. 1974	Randomized double-blind, placebo-controlled	4–6	Thiothixene 7.12 mg/day (mean), N=52 vs. Thioridazine 101.04 mg/day, N=52 vs. Placebo, N=51	No statistically significant difference in measured anxiety between the two drugs and placebo, measured at 4–6 weeks.
Pöldinger 1984	Randomized double-blind, placebo-controlled	2	Melperone 30 mg/day, N=18, vs. Melperone 75 mg/day, N=19, vs. Placebo, N=23	Reductions in Ham-A and CGI Scale scores were significantly greater in both melperone groups compared with placebo. Melperone 75 mg/day was not superior to melperone 30 mg/day.

TABLE 3–4. Randomized controlled antipsychotic augmentation trials in patients with treatment-resistant generalized anxiety disorder *(continued)*

STUDY	METHODS	DURATION OF STUDY (WEEKS)	TREATMENT ARM: DOSE (SD OR DOSE RANGE), N	OUTCOME
Mendels et al. 1986	Randomized double-blind, placebo-controlled	4	Trifluoperazine 2–6 mg/day, N=207 vs. Placebo, N=208	Trifluoperazine was superior to placebo in all anxiety outcome measures, including Ham-A.
Lehmann 1989	Randomized double-blind	6	Fluspirilene 0.5 mg/week, N=35, vs. Fluspirilene 1 mg/week, N=35, vs. Fluspirilene 1.5 mg/week, N=36	Fluspirilene 1.5 mg was superior to fluspirilene 1.0 or 0.5 mg based on measured improvement on three Ham-A scales.
Kragh-Sørensen et al. 1990	Randomized double-blind, placebo-controlled	2	Bromazepam 6 mg/day, N=97, vs. Chlorprothixene 15 mg/day, N=93, vs. Placebo, N=49	Bromazepam was superior to placebo (P<0.05) but not to chlorprothixene (P>0.10).
Pollack et al. 2006	Randomized double-blind, placebo-controlled	6	Olanzapine 8.7±7.1 mg/day, N=12, vs. Placebo, N=12	Olanzapine was superior to placebo when added to fluoxetine 20 mg/day (P<0.05). Effect size=0.58.

TABLE 3–4. Randomized controlled antipsychotic augmentation trials in patients with treatment-resistant generalized anxiety disorder *(continued)*

STUDY	METHODS	DURATION OF STUDY (WEEKS)	TREATMENT ARM: DOSE (SD OR DOSE RANGE), N	OUTCOME
Brawman-Mintzer et al. 2005	Randomized double-blind, placebo-controlled	5	Risperidone 1.1±0.4 mg/day, N=19, vs. Placebo, N=20	Risperidone was superior to placebo (P<0.05) with mean Ham-A total change scores of −9.8±5.5 in risperidone vs. −6.2±4.9 in placebo.
Simon et al. 2008	Randomized double-blind, placebo-controlled	8	Quetiapine 120.5±100.5 mg/day, N=11, vs. Placebo, N=11	There was no significant reduction in Ham-A or CGI-S score with quetiapine augmentation of Paxil CR as compared with placebo augmentation of Paxil CR.

Note. CGI=Clinical Global Impressions; CGI-S=Clinical Global Impressions—Severity scale; Ham-A=Hamilton Anxiety Scale; SD=standard deviation.

Antipsychotic Monotherapy Treatment Strategies in Treatment-Resistant GAD

We located one open-label study on atypical antipsychotic monotherapy in refractory GAD. Snyderman and colleagues (2005) reported, in a letter to the editor, pilot data from 13 patients with treatment-resistant GAD of moderate severity who received ziprasidone 20–80 mg/day (average dosage=40 mg/day). Three of the 13 patients continued taking concomitant low-dose benzodiazepine therapy, but none were receiving antidepressant therapy during the study. After 7 weeks of open-label ziprasidone treatment, patients experienced a significant decrease in Ham-A (20.31 to 11.15; $P<0.001$) and CGI-S scores (4.23 to 1.54; $P<0.001$). In this study, 54% of the patients met criteria for response, where response was defined as 50% or greater reduction in Ham-A total score, and 38% met criteria for remission, where remission was defined as a score of 7 or lower on the Ham-A. These results, although preliminary, are encouraging because SSRIs have response rates of 40%–70% in GAD. Future controlled studies, however, will need to determine how much of this response rate is due to placebo effect or pharmacological effect.

KEY CLINICAL POINTS: GENERALIZED ANXIETY DISORDER

- GAD is a common disorder, and despite efficacy of the initial pharmacotherapies, 87% of patients fail to remit with treatment at 1 year.

- Research points to the importance of both serotonergic and dopaminergic neurochemical circuits in the pathophysiology of GAD.

- Typical antipsychotics have been found to be as effective as benzodiazepines, and superior to placebo, in the treatment of a variety of anxiety symptoms.

- Trifluoperazine has FDA approval for the short-term treatment of GAD and has the strongest evidence of efficacy among antipsychotics.

- There is initial evidence for risperidone, olanzapine, and aripiprazole as augmentation treatment options in refractory

GAD, but more studies need to be done before any of these agents can be recommended.

- Limited evidence indicates that monotherapy with atypical antipsychotics is efficacious in the treatment of GAD.

- Generally, the combination of an SSRI and an antipsychotic is well tolerated, but important cytochrome P450 antidepressant-antipsychotic interactions must be considered.

Posttraumatic Stress Disorder

Psychopharmacological Treatment Strategies: Initial Treatment Options

PTSD affects approximately 9.2% of the U.S. population (Breslau et al. 1991) and is more common in women, with an estimated 12% of women being affected (Resnick et al. 1993). PTSD may occur after exposure to a traumatic event during which the patient reacts with fear or helplessness. Symptom onset can occur in close proximity to the traumatic event or with a delayed onset. As defined by DSM-IV-TR (American Psychiatric Association 2000), PTSD is characterized by the symptoms of reexperiencing of the traumatic event, efforts to persistently avoid stimuli associated with the trauma, and persistent symptoms of hyperarousal that interfere with the patient's social or occupational functioning. Patients also may describe fluctuating symptoms of panic attacks, dissociation, illusions, hallucinations, anger, agitation, or hostility (Orth and Wieland 2006). Approximately one-third of the patients with PTSD have been reported to present with comorbid schizophrenia, schizoaffective disorder, major depression with psychotic features, or atypical psychotic disorders (Sautter et al. 1999).

Initial treatment strategies include SSRIs, cognitive-behavioral therapy (focused on either repeated exposure or information processing without repeated exposure), eye movement desensitization and reprocessing therapy, education, and supportive measures. SSRIs are considered the first line treatment of PTSD for men and women because they have been shown to improve all three core symptom clusters of the disorder (Brady et al. 2000; Connor et al. 1999; Davidson et al. 2001; Marshall et al. 2001; D.J. Stein et al. 2006). Paroxetine and sertraline have received FDA approval for the treatment of PTSD in adults, but the American Psychiatric Association (2004), in its "Practice Guideline for the Treatment of Patients With Acute Stress Disorder and Posttraumatic Stress Disorder," notes that although individual SSRIs may differ in their individual pharmacokinetics and side effects, they likely have similar efficacy in PTSD. Despite the efficacy of the SSRIs, 40%–47% of the patients failed to respond to initial treatment in several randomized clinical trials (Brady et al. 2000; Davidson et al. 2001; Marshall et al. 2001), when response was defined as greater than 30% reduction from baseline in the Clinician-Administered PTSD Scale—Part 2 (CAPS-2).

When a patient achieves only a partial response or is an SSRI nonresponder, clinicians may consider off-label, non-FDA-approved augmentation strategies with anticonvulsants, antipsychotics, benzodiazepines, or adrenergic inhibitors. In this section, we discuss non-FDA-approved antipsychotic augmentation strategies for partial responders and nonresponders to the first-line PTSD therapies discussed earlier

Antipsychotic Augmentation Treatment Strategies in PTSD

Rationale

The use of augmentation agents is based on the hypothesis that neurotransmitter circuits in addition to those involving serotonin may be important in SSRI nonresponders or partial responders with PTSD. Evidence from basic and clinical research indicates that the dopaminergic and serotonergic neural networks are intricately linked both anatomically and physiologically with the glucocorticoid system during stress responses. The efficacy of atypical antipsychotics may be due to a synergistic antagonism of the serotonin receptor subtypes ($5\text{-}HT_{2A}$, $5\text{-}HT_{2C}$, $5\text{-}HT_{1A}$, $5\text{-}HT_{1D}$, and $5\text{-}HT_7$) and/or antagonism of the dopamine receptors. For an excellent review of the neural circuitry of the stress response, we refer you to Vermetten and Bremner (2002) because here we focus on serotonin and dopamine circuits as a rationale for the use of antipsychotics in PTSD.

Kaehler et al. (2000) reported that severe stress or trauma led to excessive serotonin activation in several rodent brain areas. This excessive serotonergic tone became a state of serotonergic depletion when the trauma was persistent (Matsumoto et al. 2005). Matsumoto et al. (2008) showed that exposure to early postnatal stress resulted in a reduction in $5\text{-}HT_{1A}$-mediated fear conditioning. Other studies (Czyrak et al. 2002) have found that elevated levels of corticosterone are associated with a reduction of hippocampal $5\text{-}HT_{1A}$ receptors thought to be important in the memory and dissociative symptoms of PTSD. Thus, exposure to early stress, which is associated with a sensitized corticotropin-releasing hormone neuroendocrine circuit (Gutman and Nemeroff 2003), may lead to long-lasting dysfunction of the serotonergic receptor system, which compromises fear conditioning and extinction, processes essential to the development of PTSD. Administration of tricyclic antidepressants prior to exposure to early stress has been shown to prevent stress-induced decreases in serotonin and resultant learned helplessness (Petty et al. 1992). For this reason, SSRIs are the foundation of PTSD treatment and may provide a rationale for the serotonergic pharmacological effects of the atypical antipsychotics.

In contrast to serotonin depletion, studies suggest that both acute and chronic stress increases dopamine in the prefrontal cortex and amygdala. Several neurotransmitter systems, including serotonin, modulate the stress-induced increases in mesoprefrontal cortical dopamine release (Vermetten and Bremner 2002). It has been hypothesized that the medial prefrontal cortex is involved in the inhibition of fear responses and that dysregulation of dopamine in this area may cause deficits in extinction of conditioned fear, thus causing anxiety (Morrow et al. 1999).

Acute Treatment

Earlier reports, which suggested that the typical antipsychotics perphenazine and thioridazine (Dillard et al. 1993; Thompson 1977) may be effective in the treatment of flashbacks and nightmares in PTSD, led to more recent studies of the atypical antipsychotics in PTSD treatment. The first case report of the use of clozapine (Hamner 1996) for the treatment of PTSD-related psychosis indicated that clozapine ameliorated not only psychotic symptoms, including auditory and visual hallucinations, thought disorder, and paranoid ideation, but also the core PTSD symptoms of reexperiencing, autonomic instability, and emotional numbing.

A small amount of literature indicates that atypical antipsychotic augmentation to anxiolytic therapy may be an efficacious treatment intervention in SSRI-resistant PTSD. M.B. Stein and colleagues (2002) completed the first double-blind, placebo-controlled study of adjunctive antipsychotic treatment to SSRIs for combat-related PTSD. Patients who failed to respond to 12 weeks of maximally dosed SSRIs were randomly assigned in a double-blind fashion to olanzapine (mean dosage = 15 mg/day) or placebo for 8 weeks. Olanzapine was associated with a significantly greater reduction than placebo in PTSD symptoms, as measured by the CAPS; depressive symptoms, as measured by the Center for Epidemiologic Studies Depression Scale (CES-D Scale); and sleep disturbance, as measured by the global scale on the Pittsburgh Sleep Quality Index. However, clinician-rated global response rates did not significantly differ between olanzapine and placebo, and the magnitude of effects, although statistically significant, was not clinically significant for many of the responders.

We located one study of adjunctive quetiapine treatment in PTSD. Hamner and colleagues (2003a) conducted an open trial of quetiapine augmentation (average dosage = 100 mg/day ± 70 mg/day) to a patient's current psychotropic regimen over 6 weeks in 20 combat veterans with PTSD. Adjunctive quetiapine was associated with a significant improvement in PTSD symptoms, as measured by the CAPS scores (baseline = 89.8 ± 15.7; end of study = 67.5 ± 21.0). Of the patients, 63% had a clinically significant response on the CAPS, defined as a 20% or greater reduction in CAPS composite score. Improvement on CAPS occurred in all three symptom clusters. CGI Scale ratings indicated that 58% met criteria for a significant response, 26% had minimal improvement, and 21% had no change in symptoms. The PANSS composite, positive, and general psychopathology scores also improved with quetiapine treatment. This patient sample had high levels of psychotic symptoms, as measured by the PANSS. However, both subgroups, those with high positive psychotic symptoms ratings (79%) and those with low critical symptom ratings (21%), improved with treatment. Given the open-label nature of this small study, the findings are of importance but should be replicated in larger controlled studies before quetiapine therapy can be recommended as augmentation therapy in PTSD.

Most atypical antipsychotic studies have investigated the potential efficacy of risperidone as adjunctive treatment in PTSD. A study that was primarily designed to test if risperidone adjunctive treatment reduced psychotic symptoms associated with PTSD in combat veterans found that risperidone (mean = 2.5 ± 1.25 mg/day) had only modest effects in reducing hallucinations, delusions, or thought disorder not occurring exclusively during a flashback (Hamner et al. 2003b). It is not clear if the statistically significant reduction in PANSS total scores associated with risperidone treatment (baseline 85.6 ± 14.3; end point 75.6 ± 17.2) compared with those of placebo (baseline 82.1 ± 7.9; end point 79.9 ± 16.4) was clinically significant. Risperidone did not separate from placebo on the CAPS, the secondary outcome, so there were no significant between-group differences in total PTSD symptoms. However, the authors noted that there was a trend toward greater improvement in PTSD reexperiencing symptoms, as measured by the CAPS Cluster B subscale, in the risperidone group.

Monnelly and colleagues (2003) reported that low-dose risperidone, as augmentation to antidepressant therapy, reduced irritability, as measured by the Overt Aggression Scale—Modified for Outpatients (OAS-M), and intrusive thoughts, as measured by the Patient Checklist for PTSD—Military Version (PCL-M), in combat veterans. It is unclear if the improvement was a result of the effects of risperidone alone or the combination of risperidone and antidepressants.

A larger study (Bartzokis et al. 2005) added further evidence of the effectiveness of risperidone in treating overall PTSD symptoms, with a particularly large effect size (Cohen's $d = 0.83$) for Cluster D hyperarousal symptoms (irritability, hypervigilance). This study extended the earlier findings of Monnelly and colleagues (2003) in a large cohort of severely symptomatic patients with treatment-resistant combat-related PTSD.

Two studies evaluated the efficacy of risperidone augmentation in non-combat-related PTSD. Reich and colleagues (2004) reported strongly significant reductions in CAPS-2 total scores (mean change at end point = risperidone 29.6 vs. placebo 18.6) and CAPS-2 intrusive thoughts and hyperarousal subscale scores after 8 weeks of treatment with low-dose risperidone. Rothbaum and colleagues (2008), however, did not detect a between-group difference in PTSD symptoms, as measured by the CAPS total score in a two-phase augmentation trial in civilian non-combat-related PTSD. Phase I of the trial was an 8-week open-label treatment with sertraline; patients who after 8 weeks did not remit, defined as a 70% decrease in PTSD symptoms, entered phase II, a random assignment to either placebo or risperidone augmentation for 8 additional weeks. Only in post hoc analysis did patients who received risperidone have significantly more improvement than the placebo group on the Davidson Trauma Scale sleep item. Nonsignificant trends of improvement on positive symptoms and paranoia subscales of the PANSS for the risperidone group compared with placebo also were reported. Patients may have continued to improve while taking sertraline during phase II, thus obscuring the drug–placebo difference. The authors noted that the study was not adequately powered to detect group differences.

We located one meta-analysis of the available randomized, double-blind, placebo-controlled trials of olanzapine and risperidone as monotherapy or augmentation therapy in PTSD (Pae et al. 2008). The investigators concluded that olanzapine and risperidone may have a beneficial effect in the treatment of PTSD, as suggested by significant changes from baseline in CAPS total scores and all three CAPS subscale scores (B [intrusive], C [avoidant], and D [hyperarousal]) after antipsychotic treatment.

In summary, the preliminary data for the use of atypical antipsychotics—in particular, risperidone—in the treatment of PTSD are accumulating. Current evidence is strongest for the use of risperidone in patients who have had a severe, chronic course with combat-related symptoms and a failed antidepressant trial. The recent meta-analysis suggests that the atypical antipsychotics olanzapine and risperidone may be efficacious for all three symptom clusters that define PTSD. The American Psychiatric Association (2004), in its "Practice Guideline for the Treatment of Patients With Acute Stress Disorder and Posttraumatic Stress Disorder," maintains that the preliminary studies of the second-generation antipsychotic agents suggest a potential role for these medications in pharmacological treatment, particularly when concomitant psychotic symptoms are present or when first-line approaches have been ineffective in controlling symptoms. Table 3–5 summarizes the key

TABLE 3–5. Double-blind, placebo-controlled antipsychotic augmentation trials in patients with treatment-resistant posttraumatic stress disorder (PTSD)

Study	N	Duration of study (weeks)	Antipsychotic treatment	Outcome
M.B. Stein et al. 2002	19	12 weeks of SSRI followed by 8 weeks of antipsychotic	Olanzapine 15 mg/day	Response rate of 30% (olanzapine) vs. 11% (placebo); nonsignificant
Hamner et al. 2003b	40	5	Risperidone 2.5 (±1.25) mg/day	Greater decrease in PANSS in psychotic symptoms in risperidone-treated patients compared with patients receiving placebo, $P<0.05$
Monnelly et al. 2003	15	6	Risperidone 0.57 mg/day (mean)	Greater decrease in irritability (OAS-M) and intrusive thoughts (Cluster B, PCL-M) in risperidone-treated patients compared with patients receiving placebo, $P<0.04$
Bartzokis et al. 2005	16	65	Risperidone 3 mg/day	Greater decrease in PTSD symptoms as measured by the CAPS total and CAPS-D subscale scores; Ham-A; and PANSS-P in risperidone-treated patients compared with patients receiving placebo, $P<0.05$
Reich et al. 2004	8	21	Risperidone 1.41 mg/day (mean)	Greater decrease in PTSD symptoms as measured by CAPS-2 total score and CAPS-2 intrusive thoughts and hyperarousal subscale scores in risperidone-treated patients compared with patients receiving placebo, $P<0.001$

TABLE 3–5. Double-blind, placebo-controlled antipsychotic augmentation trials in patients with treatment-resistant posttraumatic stress disorder (PTSD) *(continued)*

STUDY	N	DURATION OF STUDY (WEEKS)	ANTIPSYCHOTIC TREATMENT	OUTCOME
Rothbaum et al. 2008	45	8	Risperidone 2.1 mg/day (mean)	No significant difference in CAPS total score between groups; improved sleep combined frequency and severity item on the Davidson Trauma Scale, $P<0.03$; trends of improvement on positive symptoms and paranoia subscales of the PANSS for risperidone-treated group vs. placebo (nonsignificant)

Note. CAPS-D=Clinician-Administered PTSD Scale, D (arousal) subscale; CAPS-2=Clinician-Administered PTSD Scale—Part 2; CGI-S=Clinical Global Impression (CGI) Scale–Severity; Ham-A=Hamilton Anxiety Scale; OAS-M=Overt Aggression Scale—Modified for Outpatients; PANSS=Positive and Negative Syndrome Scale; PANSS-P=Positive and Negative Syndrome Scale—Positive Scale; PCL-M=Patient Checklist for PTSD—Military Version; SD=standard deviation; SSRI=selective serotonin reuptake inhibitor.

clinical features from the randomized controlled antipsychotic augmentation trials in patients with refractory PTSD discussed earlier.

Dosing Strategies

The reviewed evidence indicates that clinicians can consider using lower doses in augmentation than those used in primary psychotic disorders, particularly with risperidone. For example, risperidone's usual effective dosage range in the treatment of schizophrenia is 4–8 mg/day, with a maximum of 16 mg/day, but its efficacy in PTSD augmentation studies was shown at dosages of 0.5–3 mg/day. The ideal length of an antipsychotic augmentation trial has not yet been established, but data from Bartzokis and colleagues (2005) indicate that patients may continue to show benefit through 16 weeks of treatment with antipsychotic augmentation therapy.

We were not able to locate any prospective studies that evaluated the issue of maintenance treatment with antipsychotic augmentation in PTSD. It is not known how long to maintain patients who have responded to antipsychotic augmentation without precipitating relapse on antipsychotic discontinuation. Because long-term pharmacotherapy is often needed in chronic, refractory PTSD, the risks and benefits of potential long-term use of antipsychotics should be evaluated in every patient prior to initiation of augmentation treatment.

Antipsychotic Monotherapy Treatment Strategies in PTSD

A small literature has investigated the potential role of antipsychotic monotherapy for the treatment of civilian and combat-related PTSD. Two studies (Butterfield et al. 2001; Petty et al. 2001) investigated the role for olanzapine in these two PTSD subpopulations. In the study by Petty's group of male patients with chronic combat-related PTSD, 8 weeks of open-label treatment with olanzapine was associated with a 30% reduction in CAPS total score and Ham-D and Ham-A scores. Intrusive symptoms of PTSD (B cluster of the CAPS) improved independently of improvement in depression and anxiety symptoms. On the other hand, the 10-week randomized placebo-controlled study of olanzapine monotherapy in patients with noncombat PTSD by Butterfield and colleagues (2001) failed to show efficacy. In both studies, the mean dosage of olanzapine was 14 mg/day. However, important differences make comparison of these two studies difficult. According to baseline CAPS subscale scores, patients were more severely ill in the Petty and colleagues (2001) study than in the Butterfield and colleagues (2001) study, and the PTSD subpopulation differed: males with combat-related PTSD versus mostly females with rape-related PTSD. Differences in study design, gender, psychiatric comorbidity, trauma type, and chronicity could have accounted for the disparate findings.

In agreement with the results of studies by Petty and colleagues (2001) and M.B. Stein and colleagues (2002), an open-label, 6-week comparison study of olanzapine and fluphenazine in psychotic combat-related PTSD reported efficacy for both agents in reducing PTSD and psychotic symptoms (Pivac et al. 2004). Olanzapine was found to be more efficacious than fluphenazine in reducing PANSS negative, general psychopathology, and supplementary items subscale scores; scores on CGI-S, CGI-Improvement, and Patient Global Improvement Scale (PGI-I); and scores on the avoidance and increased arousal subscales of Watson's PTSD Scale. Both antipsychotics were similarly efficacious in reducing PANSS positive symptoms subscale scores and scores from the trauma reexperiencing subscale in Watson's scale. Extrapyramidal symptoms were more commonly associated with fluphenazine treatment (3 of 27 patients) than with olanzapine. Given the limitations of an open-label, nonrandomized study of a disorder with a reported high placebo response, these results should be replicated in a controlled trial.

We located two recent studies of risperidone monotherapy in PTSD. Kozaric-Kovacic and colleagues (2005) investigated the efficacy of open-label risperidone monotherapy over 6 weeks in patients with psychotic PTSD that had not responded to prior antidepressant therapy. Risperidone monotherapy was associated with consistent improvements in total PANSS scores (62% reduction from baseline) and subscale scores (44%–70%) on the PTSD Interview (PTSD-I) scale. There was no significant difference between response at 3 and 6 weeks of antipsychotic treatment. A risperidone monotherapy trial in women with abuse-related PTSD showed efficacy in a small randomized placebo-controlled trial (Padala et al. 2006). Finally, an open-label trial with quetiapine over 8 weeks in combat-related PTSD with psychotic features (Kozaric-Kovacic and Pivac 2007) found efficacy in reducing total and subscale scores on the CAPS, PANSS, and CGI-S scales.

In summary, a few small, mostly open-label studies have investigated the efficacy of the atypical antipsychotics olanzapine and risperidone as monotherapy in the treatment of PTSD. The recent meta-analysis that combined available randomized, double-blind, placebo-controlled trials of atypical antipsychotic augmentation and monotherapy suggested that the atypical antipsychotics olanzapine and risperidone may be efficacious for all three symptom clusters that define PTSD.

KEY CLINICAL POINTS: POSTTRAUMATIC STRESS DISORDER

- PTSD is a common disorder, and despite efficacy of the initial SSRI treatment, 40%–47% of patients failed to respond to initial treatment.

- The dopaminergic and serotonergic neural networks are intricately linked with the glucocorticoid system during the stress responses critical to the development of PTSD.

- Support for the use of atypical antipsychotics in the treatment of PTSD is accumulating.

- Current evidence is strongest for the use of risperidone in patients who have had a severe, chronic course with combat-related symptoms and failed an antidepressant trial.

- Clinicians can consider using lower doses in augmentation therapy for PTSD than those used for primary psychotic disorders.

- The atypical antipsychotics olanzapine and risperidone may be efficacious for all three symptom clusters that define PTSD, especially when associated with psychotic symptoms.

- Generally, the combination of an SSRI and an antipsychotic is well tolerated, but important cytochrome P450 antidepressant-antipsychotic interactions must be considered.

Safety and Tolerability of Antipsychotics in Mood and Anxiety Disorders: Fundamental Concepts

Clinicians should discuss with patients the possible side effects of antipsychotic medications and monitor the patients for the occurrence of these side effects. (For a thorough review of the possible adverse reactions with antipsychotic use, see Appendixes 7 and 8 to this book.) Generally, the combination of an SSRI and an antipsychotic is well tolerated, but there are a few

TABLE 3–6. Antipsychotics and their cytochrome P450 metabolism

TYPICAL ANTIPSYCHOTIC	CYTOCHROME P450 METABOLISM	ATYPICAL ANTIPSYCHOTIC	CYTOCHROME P450 METABOLISM
Chlorpromazine (Thorazine)	—	Clozapine (Clozaril)	1A2 substrate
Mesoridazine (Serentil)	—	Risperidone (Risperdal)	2D6 substrate
Thioridazine (Mellaril)	2D6 inhibitor	Olanzapine (Zyprexa)	1A2 substrate, 2D6 substrate
Fluphenazine (Prolixin)	2D6 substrate, 2D6 inhibitor	Quetiapine (Seroquel)	3A4 substrate
Perphenazine (Trilafon)	2D6 substrate, 2D6 inhibitor	Ziprasidone (Geodon)	3A4 substrate
Trifluoperazine (Stelazine)	—	Aripiprazole (Abilify)	2D6 substrate, 3A4 substrate
Prochlorperazine (Compazine)	—	Paliperidone (Invega)	—
Haloperidol (Haldol)	1A2 substrate, 2D6 substrate, 2D6 inhibitor	Iloperidone (Fanapt)	3A4 substrate, 2D6 substrate
Loxapine (Loxitane)	—	Asenapine (Saphris)	1A2 substrate
Molindone (Moban)	—		
Pimozide (Orap)	3A4 substrate and to a lesser extent by 2D6; CYP1A2 also may be involved as substrate		
Thiothixene (Navane)	—		

important interactions to highlight. SSRIs and selective serotonin-norepinephrine reuptake inhibitors (SNRIs), particularly fluoxetine, duloxetine, and paroxetine, can inhibit the cytochrome P450 2D6 metabolism of antipsychotic medications, resulting in the elevation of plasma antipsychotic levels. This increase in levels could lead to increased risk of antipsychotic side effects, especially orthostatic hypotension, cardiac toxicity, and extrapyramidal symptoms. Also, there is a potential toxic interaction between clozapine and fluvoxamine because fluvoxamine is known to inhibit the cytochrome P450 1A2 metabolism of clozapine, thus increasing clozapine levels. Fluvoxamine also could potentially increase aripiprazole levels through inhibition of the cytochrome P450 3A4/3A5 and 3A6 enzymes because it is a substrate. Haloperidol is a cytochrome P450 2D6 substrate and inhibitor and, as such, could increase levels of several antidepressants, including amitriptyline, clomipramine, desipramine, imipramine, paroxetine, and venlafaxine.

Generally, the combination of antipsychotics and benzodiazepines is well tolerated, but there is the potential for increased sedation and hypotension when the two are used concomitantly. Alprazolam, diazepam, midazolam, and triazolam are substrates of the cytochrome P450 3A4/3A5/3A7 enzymes, but antipsychotics are not known to be inhibitors or inducers of these enzymes, so theoretically there should be little concern with their concomitant use.

A summary of the cytochrome P450 enzymes and antipsychotic metabolic activity is shown in Table 3–6.

References

Bipolar Disorder

Asenapine [package insert]. Kenilworth, NJ, Schering-Plough, 2009

Brown EB, McElroy SI, Keck PE, et al: A 7-week, randomized, double-blind trial of olanzapine/fluoxetine combination versus lamotrigine in the treatment of bipolar I depression. J Clin Psychiatry 67:1025–1033, 2006

Calabrese JR, Keck PE Jr, McFadden W, et al: A randomized, double-blind, placebo-controlled trial of quetiapine in the treatment of bipolar I or II depression. Am J Psychiatry 162:1351–1360, 2005

Han C, Lee M-S, Pae C-U, et al: Usefulness of long-acting injectable risperidone during 12-month maintenance therapy of bipolar disorder. Prog Neuropsychopharmacol Biol Psychiatry 31:1219–1223, 2007

Hirschfield RA, Bowden CL, Gitlin MJ, et al: Practice guideline for the treatment of patients with bipolar disorder (revision). Am J Psychiatry 159:1–50, 2002

Keck PE Jr, McElroy SL, Strakowski SM, et al: Antipsychotics in the treatment of mood disorders and risk of tardive dyskinesia. J Clin Psychiatry 61 (suppl 4):33–38, 2000

Keck PE Jr, Calabrese JR, McQuade RD, et al: A randomized, double-blind, placebo-controlled 26-week trial of aripiprazole in recently manic patients with bipolar I disorder. J Clin Psychiatry 67:626–637, 2006

Keck PE Jr, Calabrese JR, McIntyre RS, et al: Aripiprazole monotherapy for maintenance therapy in bipolar I disorder: a 100-week, double-blind study versus placebo. J Clin Psychiatry 68:1480–1481, 2007

Kessler RC, Chiu WT, Demler O, et al: Prevalence, severity, and co-morbidity of twelve-month DSM-IV disorders in the National Comorbidity Survey Replication (NCS-R). Arch Gen Psychiatry 62:617–627, 2005

McElroy S, Young AH, Carlsson A, et al: Double-blind, randomized, placebo-controlled study of quetiapine and paroxetine in adults with bipolar depression (EMBO-LDEN II). Presentation at the 3rd biennial conference of the International Society for Bipolar Disorders, Delhi and Agra, India, January 27–30, 2008

Perlis RH, Welge JA, Vornik MS, et al: Atypical antipsychotics in the treatment of mania: a meta-analysis of randomized, placebo-controlled trials. J Clin Psychiatry 67:509–516, 2006

Suppes T, Dennehy EB, Swann AC, et al: Report of the Texas Consensus Conference Panel on Medication Treatment of Bipolar Disorder 2000. J Clin Psychiatry 63:288–299, 2002

Suppes T, Liu S, Paulsson B, et al: Maintenance treatment in bipolar I disorder with quetiapine concomitant with lithium or divalproex: a North American placebo-controlled, randomized multicenter trial. Poster presented at the 46th annual meeting of the American College of Neuropsychopharmacology, Boca Raton, FL, December 9–13, 2007

Thase ME, Macfadden W, Weisler RH, et al: Efficacy of quetiapine monotherapy in bipolar I and II depression: a double-blind, placebo-controlled study (the BOLDER II study). J Clin Psychopharmacol 26:600–609, 2006

Tohen M, Vieta E, Calabrese JR, et al: Efficacy of olanzapine and olanzapine-fluoxetine combination in the treatment of bipolar I depression (published erratum appears in Arch Gen Psychiatry 61:176, 2004). Arch Gen Psychiatry 60:1079–1088, 2003

Tohen M, Calabrese JR, Sachs GS, et al: Randomized, placebo-controlled trial of olanzapine as maintenance therapy in patients with bipolar I disorder responding to acute treatment with olanzapine. Am J Psychiatry 163:247–256, 2006

Traynor K: Asenapine approved for treatment of schizophrenia, bipolar disorder. Am J Health Syst Pharm 66:1596, 2009

Vieta E, Eggens I, Persson I, et al: Efficacy and safety of quetiapine in combination with lithium or divalproex as maintenance treatment for bipolar I disorder. Poster presented at the 20th European College of Neuropsychopharmacology Congress, Vienna, Austria, October 13–17, 2007

Yatham LN, Fallu A, Binder CE: A 6-month randomized open-label comparison of continuation of oral atypical antipsychotic therapy or switch to long acting injectable risperidone in patients with bipolar disorder. Acta Psychiatr Scand Suppl 434:50–56, 2007

Young AH, McElroy S, Chang W, et al: A double-blind, placebo-controlled study with acute and continuation phase of quetiapine in adults with bipolar depression (EMBOLDEN I). Presented at the 3rd biennial conference of the International Society for Bipolar Disorders, Delhi and Agra, India, January 27–30, 2008

Psychotic Depression

American Psychiatric Association: Practice guideline for the treatment of patients with major depressive disorder (revision). Am J Psychiatry 157 (4 suppl):1–45, 2000

Andreescu C, Mulsant BH, Peasley-Miklus C, et al: Persisting low use of antipsychotics in the treatment of major depressive disorder with psychotic features. STOP-PD Study Group. J Clin Psychiatry 68:194–200, 2007

Baldwin RC, Jolley DJ: The prognosis of depression in old age. Br J Psychiatry 149:574–583, 1986

Blazer D: Epidemiology of late-life depression, in Diagnosis and Treatment of Depression in Late Life. Edited by Schneider L, Reynolds C, Lebowitz B, et al. Washington, DC, American Psychiatric Press, 1994, pp 9–20

Johnson J, Horwath E, Weissman MM: The validity of major depression with psychotic features based on a community sample. Arch Gen Psychiatry 48:1075–1081, 1991

Kivela SL, Pahkala K: Delusional depression in the elderly: a community study. Z Gerontol 22:236–241, 1989

Meyers BS, Flint AJ, Rothschild AJ, et al: A double-blind randomized controlled trial of olanzapine plus sertraline versus olanzapine plus placebo for psychotic depression—the Stop-PD Study. STOP-PD Study Group. Arch Gen Psychiatry 66:838–847, 2009

Muller-Siecheneder F, Muller MJ, Hiller A, et al: Risperidone versus haloperidol and amitriptyline in the treatment of patients with a combined psychotic and depressive syndrome. J Clin Psychopharmacol 18:111–120, 1998

Mulsant BH, Haskett RF, Prudic J, et al: Low use of neuroleptic drugs in the treatment of psychotic major depression. Am J Psychiatry 154:559–561, 1997

Ohayon MM, Schatzberg AF: Prevalence of depressive episodes with psychotic features in the general population. Am J Psychiatry 159:1855–1861, 2002

Rothschild AJ (ed): Clinical Manual for Diagnosis and Treatment of Psychotic Depression. Washington, DC, American Psychiatric Publishing, 2009

Rothschild AJ, Williamson DJ, Tohen MF, et al: A double-blind, randomized study of olanzapine and olanzapine/fluoxetine combination for major depression with psychotic features. J Clin Psychopharmacol 24:365–373, 2004

Ryan ND, Puig-Antich J, Ambrosini P, et al: The clinical picture of major depression in children and adolescents. Arch Gen Psychiatry 44:854–861, 1987

Smith E, Rothschild AJ, Heo M, et al: Weight gain during olanzapine treatment for psychotic depression: effects of dose and age. STOP-PD Collaborative Study Group. Int Clin Psychopharmacol 23:130–137, 2008

Spiker DG, Weiss JC, Dealy RS, et al: The pharmacological treatment of delusional depression. Am J Psychiatry 142:430–436, 1985

Wijkstra J, Lljmer J, Balk FJ, et al: Pharmacological treatment for unipolar psychotic depression. Br J Psychiatry 188:410–415, 2006

Wijkstra J, Burger H, van den Broek WW, et al: Treatment of unipolar psychotic depression: a randomized, double-blind study comparing imipramine, venlafaxine, and venlafaxine plus quetiapine. Acta Psychiatr Scand August 19, 2009 (Epub ahead of print)

Treatment-Resistant Depression

Corya SA, Williamson D, Sanger TM, et al: A randomized, double-blind comparison of olanzapine/fluoxetine combination, olanzapine, fluoxetine, and venlafaxine in treatment-resistant depression. Depress Anxiety 23:364–372, 2006

Nelson JC, Papakostas GI: Atypical antipsychotic augmentation in major depressive disorder: a meta-analysis of placebo-controlled randomized trials. Am J Psychiatry 166:980–991, 2009

Papakostas GI, Shelton RC: Use of atypical antipsychotics for treatment-resistant major depressive disorder. Curr Psychiatry Rep 10:481–486, 2008

Shelton RC, Tollefson GD, Tohen M, et al: A novel augmentation strategy for treating resistant major depression. Am J Psychiatry 158:131–134, 2001

Shelton RC, Williamson DJ, Corya SA, et al: Olanzapine/fluoxetine combination for treatment-resistant depression: a controlled study of SSRI and nortriptyline resistance. J Clin Psychiatry 66:1289–1297, 2005

Thase ME, Corya SA, Osuntokun O, et al: A randomized, double-blind comparison of olanzapine/fluoxetine combination, olanzapine, and fluoxetine in treatment-resistant major depressive disorder. J Clin Psychiatry 68:224–236, 2007

Nonpsychotic Depression

Berman RM, Marcus RN, Swanink R, et al: The efficacy and safety of aripiprazole as adjunctive therapy in major depressive disorder: a multicenter, randomized, double-blind, placebo-controlled study. J Clin Psychiatry 68:843–853, 2007

Marcus RN, McQuade RD, Carson WH, et al: The efficacy and safety of aripiprazole as adjunctive therapy in major depressive disorder: a second multicenter, randomized, double-blind, placebo-controlled study. J Clin Psychopharmacol 28:156–165, 2008

Obsessive-Compulsive Disorder

American Psychiatric Association: Practice Guideline for the Treatment of Patients With Obsessive-Compulsive Disorder. July 2007. Available at: http://www.psychiatryonline.com/pracGuide/pracGuideChapToc_10.aspx. Accessed December 2008.

Atmaca M, Kuloglu M, Tezcan E, et al: Quetiapine augmentation in patients with treatment resistant obsessive-compulsive disorder: a single-blind, placebo-controlled study. Int Clin Psychopharmacol 17:115–119, 2002

Baer L: Factor analysis of symptom subtypes of obsessive compulsive disorder and their relation to personality and tic disorders. J Clin Psychiatry 55 (suppl):18–23, 1994

Baker RW, Chengappa KNR, Baird JW, et al: Emergence of obsessive-compulsive symptoms during treatment with clozapine. J Clin Psychiatry 53:439–442, 1992

Bloch MH, Landeros-Weisenberger A, Kelmendi B, et al: A systematic review: antipsychotic augmentation with treatment refractory obsessive-compulsive disorder. Mol Psychiatry 11:622–632, 2006

Bystritsky A, Ackerman DL, Rosen RM, et al: Augmentation of serotonin reuptake inhibitors in refractory obsessive-compulsive disorder using adjunctive olanzapine: a placebo-controlled trial. J Clin Psychiatry 65:565–568, 2004

Carey PD, Vythilingum B, Seedat S, et al: Quetiapine augmentation of SRIs in treatment refractory obsessive-compulsive disorder: a double-blind, randomised, placebo-controlled study. BMC Psychiatry 5:5, 2005

Connor KM, Payne VM, Gadde KM, et al: The use of aripiprazole in obsessive-compulsive disorder: preliminary observations in 8 patients. J Clin Psychiatry 66:49–51, 2005

Denys D, de Geus F, van Megan HJGM, et al: A double-blind, randomized, placebo-controlled trial of quetiapine addition in patients with obsessive-compulsive disorder refractory to serotonin reuptake inhibitors. J Clin Psychiatry 65:1040–1048, 2004

Erzegovesi S, Cavallini MC, Cadini P, et al: Clinical predictors of drug response in obsessive-compulsive disorder. J Clin Psychopharmacol 21:488–492, 2001

Erzegovesi S, Guglielmo E, Siliprandi F, et al: Low-dose risperidone augmentation of fluvoxamine treatment in obsessive-compulsive disorder: a double-blind, placebo-controlled study. Eur Neuropsychopharmacol 15:69–74, 2005

Fineberg NA, Sivakumaran T, Roberts A, et al: Adding quetiapine to SRI in treatment-resistant obsessive-compulsive disorder: a randomized controlled treatment study. Int Clin Psychopharmacol 20:223–226, 2005

Goodman WK, McDougle CJ, Price LH, et al: Beyond the serotonin hypothesis: a role for dopamine in some forms of obsessive-compulsive disorder? J Clin Psychiatry 51:36–43, 1990

Goodman WK, McDougle CJ, Barr LC, et al: Biological approaches to treatment-resistant OCD. J Clin Psychiatry 54:16–26, 1993

Hollander E, Baldini Rossi N, Sood E, et al: Risperidone augmentation in treatment-resistant obsessive-compulsive disorder: a double-blind, placebo-controlled study. Int J Neuropsychopharmacol 6:397–401, 2003

Kaplan A, Hollander E: A review of pharmacologic treatments for obsessive-compulsive disorder. Psychiatr Serv 54:1111–1118, 2003

Karno M, Golding JM: Obsessive compulsive disorder, in Psychiatric Disorders in America: The Epidemiologic Catchment Area Study. Edited by Robins SL, Regier DA. New York, Free Press, 1991, pp 204–219

Kordon A, Wahl K, Koch N, et al: Quetiapine addition to serotonin reuptake inhibitors in patients with severe obsessive compulsive disorder. J Clin Psychopharmacol 28:550–555, 2008

Li X, May RS, Tolbert LC, et al: Risperidone and haloperidol augmentation of serotonin reuptake inhibitors in refractory obsessive-compulsive disorder: a crossover study. J Clin Psychiatry 66:736–743, 2005

Lipsman N, Neimat JS, Lozano AM: Deep brain stimulation for treatment refractory obsessive compulsive disorder: the search for a valid target. Neurosurgery 61:1–13, 2007

Lykouras L, Zeruas IM, Gournellis R, et al: Olanzapine and obsessive-compulsive symptoms. Eur Neuropsychiatry 10:385–387, 2000

Maina G, Albert U, Ziero S, et al: Antipsychotic augmentation for treatment resistant obsessive-compulsive disorder: what if antipsychotic is discontinued? Int Clin Psychopharmacol 18:23–28, 2003

Maina G, Pessina E, Albert U, et al: 8-Week, single-blind, randomized trial comparing risperidone versus olanzapine augmentation of serotonin reuptake inhibitors in treatment-resistant obsessive-compulsive disorder. Eur Neuropsychopharmacol 18:364–372, 2008

Matsunaga H, Nagata T, Hayashida K, et al: A long-term trial of the effectiveness and safety of atypical antipsychotic agents in augmenting SSRI-refractory obsessive-compulsive disorder. J Clin Psychiatry 70:863–868, 2009

Mataix-Cols D, Rosario-Campos MC, Leckman JF: A multidimensional model of obsessive-compulsive disorder. Am J Psychiatry 162:222–238, 2005

McDonough M, Kennedy N: Pharmacological management of obsessive compulsive disorder: a review for clinicians. Harv Rev Psychiatry 10:127–137, 2002

McDougle CJ, Goodman WK, Leckman JF, et al: Haloperidol addition in fluvoxamine-refractory obsessive-compulsive disorder: a double-blind, placebo-controlled study in patients with and without tics. Arch Gen Psychiatry 51:302–308, 1994

McDougle CJ, Barr LC, Goodman WK, et al: Lack of efficacy of clozapine monotherapy in refractory obsessive-compulsive disorder. Am J Psychiatry 152:1812–1814, 1995

McDougle CJ, Epperson N, Pelton G, et al: A double-blind, placebo controlled study of risperidone addition in serotonin reuptake inhibitor-refractory obsessive-compulsive disorder. Arch Gen Psychiatry 57:794–901, 2000

Moresco RM, Pietra L, Henin M, et al: Fluvoxamine treatment and D2 receptors: a PET study on OCD drug-naïve patients. Neuropsychopharmacology 1:1–9, 2006

Olver JS, O'Keefe G, Jones GR, et al: Dopamine D1 receptor binding in the striatum of patients with obsessive-compulsive disorder. J Affect Disord 114:321–326, 2009

Pallanti S, Quercioli L: Treatment-refractory obsessive-compulsive disorder: methodological issues, operational difficulties and therapeutic lines. Prog Neuropsychopharmacol Biol Psychiatry 30:400–412, 2006

Poyurovsky M, Hermesh H, Weizman A: Fluvoxamine treatment in clozapine-induced obsessive-compulsive symptoms in schizophrenic patients. Clin Neuropharmacol 19:305–313, 1996

Scahill L, Lechman JF, Schultz RT, et al: A placebo-controlled trial of risperidone in Tourette syndrome. Neurology 60:1130–1135, 2003

Shapira NA, Ward HE, Mandoki M, et al: A double-blind, placebo-controlled trial of olanzapine addition in fluoxetine refractory obsessive-compulsive disorder. Biol Psychiatry 550:553–555, 2004

Shapiro E, Shapiro AK, Fulop G, et al: Controlled study of haloperidol, pimozide and placebo for the treatment of Gilles de la Tourette's syndrome. Arch Gen Psychiatry 46:722–730, 1989

Skapinakis P, Papatheordorou T, Venetsanos M: Antipsychotic augmentation of serotonergic antidepressants in treatment-resistant obsessive-compulsive disorder: a meta-analysis of the randomized controlled trials. Eur Neuropsychopharmacol 17:79–93, 2007

Generalized Anxiety Disorder

Brawman-Mintzer O, Knapp RG, Nietert PJ: Adjunctive risperidone in generalized anxiety disorder: a double-blind, placebo-controlled study. J Clin Psychiatry 66:1321–1325, 2005

Doongagi DR, Sheth AS, Ramesh SP, et al: A double blind study of pimozide versus chlordiazepoxide in anxiety neuroses. Acta Psychiatr Belg 76:632–643, 1976

Gelenberg AJ, Lydiard RB, Rudolph RL, et al: Efficacy of venlafaxine extended-release capsules in nondepressed outpatients with generalized anxiety disorder: a 6-month randomized controlled trial. JAMA 283:3082–3088, 2000

Hoge EA, Worthingon JJ, Kaufman RE, et al: Aripiprazole as augmentation treatment of refractory generalized anxiety disorder and panic disorder. CNS Spectr 13:522–527, 2008

Kragh-Sørensen P, Holm P, Fynboe C, et al: Bromazepam in generalized anxiety: randomized multi-practice comparisons with both chlorprothixene and placebo. Psychopharmacology 100:383–386, 1990

Lehmann E: The dose-effect relationship of 0.5, 1.0 and 1.5mg fluspirilene on anxious patients. Neuropsychobiology 21:197–204, 1989

Mendels J, Krajewski TF, Huffer V, et al: Effective short-term treatment of generalized anxiety disorder with trifluoperazine. J Clin Psychiatry 47:170–174, 1986

Pezze MA, Feldon J: Mesolimbic dopaminergic pathways in fear conditioning. Prog Neurobiol 74:301–320, 2004

Pöldinger WJ: Melperone in low doses in anxious neurotic patients: a double-blind placebo-controlled clinical study. Neuropsychobiology 11:171–186, 1984

Pollack MH, Zaninelli R, Goddard A, et al: Paroxetine in the treatment of generalized anxiety disorder: results of a placebo-controlled, flexible-dosage trial. J Clin Psychiatry 62:350–357, 2001

Pollack MH, Simon NM, Zalta AK, et al: Olanzapine augmentation of fluoxetine for refractory generalized anxiety disorder: a placebo controlled study. Biol Psychiatry 59:211–215, 2006

Rickels K, Weise CC, Clark EL, et al: Thiothixene and thioridazine in anxiety. Br J Psychiatry 125:79–87, 1974

Salzman C, Miyawaki EK, le Bars P, et al: Neurobiologic basis of anxiety and its treatment. Harv Rev Psychiatry 1:197–206, 1993

Simon NM, Hoge EA, Fischmann D, et al: An open-label trial of risperidone augmentation for refractory anxiety disorders. J Clin Psychiatry 67:381–385, 2006

Simon NM, Connor KM, LeBeau RT, et al: Quetiapine augmentation of paroxetine CR for the treatment of refractory generalized anxiety disorder: preliminary findings. Psychopharmacology 197:675–681, 2008

Snyderman SH, Rynn MA, Rickels K: Open-label pilot study of ziprasidone for refractory generalized anxiety disorder. J Clin Psychopharmacol 25:497–499, 2005

Wittchen H-U, Zhao S, Kessler RC, et al: DSM-III-R generalized anxiety disorder in the National Comorbidity Survey. Arch Gen Psychiatry 51:355–364, 1994

Yamamoto J, Kline FM, Burgoyne RW: The treatment of severe anxiety in outpatients: a controlled study comparing chlordiazepoxide and chlorpromazine. Psychosomatics 14:46–51, 1973

Yonkers KA, Warshaw MD, Massion AO, et al: Phenomenology and course of generalized anxiety disorder. Br J Psychiatry 168:308–313, 1996

Yonkers KA, Bruce SE, Dyck IR, et al: Chronicity, relapse, and illness—course of panic disorder, social phobia and generalized anxiety disorder: findings in men and women from 8 years of follow-up. Depress Anxiety 17:173–179, 2003

Posttraumatic Stress Disorder

American Psychiatric Association: Diagnostic and Statistical Manual of Mental Disorders, 4th Edition, Text Revision. Washington, DC, American Psychiatric Association, 2000

American Psychiatric Association: Treatment of Patients With Acute Stress Disorder and Posttraumatic Stress Disorder. November 2004. Available at: http://www.psychiatryonline.com/pracGuide/pracGuideChapToc_11.aspx. Accessed August 21, 2009.

Bartzokis G, Lu PH, Turner J, et al: Adjunctive risperidone in the treatment of chronic combat-related posttraumatic stress disorder. Biol Psychiatry 57:474–479, 2005

Brady K, Pearlstein T, Asnis GM, et al: Efficacy and safety of sertraline treatment of posttraumatic stress disorder: a randomized trial. JAMA 283:1837–1844, 2000

Breslau N, Davis GC, Andreski P, et al: Traumatic events and posttraumatic stress disorder in an urban population of young adults. Arch Gen Psychiatry 48:216–222, 1991

Butterfield MI, Becker ME, Connor KM, et al: Olanzapine in the treatment of post-traumatic stress disorder: a pilot study. Int Clin Psychopharmacol 16:197–203, 2001

Connor KM, Sutherland SM, Tupler LA, et al: Fluoxetine in post-traumatic stress disorder: randomized, double-blind study. Br J Psychiatry 175:17–22, 1999

Czyrak A, Mackowiak M, Chocyk A, et al: Prolonged corticosterone treatment alters the responsiveness of 5-HT-1A receptors to 8-OH-DPAT in rat CA1 hippocampal neurons. Naunyn Schmiedebergs Arch Pharmacol 366:357–367, 2002

Davidson JT, Rothbaum BO, van der Kolk BA, et al: Multicenter, double-blind comparison of sertraline and placebo in the treatment of posttraumatic stress disorder. Arch Gen Psychiatry 58:485–492, 2001

Dillard ML, Bendfeldt F, Jernigan P: Use of thioridazine in posttraumatic stress disorder. South Med J 86:1276–1278, 1993

Gutman DA, Nemeroff CB: Persistent central nervous system effects of an adverse early environment: clinical and preclinical studies. Physiol Behav 79:471–478, 2003

Hamner MB: Clozapine treatment for a veteran with comorbid psychosis and PTSD. Am J Psychiatry 153:841, 1996

Hamner MB, Deitsch SE, Brodrick PS, et al: Quetiapine treatment in patients with posttraumatic stress disorder: an open trial of adjunctive treatment. J Clin Psychopharmacol 23:15–20, 2003a

Hamner MB, Faldowski RA, Ulmer HG, et al: Adjunctive risperidone treatment in post-traumatic stress disorder: a preliminary controlled trial of effects on comorbid psychotic symptoms. Int Clin Psychopharmacol 18:1–8, 2003b

Kaehler S, Singewald N, Sinner C, et al: Conditioned fear and inescapable shock modify the release of serotonin in the locus coeruleus. Brain Res 859:249–254, 2000

Kozaric-Kovacic D, Pivac N: Quetiapine treatment in an open trial in combat-related post-traumatic stress disorder with psychotic features. Int J Neuropsychopharmacol 10:253–262, 2007

Kozaric-Kovacic D, Pivac N, Muck-Seler D, et al: Risperidone in psychotic combat-related posttraumatic stress disorder. J Clin Psychiatry 66:922–927, 2005

Marshall RD, Beebe KL, Oldham M, et al: Efficacy and safety of paroxetine treatment for chronic PTSD: a fixed-dose, placebo-controlled study. Am J Psychiatry 158:1982–1988, 2001

Matsumoto M, Higuchi K, Togashi H, et al: Early postnatal stress alters the 5-HTergic modulation to emotional stress at postadolescent periods of rats. Hippocampus 15:775–781, 2005

Matsumoto M, Togashi J, Konno K, et al: Early postnatal stress alters the extinction of context-dependent conditioned fear in adult rats. Pharmacol Biochem Behav 89:247–252, 2008

Monnelly EP, Ciraulo DA, Knapp C, et al: Low-dose risperidone as adjunctive therapy for irritable aggression in posttraumatic stress disorder. J Clin Psychopharmacol 23:193–196, 2003

Morrow BA, Elsworth JD, Rasmusson AM, et al: The role of mesoprefrontal neurons in the acquisition and expression of conditioned fear in the rat. Neuroscience 92:553–564, 1999

Orth U, Wieland E: Anger, hostility and posttraumatic stress disorder in trauma-exposed adults: a meta-analysis. J Consult Clin Psychol 74:698–706, 2006

Padala PR, Madison J, Monnahan M, et al: Risperidone monotherapy for post-traumatic stress disorder related to sexual assault and domestic abuse in women. Int Clin Psychopharmacol 21:275–280, 2006

Pae C, Lim H, Peindl K, et al: The atypical antipsychotics olanzapine and risperidone in the treatment of posttraumatic stress disorder: a meta-analysis of randomized, double-blind, placebo-controlled clinical trials. Int Clin Psychopharmacol 23:1–8, 2008

Petty F, Kramer G, Wilson L: Prevention of learned helplessness: in vivo correlation with cortical serotonin. Pharmacol Biochem Behav 43:361–367, 1992

Petty F, Brannan S, Casada J, et al: Olanzapine treatment for posttraumatic stress disorder: an open-label study. Int Clin Psychopharmacol 16:331–337, 2001

Pivac N, Kozaric-Kovacic D, Muck-Seir D: Olanzapine versus fluphenazine in an open trial in patients with psychotic combat-related posttraumatic stress disorder. Psychopharmacology 175:451–456, 2004

Reich DB, Winternitz S, Hennen J, et al: A preliminary study of risperidone in the treatment of posttraumatic stress disorder related to childhood abuse in women. J Clin Psychiatry 65:1601–1606, 2004

Resnick HS, Kilpatrick DG, Dansky BS, et al: Prevalence of civilian trauma and post-traumatic stress disorder in a representative national sample of women. J Consult Clin Psychol 61:984–991, 1993

Rothbaum BO, Killeen TK, Davidson JRT, et al: Placebo-controlled trial of risperidone augmentation for selective reuptake inhibitor-resistant civilian posttraumatic stress disorder. J Clin Psychiatry 69:520–525, 2008

Sautter FJ, Brailey K, Uddo MM, et al: PTSD and comorbid psychotic disorder: comparison with veterans diagnosed with PTSD or psychotic disorder. J Trauma Stress 12:73–88, 1999

Stein DJ, Ipser JC, Seedat S: Pharmacotherapy for posttraumatic stress disorder (PTSD). Cochrane Database Syst Rev (1):CD002795, 2006

Stein MB, Kline NA, Matloff JL: Adjunctive olanzapine for SSRI-resistant combat-related PTSD: a double-blind, placebo-controlled trial. Am J Psychiatry 159:10, 2002

Thompson GN: Posttraumatic psychoneurosis: evaluation of drug therapy. Dis Nerv Syst 38:617–619, 1977

Vermetten E, Bremner JD: Circuits and systems in stress: preclinical studies, I: preclinical studies. Depress Anxiety 15:126–147, 2002

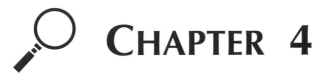

CHAPTER 4

Personality Disorders

Kenneth R. Silk, M.D.
Michael D. Jibson, M.D., Ph.D.

THE ROLE OF ANTIPSYCHOTIC MEDICATIONS in patients with personality disorders has been studied since the mid-1970s. In the personality disorders, antipsychotics are used for a wide array of symptoms in addition to their use in psychotic or psychotic-like states. Recent evidence indicates that some of the atypical antipsychotics have a role in the treatment of treatment-resistant depression, especially in the depression of bipolar disorder (see Chapter 3, "Mood and Anxiety Disorders," in this volume). We are confident that there will be further explorations into the efficacy of antipsychotic medications, both typical and atypical, in personality disorders, particularly because affective disturbances and dysphoria often occur in patients with personality disorders. In fact, it is often depression and dysphoria that bring patients with personality disorders to clinical attention.

In this chapter, we briefly describe how psychosis or peripsychotic experiences are thought of in the personality disorders. Then we discuss the use of antipsychotic medication, both typical and atypical, in the personality disorders in general. We describe the range of symptoms that have been considered to be possibly responsive to antipsychotic medication. We then turn to borderline personality disorder (BPD) and schizotypal personality disorder (STPD) to discuss the use of these medications in these particular diagnostic groupings. Finally, we discuss very briefly the purported use of antipsychotic medication in other personality disorders; we say purported because few empirical data exist for their use outside of BPD and STPD.

How Psychosis Is Viewed in Personality Disorder

The definition of *psychosis* is a loss of contact with reality, including false ideas about what is taking place or who one is (delusions) and seeing or hearing things that are not there (U.S. National Library of Medicine 2008). This concept is usually applied to disorders such as schizophrenia, bipolar disorder, and psychotic depression; states of dementia or intoxication; or certain organic conditions in which hallucinations and/or delusions are prominent parts of the clinical picture. Many of these disorders are discussed in other chapters within this book.

However, the idea of psychosis in personality disorders takes on several significant differences. First, the psychosis or the psychotic state is transient, and although the length of time spent in psychosis may be interpreted differently among clinicians and researchers, the psychosis is not continuous and rarely lasts for more than a few hours and certainly not for more than a few days. Second, the psychosis is often thought to be the result of stress—that is, when the patient experiences significant stress, then psychotic-like thinking and/or hallucinatory-like phenomena occur (Chopra and Beatson 1986)— but these states can result from sleep deprivation, substance misuse, or comorbid mood disorder. These psychotic-like phenomena may take the form of hearing a voice in the distance or some sound that seems as if it is a voice but lacks clarity, so the "words" of the voice are not understandable. Or the psychotic-like phenomena manifest as illusions or in experiences when patients feel a "distance" between themselves and the world (derealization) as if they were looking at the rest of the world through a pane of glass or when patients feel like they are outside of themselves viewing and even experiencing themselves from a distance (depersonalization). Third, even when the patient hears voices, the words spoken by the voice are very few, often in a short phrase that is repeatedly heard, and are unlike those often thought of as Schneiderian first-rank symptoms—namely, two or more voices talking to the patient (giving commands) or giving a running commentary of the patient's behavior, either behavior that has occurred in the immediate past or behavior that is about to occur (a command hallucination) (Silverstein and Harrow 1989). Fourth, the patient is aware that the "psychotic" phenomena are unusual and are not supposed to be there, and the presence of these phenomena creates a good deal of anxiety in the patient. This is because even though these patients have distorted reality and may be experiencing a modification in relation to reality, they have not lost their ability to test reality (Frosch 1964). These points are summarized in Table 4–1.

Historical Considerations

Antipsychotic medication was actually the first medication class "tested" in the treatment of various personality disorders. Trials of antipsychotic medication were given to patients who were thought to be "borderline," even though, especially before DSM-III (American Psychiatric Association 1980), the group of patients referred to as "borderline" probably contained many patients who would now be better classified as having STPD (Spitzer et al. 1979). However, the group of disorders in the borderline spectrum included not only those classified as schizotypal but also those called by terms such as *ambulatory schizophrenia, pseudo-neurotic schizophrenia,* and *borderline states.* It made sense then that patients with these disorders, being thought of as "atypical schizophrenic patients," would be given a trial of antipsychotic medication. In these instances, the antipsychotic medications used were the first-generation antipsychotics (FGAs)—namely, the neuroleptics (phenothiazines), butyrophenone derivatives such as haloperidol, and thioxanthenes.

TABLE 4–1. Psychotic symptoms in personality disorders

The psychotic state is usually quite transient, lasting only a few moments to at most a few hours.

The psychotic state is usually the result of external forces (i.e., increased stress, lack of sleep, drug use, or comorbid mood disorder).

Hallucinatory experiences often consist of vague sounds or indistinguishable voices or a single voice repeating the same short phrase, often of a self-deprecating nature.

Depersonalization, derealization, and illusions are included here.

The patient is aware that the psychotic phenomena are not supposed to occur, and their presence causes a good deal of anxiety. Usually a delusional elaboration cannot explain these phenomena.

Mechanism of Action

Antipsychotic medications are rich in both pharmacological activity and clinical efficacy. Because they bind to a variety of receptors beyond the dopamine family, they show a range of clinical activities beyond the ability to reduce delusions, hallucinations, and thought disorganization. As a group, they have excellent efficacy in the treatment of bipolar mania, they all reduce acute agitation and impulsive aggression, several of them show anxiolytic properties, and a few of them improve mood in unipolar or bipolar depression (see Chapter 3).

Personality disorders arise from a complex mix of biological and psychological factors, some of which appear related to the pharmacological and clinical properties of antipsychotics. Although it is premature to suggest a precise mechanism by which these medications benefit personality disorders, the outline of a model for their actions has emerged (New et al. 2008).

Antagonist or partial agonist activity at dopamine D_2 receptors appears essential to the activity of both FGA and second-generation antipsychotic (SGA) medications. This corresponds well with the biology of schizophrenia that is known to involve aberrations of dopamine function (see Chapter 2, "Schizophrenia and Schizoaffective Disorder," in this volume). Both STPD and schizophrenia include oddities of thought and speech, blunted and atypical affect, unusual interests and beliefs, a broad range of interpersonal deficits, and risk for overt psychotic symptoms. Family studies show strong genetic interplay between the disorders, with both diagnoses tending to cluster within the same families. Psychological factors typical of schizophrenia, such as abnormal information processing, impaired attention, and deficient executive function, are similarly prevalent in STPD. The characteristic structural changes in the brains of schizophrenia patients, such as enlarged lateral ventricles and increased ventricular-to-brain ratios, have been reported in STPD patients as well. Most important from the perspective of pharmacological treatment, STPD patients show the same increased dopamine activity that is found in schizophrenia (Siever et al. 1993). Regulation of dopamine pathways therefore appears essential for the pharmacological treatment of schizotypal traits.

BPD is a more complex mix of pathologies, involving affective dysregulation, impulsivity, and self-directed aggression, in addition to transient psychotic states. A biological model for borderline traits is justified by its high heritability and a variety of studies showing abnormalities of brain structure and neurotransmitter function (New et al. 2008; Putnam and Silk 2005). Most striking among these studies is the role of serotonergic function, which has been implicated in emotional dysregulation, misinterpretation of affective communication, and impulsive acts of aggression. Evidence of decreased serotonin levels has been found by direct measurement in suicidal BPD patients. Functional imaging shows decreased serotonin metabolism in the frontal cortex of similar patients. Genetic studies have detected specific abnormalities in genes coding for various enzymes involved in serotonin metabolism. Emotional dysregulation is correlated with decreased serotonin levels in frontal and limbic regions. It is likely, therefore, that antipsychotic medications reduce the mood instability, impulsivity, and self-destructive tendencies of BPD patients through modulation of serotonin pathways.

A specific mechanism for this activity has been described in greatest detail for impulsive aggression (Siever 2008). Although not specific to BPD, impulsive acts of violence, particularly toward oneself, are characteristic of the disorder. A model of limbic irritability or hyperactivity that creates impulsive urges to act aggressively, paired with dysfunction of inhibitory responses from the prefrontal cortex, has emerged from a growing body of evidence. Limbic dysregulation is associated with decreased γ-aminobutyric acid (GABA) activity, increased glutaminergic function, and increased acetylcholine transmission. Increased dopaminergic activity in subcortical areas may contribute to the cognitive distortions often seen in these episodes but otherwise appears to have limited involvement. The most compelling evidence for this model is found in the decreased serotonergic activity of the prefrontal cortex, indicated by direct measurement of serotonin levels and functional imaging of serotonin pathways. The serotonin story is not entirely consistent, however, because both serotonin-enhancing selective serotonin reuptake inhibitors (SSRIs) and antagonist antipsychotics reduce impulsive aggression. This may be related to different functions of serotonin receptor subtypes because clinical benefits have been documented with antagonists at serotonin type 2A ($5\text{-}HT_{2A}$) receptors and agonists at $5\text{-}HT_{2C}$ sites.

Indications and Efficacy

The only controlled studies for the use of antipsychotic medications, both typical and atypical, are in BPD and STPD. The bulk of randomized controlled trials (RCTs) have been with people with BPD. Although one might assume that there should be some controlled trials for their use in antisocial personality disorder, none are found. Some open trials and some single case studies have been done in this population, but we have decided to restrict the discussion (and the listing of relevant studies in the tables) to controlled studies. Furthermore, data for the use of antipsychotic medications in BPD and STPD are inconsistent and have several problems that make it difficult to generalize. Despite all the controlled trials, no medication or medication class has been approved for the treatment of any personality disorder; thus, the discussion that follows would fall into the category of the "off-label" use of these drugs.

Even though both typical and atypical antipsychotics have been studied, no prototypical antipsychotic, typical or atypical, has been studied. Because many of the studies involved small numbers of subjects, the reader will appreciate that most of these studies produced preliminary evidence at best, even if the study was well designed and would qualify as a true RCT.

Another source of inconsistency is that different instruments are used to measure the same outcome in different studies, or more than one outcome measurement may be used for the same outcome parameter. Often, the two do not agree. We are then left with trying to figure out the subtle (or sometimes not so subtle) distinction between two instruments that essentially study the same outcome or improvement in a specific outcome parameter. This leads to a variation in outcomes across studies that is difficult to explain and leaves the field not much better informed than before the study was initiated. For example, in a review of RCTs for BPD, Saunders and Silk (in press) attempted to separate the various outcomes into categories broader than specific symptoms to consolidate some of the findings from different studies. They tried to classify outcome according to the following dimensions: 1) affective instability, 2) anxiety or inhibition, 3) impulsivity or aggression, and 4) cognition or perception (Siever and Davis 1991). In this review, they found that in BPD

- More RCTs involved antipsychotic (both typical and atypical) medications than any other drug class across these four dimensions.
- Evidence from some studies suggested that antipsychotics might be useful in each of the four dimensions.
- Evidence for the effectiveness of antipsychotics in each of the dimensions was as strong as, if not stronger than, that for other classes of drugs (mood stabilizers, SSRIs, monoamine oxidase inhibitors) in each of these dimensions.
- There was no evidence (pro or con) regarding the long-term use of these medications in these patients.

Clinical Use

In general, the dosage of antipsychotic medication used in patients with BPD (and in STPD) is lower than that used in psychotic patients. The medication should be started at a low dosage, and the dosage should be kept low for 2–6 weeks to determine whether the medication is having an effect. In some cases, the effect is seen early, and in other cases, the patient improves only gradually. If the medication does not appear to be working, then the dose can be doubled from its original low dose, and it may be another 4 weeks until an effect is noticed. It is important to identify the symptom, symptom complex, or behavior that one is expecting or hoping to improve with the medication, but one must not fail to notice if improvements occur in other areas that were not expected. As explained earlier in the "Mechanism of Action" section, and as reviewed later in this chapter, antipsychotic medication may affect a broad array of symptoms, especially in BPD. If after this time the particular medication still does not appear to be working, it is best to discontinue that antipsychotic and start with a different antipsychotic medication. A second antipsychotic should not be added to augment the first antipsychotic. These patients may have a tendency to use polypharmacy, and there is no evidence for such prescribing practices in patients with personality disorders.

The antipsychotic medications have been used in patients with personality disorders for a wide variety of symptomatic outcomes. In a recent review, Duggan and colleagues (2008) found that antipsychotic medication had been used for and been found to be somewhat effective for (although often not impressively so and often not in all studies) the following:

- Cognitive perceptual symptoms such as paranoid thinking and psychoticism (haloperidol, thioridazine, thiothixene, aripiprazole)
- Affective symptoms (and symptoms of affective dysregulation) such as depression (haloperidol, loxapine, trifluoperazine, aripiprazole)
- Anger or hostility (haloperidol, aripiprazole, olanzapine)
- General anxiety (with marginal results for loxapine, thiothixene, trifluoperazine, aripiprazole, olanzapine)
- Phobic anxiety (thiothixene, aripiprazole)
- Social anxiety (aripiprazole) (see Table 4–2)

Antipsychotic medications have been studied in impulse dyscontrol, even though little evidence points to their effectiveness (except for one study that suggested that haloperidol may have a role here and another that suggested olanzapine); however, they have a good track record in improving global functioning (haloperidol, risperidone, olanzapine, and aripiprazole). This listing does not mean that only these particular antipsychotic agents are effective, but they are the only ones that have shown such effectiveness in RCTs. In most studies, they have been used to improve overall global functioning, and more data probably support the effectiveness of antipsychotics for this outcome measure than for any other measure. But as shown in Table 4–2, they have been used successfully to reduce different forms of anxiety; improve dissociative states; decrease impulsivity, aggression, and mood lability (often referred to as *emotional dysegulation*); or "soften" paranoid thoughts. In one of the earliest controlled studies, a typical antipsychotic (haloperidol) was shown to be better at treating the "depression" of BPD than a comparison tricyclic antidepressant (amitriptyline) (Soloff et al. 1986a). However, later it appeared that the antipsychotic used in this study was not a better antidepressant than amitriptyline (Soloff et al. 1989) and was inferior to a monoamine oxidase inhibitor antidepressant (Soloff et al. 1993).

Table 4–2 lists the antipsychotic medications that have been subjected to RCTs to explore their use in the treatment of some of the symptoms in BPD and STPD. We reemphasize that these medications are not used solely to treat psychotic or psychotic-like symptoms in BPD.

Guidelines for Selection and Use

No specific guidelines indicate which antipsychotic medication to use preferentially for any given personality disorder, but one might wish that use be restricted to those that have been shown to be effective in an RCT. Choice of an antipsychotic medication might be based on side-effect profile. For example, many patients with BPD are young women who are strongly invested in their physical appearance, and weight gain in these people may create more stress and increase symptomatology. In these circumstances, it could be difficult to appreciate if the medication might be making some (positive) difference in the patient's symptoms or in the patient's ability to deal with and not be overwhelmed by life if substantial weight gain had occurred. Thus, in these circumstances, one might wish to avoid the SGAs olanzapine and quetiapine and perhaps clozapine.

RCTs have been done on the use of antipsychotic medications in the BPD and STPD population since the late 1970s. The first-generation, or typical, antipsychotic medications that have been used in this population include chlorpromazine, haloperidol, loxapine, thioridazine, thiothixene, and trifluoperazine; the second-generation, or atypical, agents that have been studied include aripiprazole, olanzapine, and risperidone (see Table 4–2). In general, both the typical and the atypical antipsychotics, as a group, have been shown to be effective in this patient population, although their effectiveness is inconsistent across studies. This may be a result of how the patients were selected, as well as what the target symptoms were that were being measured for outcome. As shown in Table 4–2, antipsychotic medications have been used in RCTs to treat a variety of symptoms from depression through transient psychosis.

No studies on the long-term use of these medications have been done in these patients. Long-term use, especially of the FGAs, can lead to movement disorders such as tardive dyskinesia, which in some small minority can become so severe that they can result in significant disability greater than the

TABLE 4–2. Symptoms that have been found to respond to antipsychotic medications in patients with personality disorder

MEDICATION	SYMPTOM(S)
Chlorpromazine	Global
Haloperidol	Global, paranoid thinking, psychoticism, depression (±), anger or hostility, impulse control (±)
Loxapine	Global, depression, anxiety
Trifluoperazine	Depression, general anxiety
Thiothixene	Global, cognitive symptoms, anxiety, derealization, phobic anxiety
Thioridazine	Global, paranoid thinking
Aripiprazole	Global, psychoticism, paranoia, depression, anger or hostility, general and phobic and social anxiety
Olanzapine	Global, general anxiety, anger, aggression, impulsivity
Risperidone	Global, schizotypal symptoms

Note. ± reflects that evidence is weak or has been contradicted by other studies.
Source. Expanded from summary in Duggan et al. 2008.

disability that can be directly attributed to the primary psychiatric disorder. Women who have been taking these medications, especially the FGAs, have the greatest tendency to develop tardive dyskinesia. At least in BPD, this should not be a very prominent problem because these medications should be used only for a limited amount of time; however, in treating STPD, there are probably good reasons to continue these medications for longer periods (see subsection "Side Effects and Their Management" below). However, if the medication does not appear to be affecting the identified target symptoms or, by extension, other symptoms, then the medication should be stopped, and consideration should be given to using another antipsychotic medication, some other class of medication, or no medication at all.

The choice of medication may depend on several factors: 1) the actual cost of the medication to the patient, 2) the side-effect profile of the medication, 3) the potential or actual interactions of the medication with other medications that the patient is currently taking, and 4) the coexisting medical problems or medical status of the patient (see Table 4–3). For example, a patient who has diabetes or a strong family history of diabetes may not be someone for whom the clinician would want to prescribe olanzapine or quetiapine but might benefit from an FGA that has less of a chance of interfering with glucose metabolism and promoting weight gain. A geriatric patient with multiple medical problems taking multiple

---

TABLE 4–3. Factors to consider in choosing a specific antipsychotic medication

---

Actual cost of the medication to the patient

Side-effect profile of the medication and its effect on patients of a specific gender and age

Potential interactions of the medication with the medication(s) the patient is already taking

Coexisting medical problems or the medical status of the patient

Some evidence, provided through a randomized controlled trial, that the medication affects the specific symptom or behavior being targeted

---

medications would not be someone for whom the clinician would choose an antipsychotic medication that has hypotension as a side effect.

Side Effects and Their Management

The side effects of these medications in this patient population are no different from the side effects that these medications might induce among patients with any diagnosis (and probably among nonpatients as well) (see Appendix 7). Young men have a high chance of developing dyskinesias and akinesias, especially young males exposed to the older antipsychotics (haloperidol, trifluoperazine, thiothixene). Chronic use of these medications, again particularly the older antipsychotics or FGAs, can lead to tardive dyskinesia, especially among women. But there is little evidence one way or another as to the effectiveness of these medications over the long term, and thus we recommend against continuing any antipsychotic medication (either FGA or SGA) in someone with BPD for an indefinite multiyear period. This would not necessarily apply to STPD because of its relation to schizophrenia and to the idea that it is a schizophrenia spectrum disorder.

Borderline Personality Disorder

Typical Versus Atypical Antipsychotics

RCTs with both typical (FGAs) and atypical (SGAs) antipsychotics have been conducted in patients with BPD (see Table 4–4). One might make the argument to restrict use of these antipsychotic medications to only those specific medications that have actual RCTs that explored their effectiveness and to restrict the specific medication to only those symptoms or symptom complexes that have been shown to have been reduced by their use. The data for effectiveness overall are often quite weak and the sample sizes quite small. Perhaps a good rule of thumb, in light of such "weak" data, is to choose the medication according to its side-effect profile.

Indications and Efficacy

Many different outcome measures have been used to study the typical antipsychotics (FGAs) in BPD, although most of the studies looked at improvement in overall (global) functioning (Table 4–2). The FGAs that have been studied in BPD include chlorpromazine, haloperidol, loxapine, trifluoperazine, thioridazine, and thiothixene and have shown effectiveness in improving not only overall functioning but also paranoid thinking, psychotic thinking (mild), general anxiety, and anger or hostility. There is less evidence for an effect in improving depression and impulsivity. The atypical antipsychotics (SGAs) that have been studied in BPD are aripiprazole and olanzapine. Other medications in these classes have been studied, but under conditions of open-label studies or if involving an RCT, they were not found to be effective. In addition to improvement in global functioning, the SGAs have been shown to improve paranoid thinking, psychotic thinking (mild), general anxiety, and anger or hostility. In addition, some evidence indicates that they can improve depression, general anxiety, phobic anxiety, and social anxiety. There is less evidence for improvement in impulse control (see Table 4–2).

Agitation and Aggression

In addition to the above "outcomes," these medications can be used when the patient is agitated or aggressive. However, these medications should be used, at least initially, in doses lower than one might use with a psychotic patient. One might also, in lieu of treating the symptoms with an antipsychotic, try using a benzodiazepine in situations of significant agitation. Of course, when the behavior appears severe and not controllable through oral medication, an injectable antipsychotic or benzodiazepine should be used. In these circumstances, issues of weight gain are not a consideration because it should take only one or two doses to quell the agitation or aggression.

Clinical Use

The clinical use of antipsychotic medications in these patients may require time for the clinician to familiarize himself or herself with the patient before

TABLE 4–4. Randomized controlled trials (RCTs) involving patients with borderline personality disorder (BPD)

STUDY	METHODS	OUTCOME
Leone 1982	6-week RCT of loxapine vs. chlorpromazine in 80 patients with BPD	Both groups improved with loxapine more than with chlorpromazine in reducing depression and anger or hostility.
Serban and Siegel 1984	3-month RCT of thiothixene 9.4 mg/day vs. haloperidol 3 mg/day in 16 patients with BPD (plus 16 with STPD and 16 with mixed personality disorders)	Patients showed improvement in ideas of reference, paranoia, derealization, anxiety, and depression.
Soloff et al. 1986a	5-week RCT of haloperidol 7.2 mg/day vs. amitriptyline vs. placebo in 36 schizotypal and mixed schizotypal and borderline patients	Haloperidol-treated patients improved more than patients taking placebo or amitriptyline for depressive and anxiety symptoms, hostility, paranoia, and psychotic and other behavioral symptoms, but follow-up did not find this advantage for haloperidol over amitriptyline or over the antidepressant phenelzine sulfate (Soloff et al. 1989, 1993).
Goldberg et al. 1986	12-week randomized trial of thiothixene 8.7 mg/day vs. placebo in 37 BPD and mixed schizotypal and borderline patients	Significant drug-placebo differences in effect on illusions, ideas of reference, psychoticism, obsessive-compulsive symptoms, and phobic anxiety but not on depression.

TABLE 4–4. Randomized controlled trials (RCTs) involving patients with borderline personality disorder (BPD) *(continued)*

STUDY	METHODS	OUTCOME
Cowdry and Gardner 1988	6-week randomized two-phase trial; phase 1: alprazolam 4.7 mg/day vs. carbamazepine 820 mg/day; phase 2: trifluoperazine HCl 7.8 mg/day vs. tranylcypromine sulfate 40 mg/day in 16 female outpatients with BPD	Among patients who tolerated trifluoperazine: trifluoperazine was more effective than placebo in reduction of depressive and anxiety symptoms. No improvement was seen in overall global functioning.
Zanarini and Frankenburg 2001	24-week RCT of olanzapine 5.3 mg/day vs. placebo in 28 females with BPD	Olanzapine was more effective than placebo in reducing anxiety, impulsivity, anger, and interpersonal sensitivity.
Zanarini et al. 2004	8-week RCT of olanzapine 3 3 mg/day vs. fluoxetine 15 mg/day vs. olanzapine+fluoxetine in 45 females	Olanzapine and olanzapine+fluoxetine were more effective than fluoxetine in reducing depression, impulsivity, and impulsive aggression.
Bogenschutz and Nurrberg 2004	8-week RCT of olanzapine 6.9 mg/day vs. placebo in 40 females with BPD	Olanzapine was better than placebo in reducing global pathology and anger but not psychotic symptoms, anxiety, or aggression.
Soler et al. 2005	12-week RCT of olanzapine 8.8 mg/day+DBT vs. placebo+DBT in 60 females with BPD	Olanzapine assisted in improvement in anxiety, depression, and impulsive-aggressive behavior.
Nickel et al. 2006	8-week RCT plus 18-month follow-up of aripiprazole 15 mg/day vs. placebo in 52 BPD subjects	Aripiprazole was better than placebo in improving global functioning, anxiety, depression, anger, aggression, and paranoia.

Note. All doses are average doses. DBT=dialectical behavior therapy; STPD=schizotypal personality disorder.

deciding on the use of an antipsychotic (or perhaps any medication). Patients with BPD present with a wide array of symptoms of varying severity, and the symptoms may come and go and the severity may change dramatically from session to session. It may be wise to wait until a reasonably confident picture emerges of what symptoms or symptom complexes appear to be most persistent in a particular patient or vary the least from session to session before deciding on a pharmacological strategy. Once identified (not always an easy task), these symptoms or symptom complexes can become the target for the pharmacological intervention.

As stated earlier, antipsychotic medication can be used for a variety of symptoms that are experienced by patients with BPD (see Table 4–5). Some RCTs reported effectiveness (although more often a modest rather than a strong effect) on impulsivity, aggression and hostility (especially when accompanied by paranoid ideation), transient psychotic episodes, transient paranoid experiences, derealization, and anxiety (general, phobic, and social). Open-label studies support effectiveness with depersonalization, chronic self-destructive behavior, emotion dysregulation, and overall mood lability. Some evidence indicates effectiveness against the chronic dysphoria (depression) found in patients with BPD. This latter comment is controversial because these medications will not affect the chronic loneliness, emptiness, and fear of abandonment—states or symptoms often mistaken for depression in these patients.

Whatever the symptom or symptom complex, the medication should be given in a reasonable dose (a lower dose often is given in BPD than in psychosis). Doses determined by extrapolating from RCTs and clinical experience from treating physicians would suggest haloperidol 5–10 mg/day, thiothixene and trifluoperazine 3–7.5 mg/day (same range as for olanzapine), and aripiprazole 5–15 mg/day. The medication needs to be given for a sufficient period, somewhere between 1 and 2 months, to determine whether there has been a change. If no change has occurred, then the medication should be discontinued and replaced by a different medication. Augmentation, as stated earlier, should be avoided to mitigate against polypharmacy.

Guidelines for Selection and Use

No formal guidelines for selection are available; however, within each of the categories of FGAs and SGAs, specific medications have been subjected to RCTs and have been shown to be effective against specific symptoms in those RCTs (see Tables 4–2 and 4–4). In general, the best advice is to choose the medication primarily by the side-effect profile. How much sedation would you want the medication to have? How much orthostasis might it induce? How much will it cost (considering both the health plan and the patient)? Will it interact with other medications the patient is currently taking? Obviously, in patients who are older

TABLE 4–5. Symptoms of borderline personality disorder that have been shown to be responsive to antipsychotic medication

Symptoms that have been shown to be reduced by antipsychotic medications in randomized controlled trials

Impulsivity

Aggression and hostility (especially when accompanied by paranoid ideation)

Transient psychotic episodes

Transient paranoid experiences

General anxiety

Social anxiety

Phobic anxiety

Depression (although results are contradictory)

Derealization

Symptoms that have been shown to be reduced by antipsychotic medications in open studies

Depersonalization

Chronic self-destructive behavior

Emotion dysregulation

Mood lability

or medically frail, issues such as orthostasis and sedation may be more important (making the medication less likely to be used) than in patients who are young and medically healthy. Again, in this patient population, these medications should be used in doses lower than a "standard" dose used in a person with ongoing psychosis or even an acute psychosis in the face of a chronically psychotic condition.

Pretreatment

The advantages and disadvantages, as well as the side effects, of the medication should be discussed thoroughly with the patient with adequate opportunity and encouragement for the patient to ask questions. The patient may want to read about the particular medication on the Internet, but the reliability of the information on the Internet is always questionable. Nonetheless, this collaborative approach is important to establish, especially in patients with BPD who also may have experienced significant abuse in their past.

It is always prudent to have some screening blood tests before initiating any medications. When antipsychotic medication is being initiating, it is useful to administer the tests listed in Appendixes 4 and 5, if only to have some baseline measures and to rule out any baseline abnormalities. The prescriber also should monitor the patient as outlined in those appendixes.

Side Effects, Drug-Drug Interactions, and Other Adverse Events

The side effects of these medications are no different in patients with BPD than the side effects in general (see Appendixes 7 and 8). No specific unusual, untoward events might or should occur because of the BPD diagnosis. Nonetheless, mention needs to be made that patients with BPD are thought to be very sensitive to the side effects of psychotropic medication, although no empirical studies support this observation. The management of these side effects is no different in this patient population than in any other patient population.

Because these patients often receive polypharmacy, drug-drug interactions are important to consider (see Table 3–6 in Chapter 3). One should always ensure that patients who are taking a mood stabilizer and/or an SSRI will not have interactions with these antipsychotic medications. Caution is urged in using antipsychotic medication concomitantly with carbamazepine or valproic acid.

Fortunately, most of these drugs are reasonably safe in overdose. However, that does not mean that one should simply ignore an overdose. First, of course, the patient may have become so obtunded that he or she could aspirate. Perhaps he or she had been using (and maybe overdosed on) illicit substances and/or alcohol, because comorbid substance misuse is not uncommon among these patients. Furthermore, in light of the fact that these patients are often taking multiple psychopharmacological agents, some of which may be more dangerous in overdose than the antipsychotic medications, the clinician must make sure that the patient did not overdose with other medications. Even in a situation when the patient is medically safe after an overdose, the act and the behavior leading up to the act should not be ignored. It is very important to discuss the proper use of medications; that prescribing them means that the patient will be serious and conscientious in their use. Patients must be honest with the clinician when they have been noncompliant with how the medications have been prescribed, they should not stop the medications without letting the clinician know, and they should inform the clinician immediately if they take more than the prescribed dosage.

Schizotypal Personality Disorder

The delineation of STPD as a unique entity within the broader category of borderline personality or "pseudoneurotic schizophrenia" was first proposed by

Spitzer et al. (1979) on the eve of the publication of DSM-III, which officially recognized the disorder for the first time. The utility of this distinction soon became apparent as evidence for similarities between schizotypal and schizophrenic patients multiplied (Spitzer et al. 1979), in contrast to the more prominent mood instability of borderline personality patients, as defined by DSM-III.

The rationale for the use of antipsychotic medications in the treatment of STPD is based on three approaches to the disorder. First, schizophrenia and STPD may be variants within the same spectrum of brain dysfunction. Their similar presentations and overlapping courses, with schizotypal personality virtually indistinguishable from prodromal or residual schizophrenia, and the greatly increased risk for schizophrenia in schizotypal patients (Fenton and McGlashan 1989) are consistent with this hypothesis. Antipsychotic medications have therefore been suggested as an appropriate treatment because of their overall efficacy for schizophrenia.

Second, antipsychotic medications provide symptomatic rather than curative treatment by addressing manifestations of illness rather than underlying pathology. The similar manifestations of STPD and schizophrenia would suggest that symptomatic treatment of the two disorders should overlap.

Third, it has been proposed that schizotypal personality traits are a schizophrenia prodrome, and although not all schizotypal patients will go on to develop schizophrenia, all are at risk and should be treated prophylactically. These models indicate that the goals of antipsychotic treatment should be reduced oddities of thought, modest reduction in negative symptoms, reduced risk for development of active psychosis, and overall improvement in level of function.

Typical Versus Atypical Antipsychotics

Early studies of antipsychotic medications for treatment of personality disorders typically involved a mix of patient groups but included descriptions of patients that allowed for some conclusions regarding their effectiveness with a more narrowly defined schizotypal population. Pimozide (Reyntjens 1972), thiothixene (Goldberg et al. 1986; Serban and Siegel 1984), and haloperidol (Serban and Siegel 1984; Soloff et al. 1986a) at doses well below those usually seen in schizophrenia treatment have been effective for at least some schizotypal symptoms. Patients showed improvement not only in ideas of reference, paranoia, and derealization but also in anxiety, depression, and obsessive-compulsive symptoms. In fact, patients tended to improve about as much on the Hamilton Rating Scale for Depression (Ham-D) as on the Psychotic Assessment Interview. Amitriptyline, in contrast, had no effect on mood, anxiety, or psychotic symptoms in the same patients (Soloff et al. 1986b). Most of these studies showed comparable levels of improvement among all patient groups, not a preferential response among schizotypal patients compared with borderline or other personality disorders (Serban and Siegal 1984; Soloff et al. 1986a).

More recent studies of antipsychotics in the treatment of STPD have focused on atypical drugs and more homogeneous patient populations. Studies of low doses of risperidone (Koenigsberg et al. 2003; Rybakowski et al. 2007) and olanzapine (Keshevan et al. 2004) ranging from 7 weeks to 7 years have shown 30%–40% improvement across the full spectrum of symptoms represented by the Positive and Negative Syndrome Scale (PANSS), Brief Psychiatric Rating Scale (BPRS), Global Assessment of Functioning (GAF), and Ham-D. Improvements in cognitive, social, and vocational functioning were maintained even after the medication was discontinued.

There is little basis in these studies for comparison among agents or even classes of antipsychotic medication. All of the drugs tested have proved to be effective across a broad range of pertinent symptoms. As with schizophrenia treatment, the major differences among these medications appear to be in side-effect profiles, rather than efficacy, and most treatment decisions will be based on tolerability.

RCTs involving antipsychotic medication and STPD are listed in Table 4–6.

Indications and Efficacy

Studies of antipsychotic treatment for STPD are striking in several regards. First, low doses of antipsychotic medications appeared fully effective. Second, improvements in schizotypal patients were not limited to thought disorder or reality testing but included comparable resolution of mood and anxiety symptoms as well. Third, in the early studies involving conventional neuroleptics, diagnosis did not predict response to treatment.

As a result of the observed efficacy of antipsychotics in these studies, appropriate indications for treatment would include psychotic and near-psychotic symptoms; mood and anxiety symptoms; and functional impairment in work, relationships, and cognitive processing.

Antipsychotics also may be appropriate as prophylactic agents to avoid, delay, or ameliorate the onset of frank psychotic symptoms that would herald a transition from prodromal to acute schizophrenia. Risperidone (McGorry et al. 2002) and olanzapine (McGlashan et al. 2006) have each shown efficacy in reducing the risk of onset of schizophrenia in high-risk populations meeting most criteria for STPD. An overall reduction of risk by a factor of 2.5–3.5 during these studies was partially offset by a gradual reduction in effectiveness over time and a loss of detectable benefit within 1 year of treatment discontinuation. These latter findings suggest that the antipsychotic medication delayed, rather than prevented, onset of overt psychosis. These studies support sustained, rather than short-term, use of the medications.

TABLE 4–6. Randomized controlled trials (RCTs) involving patients with schizotypal personality disorder (STPD)

AUTHORS	METHODS	OUTCOME
Serban and Siegel 1984	3-month RCT of thiothixene 9.4 mg/day vs. haloperidol 3 mg/day in 16 patients with STPD (plus 16 with BPD and 16 with mixed personality disorders)	Patients showed improvement in ideas of reference, paranoia, derealization, anxiety, and depression.
Soloff et al. 1986a	5-week RCT of haloperidol 7.2 mg/day vs. amitriptyline vs. placebo in 36 schizotypal and mixed schizotypal and borderline patients	Haloperidol-treated patients improved in neurotic, psychotic, depressive, and behavioral symptoms.
Goldberg et al. 1986	12-week randomized trial of thiothixene 8.7 mg/day vs. placebo in 33 schizotypal and mixed schizotypal and borderline patients	There were significant drug-placebo differences in effect on illusions, ideas of reference, psychoticism, obsessive-compulsive symptoms, and phobic anxiety but not on depression.
Koenigsberg et al. 2003	9-week randomized, double-blind titration of risperidone from 0.25 to 2 mg vs. placebo in 29 schizotypal patients	Lower scores on PANSS Positive Symptom scale were obtained.

Note. All doses are average doses. BPD=borderline personality disorder; PANSS=Positive and Negative Syndrome Scale.

Agitation and Aggression

Treatment of agitation and aggression in STPD, in essence, does not differ from treatment of agitation and aggression in BPD. One should evaluate, at these times, how psychotic the patient actually is. Is there a breakthrough of psychotic thought? Or of hallucinations? Or is the patient's increase in agitation primarily related to anxiety rather than to a breakthrough of psychotic material? These situations are considered because a breakthrough of more severe psychotic thinking may require larger doses of medication than if the patient simply had an increase in anxiety, which can be quite substantial in STPD. But in either instance, it appears that benzodiazepines are not as useful for treating these situations; however, in some instances, benzodiazepines might be useful, especially if the symptoms are accompanied by a panic attack.

Clinical Use

The decision to begin medication treatment in STPD may reasonably be based on the degree of the patient's subjective distress with symptoms, functional impairment in relationships or occupation, or risk of development of schizophrenia. In general, treatment should be ongoing rather than episodic, and patients should anticipate medication use over years, not weeks.

The few available studies that focused on schizotypal symptoms consistently pointed to the use of lower doses of medication than are required for schizophrenia or other psychotic disorders. Specifically, studies have involved haloperidol 3 and 7 mg/day, thiothixene 8–10 mg/day, risperidone 0.25–2 mg/day, and olanzapine 2.5–12.5 mg/day. The risperidone study involved a systematic dose titration over several weeks that showed most improvement by week 3, before the dose was increased to more than 0.5 mg/day. Only positive symptoms, as measured with the PANSS Positive Symptom scale, improved at a higher dosage (1.5 mg/day) and with longer exposure (7 weeks) before improvement became significant; no additional symptoms improved with continued titration to 2 mg/day.

Similarly low doses of antipsychotics were used in studies of schizophrenia prevention. Risperidone was effective at 1–2 mg/day and olanzapine at 5–15 mg/day. It is noteworthy that even in these long-term studies, dropout rates were well below those seen with schizophrenia, possibly related to the better tolerability of low-dose medication.

Guidelines for Selection and Use

The limited studies available do not provide sufficient data to detect differences in antipsychotic efficacy and suggest that effectiveness is comparable among all available antipsychotics, both conventional and atypical. In general, treatment selection will be based on tolerability, patient preference, insurance coverage, and oral versus depot administration.

As noted earlier, low doses and gradual titration have been used successfully and are recommended for most patients. This approach has the advantage of minimizing side-effect risk and encouraging continued adherence to treatment.

Pretreatment

Patients should be instructed in the expected benefits and limitations of medication treatment, side-effect risks, and importance of continuity of care. Among other issues, clarity regarding the limitations of antipsychotic use and the importance of other modalities of treatment should be discussed. For schizotypal patients, a discussion of their elevated risk for schizophrenia and possible benefits of medications in delaying or avoiding the disorder is appropriate.

As with all disorders that carry a high risk of psychosis, medical evaluation is essential, including a screening history and physical examination, comprehensive chemistry panel, drug screen, urinalysis, and complete blood count. Positive findings should be further evaluated with specific tests. Guidelines regarding initial evaluation and follow-up monitoring of patients taking antipsychotic medications are shown in Appendixes 4 and 5. Depending on the clinical setting, brain imaging may be appropriate.

Side Effects, Drug-Drug Interactions, and Management of Overdose

Side effects, drug-drug interactions, and management of overdose in this diagnostic group are no different from those in other patients. The lower doses of medications used for treating patients with personality disorders reduce but do not eliminate side-effect risks.

Other Personality Disorders

No data are available for the use of antipsychotic medication in the treatment of other personality disorders, including antisocial personality disorder. Obviously, patients with other personality disorders may experience transient psychotic episodes (or maybe even longer-lasting episodes or severe anxiety or resistant depression in the face of emotional lability). In these instances, there may be some wisdom in the use of antipsychotic medication, but there is no support, pro or con, for the use of these medications in this patient population, even under these circumstances.

KEY CLINICAL POINTS

- There are no indications for the use of any psychotropic medication in any specific personality disorder or in the group as a whole.

- There are no indications for the use of any specific antipsychotic medications for any personality disorder; thus, treatment of personality disorder with antipsychotic medication is off-label use.

- Although RCTs have examined the use of FGAs and SGAs in BPD and STPD, no RCTs have been done for the other personality disorders.

- No studies would suggest that there is any difference in effectiveness between FGAs and SGAs in these patients.

- In BPD, antipsychotic medications have been found in some studies to be effective for a wide array of symptoms and behaviors, including global functioning, cognitive symptoms, aggression, hostility, and anxiety and, in some studies, impulsivity, mood lability, and depression.

- In STPD, antipsychotic medications have been found in some studies to be effective primarily for cognitive-perceptual symptoms, although some evidence indicates usefulness for anxiety and some depressive affect.

- When using antipsychotic medication in patients with either STPD or BPD, the doses used are usually much smaller than those used in the treatment of psychosis.

- The antipsychotic medication can be used for the treatment of agitation and aggression in this patient population.

- The side effects of antipsychotic medication in patients with personality disorders are no different from the side effects of these medications in any patient population.

- The laboratory tests and other screening tests (such as electrocardiograms) that are recommended prior to using these medications in this population are no different from those needed prior to their use in any clinical population.

- No studies of the long-term use of these medications in patients with personality disorder have been done.

References

American Psychiatric Association: Diagnostic and Statistical Manual of Mental Disorders, 3rd Edition. Washington, DC, American Psychiatric Association, 1980

Bogenschutz MP, Nurnberg HG: Olanzapine versus placebo in the treatment of borderline personality disorder. J Clin Psychiatry 54:104–109, 2004

Chopra HD, Beatson JA: Psychotic symptoms in borderline personality disorder. Am J Psychiatry 143:1605–1607, 1986

Cowdry RW, Gardner DL: Pharmacotherapy of borderline personality disorder: alprazolam, carbamazepine, trifluoperazine, and tranylcypromine. Arch Gen Psychiatry 45:111–119, 1988

Duggan C, Huband N, Smailagic N, et al: The use of pharmacological treatments for people with personality disorder: a systematic review of randomized controlled trials. Personality Ment Health 2:119–170, 2008

Fenton WS, McGlashan TH: Risk of schizophrenia in character disordered patients. Am J Psychiatry 146:1280–1284, 1989

Frosch J: The psychotic character: clinical psychiatric considerations. Psychiatr Q 38:81–96, 1964

Goldberg SC, Schulz SC, Schulz PM, et al: Borderline and schizotypal personality disorders treated with low-dose thiothixene vs placebo. Arch Gen Psychiatry 43:680 686, 1986

Keshavan M, Shad M, Soloff P, et al: Efficacy and tolerability of olanzapine in the treatment of schizotypal personality disorder. Schizophr Res 71:97–101, 2004

Koenigsberg HW, Reynolds D, Goodman M, et al: Risperidone in the treatment of schizotypal personality disorder. J Clin Psychiatry 64:628–634, 2003

Leone NF: Response of borderline patients to loxapine and chlorpromazine. J Clin Psychiatry 43:148–150, 1982

McGlashan TH, Zipursky RB, Perkins D, et al: Randomized, double-blind trial of olanzapine versus placebo in patients prodromally symptomatic for psychosis. Am J Psychiatry 163:790–799, 2006

McGorry PD, Yung AR, Phillips LJ, et al: Randomized controlled trial of interventions designed to reduce the risk of progression to first-episode psychosis in a clinical sample with subthreshold symptoms. Arch Gen Psychiatry 59:921–928, 2002

New AS, Goodman M, Triebwasser J, et al: Recent advances in the biological study of personality disorders. Psychiatr Clin No Am 31:441–461, 2008

Nickel MK, Muechlacher M, Nickel C, et al: Aripiprazole in the treatment of patients with borderline personality disorder: a double-blind, placebo-controlled study. Am J Psychiatry 163:833–838, 2006

Putnam KM, Silk KR: Emotion dysregulation and the development of borderline personality disorder. Dev Psychopathol 17:899–925, 2005

Reyntjens AM: A series of multicentric pilot trials with pimozide in psychiatric practice, I: pimozide in the treatment of personality disorders. Acta Psychiatr Belg 72:653–666, 1972

Rybakowski JK, Drozdz W, Borkowska A: Long-term administration of the low-dose risperidone in schizotaxia subjects. Hum Psychopharmacol 22:407–412, 2007

Saunders EFH, Silk KR: Personality trait dimensions and the pharmacologic treatment of borderline personality disorder. J Clin Psychopharmacol (in press)

Serban G, Siegel S: Response of borderline and schizotypal patients to small doses of thiothixene and haloperidol. Am J Psychiatry 141:1455–1458, 1984

Siever LJ: Neurobiology of aggression and violence. Am J Psychiatry 165:429–442, 2008

Siever LJ, Davis KL: A psychobiological perspective on the personality disorders. Am J Psychiatry 148:1647–1658, 1991

Siever LJ, Kalus OF, Keefe RSE: The boundaries of schizophrenia. Psychiatr Clin No Am 16:217–244, 1993

Silverstein ML, Harrow M: Schneiderian first-rank symptoms in schizophrenia. Arch Gen Psychiatry 38:288–293, 1989

Soler J, Pascual JC, Camoins J, et al: Double-blind, placebo-controlled study of dialectical behavior therapy plus olanzapine for borderline personality disorder. Am J Psychiatry 162:1221–1224, 2005

Soloff PH, George A, Nathan RS, et al: Progress in pharmacotherapy of borderline disorders: a double-blind study of amitriptyline, haloperidol, and placebo. Arch Gen Psychiatry 43:691–697, 1986a

Soloff PH, George A, Nathan S, et al: Amitriptyline and haloperidol in unstable and schizotypal borderline disorders. Psychopharmacol Bull 22:177–182, 1986b

Soloff PH, George A, Nathan S, et al: Amitriptyline versus haloperidol in borderlines: final outcomes and predictors of response. J Clin Psychopharmacol 9:238–246, 1989

Soloff PH, Cornelius J, George A, et al: Efficacy of phenelzine and haloperidol in borderline personality disorder. Arch Gen Psychiatry 50:377–385, 1993

Spitzer RL, Endicott J, Gibbon M: Crossing the border into borderline personality and borderline schizophrenia. Arch Gen Psychiatry 36:17–24, 1979

U.S. National Library of Medicine: Medical Encyclopedia: Psychosis. February 6, 2008. Available at: http://www.nlm.nih.gov/medlineplus/ency/article/001553.htm#Definition. Accessed November 7, 2008.

Zanarini MC, Frankenburg FR: Olanzapine treatment of female borderline personality disorder patients: a double-blind, placebo-controlled pilot study. J Clin Psychiatry 62:849–854, 2001

Zanarini MC, Frankenburg FR, Parachini EA: A preliminary, randomized trial of fluoxetine, olanzapine, and the olanzapine-fluoxetine combination in women with borderline personality disorder. Am J Psychiatry 160:167–169, 2004

CHAPTER 5

Substance Abuse Disorders

Gerardo Gonzalez, M.D.
Ruben Miozzo, M.D., M.P.H.
Douglas Ziedonis, M.D., M.P.H.

ANTIPSYCHOTIC MEDICATIONS have been found to be efficacious in numerous clinical trials for individuals with a range of major primary psychiatric disorders, including schizophrenia, bipolar disorder, and major depression. Although these medications have been approved by the U.S. Food and Drug Administration (FDA) for many of these disorders, they also have important side effects, and better and safer medication interventions need to be developed. Because of their unique pharmacological properties, this class of medications also has been hypothesized and tested for use in a variety of specific substance use disorders, particularly cocaine addiction. Currently, these medications have no FDA-approved indication for this use; however, some clinicians do use these medications "off label" for treating addiction and have found that particular choices of antipsychotics might have advantages in patients with co-occurring serious mental illness and addiction. First-generation, or typical, antipsychotics (FGAs) and second-generation, or atypical, antipsychotics (SGAs) have been reported to be used in four clinical situations either alone or more typically in combination with other medications:

1. Psychomotor agitation syndrome during intoxication or withdrawal from different substances
2. Psychotic syndromes that emerge in the context of substance use usually associated with stimulants and cannabis
3. Co-occurring primary psychotic disorders such as schizophrenia, schizoaffective disorder, and bipolar disorder and substance use disorders
4. Treatment of primary substance use disorders, particularly stimulants

In this chapter, we review the FGAs and SGAs most commonly used within the framework of each of these clinical situations and then focus on the specific substance use disorders and substance-related syndromes in which the use of this class of medication may be useful and need additional research study. We suggest guidelines for their use and monitoring based on clinical experience, including a review of the limited studies supporting their use for these indications. The potential uses of antipsychotic medications for patients with substance abuse are outlined in Table 5–1.

Substance-Related Psychomotor Agitation

General Approach

Psychomotor agitation in patients presenting to emergency departments may have a variety of etiologies. In general, clarifying the etiology may be critical to treat the underlying cause of this behavioral disruption, but the initial approach should optimize the safety of the patient and staff. De-escalation techniques with active listening and calm reassurance are key elements for all patients. Physically threatening patients may need to be approached with standard behavioral control measures, which may include the use of seclusion or restraints.

An important issue to assess is whether the individual presents with substance intoxication or withdrawal. This is important in determining which specific substance (and likely polysubstances) has been consumed. There may be situations in which an individual is in withdrawal from one substance while simultaneously being intoxicated with another. Because alcohol and other sedative withdrawal can be life-threatening, determining whether these substances are part of the clinical situation is very important. Obviously, after

TABLE 5–1. Antipsychotic medications and their indications for substance use disorders

Medication	Indication	Dosage or Dosage Range	Monitoring	Evidence
Aripiprazole	Psychomotor agitation	9.75 mg IM	Urine toxicology	+
	Schizophrenia and cocaine abuse	10–30 mg/day	Metabolic syndrome; urine toxicology	+++
Clozapine	Schizophrenia, alcohol and cocaine abuse	416–550 mg/day[a]	WBC monitoring; metabolic syndrome; urine toxicology	+++
Haloperidol	Psychomotor agitation	0.5–5 mg IM	QT prolongation; acute EPS; urine toxicology	+++
	Stimulant-associated psychosis	5–20 mg/day[a]	QT prolongation; EPS; urine toxicology	++++
Olanzapine	Psychomotor agitation	10 mg IM	Urine toxicology	+
	Stimulant-associated psychosis	5–20 mg/day[a]	Metabolic syndrome; urine toxicology	++++
	Schizophrenia and cocaine abuse	15–25 mg/day[a]	Metabolic syndrome; urine toxicology	++++
Quetiapine	Schizophrenia and substance abuse (including alcohol)	300–800 mg/day	Metabolic syndrome; urine toxicology; Breathalyzer	++
	Bipolar disorder and substance abuse	50–400 mg/day[a]	Metabolic syndrome; urine toxicology	+++
	Alcohol (type B)	400 mg/day[a]	Metabolic syndrome; Breathalyzer	++++
	Cocaine	300–600 mg/day[a]	Metabolic syndrome; urine toxicology	+++

TABLE 5–1. Antipsychotic medications and their indications for substance use disorders *(continued)*

MEDICATION	INDICATION	DOSAGE OR DOSAGE RANGE	MONITORING	EVIDENCE
Risperidone	Schizophrenia and cocaine abuse	4–6 mg/day[a]	Metabolic syndrome; urine toxicology	+++
	Schizophrenia and cocaine abuse	47.2 mg IM per 15 days and 2–6 mg/day oral risperidone[a]	Metabolic syndrome; urine toxicology	++++
Ziprasidone	Schizophrenia and substance abuse	60–160 mg/day[a]	Metabolic syndrome; urine toxicology	+++

Note. EPS=extrapyramidal symptoms; IM=intramuscular; WBC=white blood cell. Evidence key: +=no clear evidence; ++=case report; +++=open-label study; ++++=randomized controlled study.

[a]Dosage or dosage range used during a study.

intoxication comes withdrawal, so the clinical picture will change as the drug-induced state changes. Psychomotor agitation can be seen in both intoxication and withdrawal; however, the causes and treatments in these two clinically different states are important to consider. Treating the withdrawal symptoms of alcohol or other sedatives with the gold standard of benzodiazepines is likely to reduce psychomotor agitation (a symptom of withdrawal).

In many cases of intoxication and withdrawal, pharmacological treatment with benzodiazepines, with and without antipsychotic medications, is used in the emergency department setting (Huf et al. 2005). If the patient has a major psychiatric disorder and is already taking antipsychotic medication, then resuming or continuing the same medication would be part of the treatment in this setting; however, managing the acute withdrawal or intoxication is a priority that must occur simultaneously. Part of the difficulty in managing a patient with co-occurring serious mental illness and acute intoxication and withdrawal is determining how many of the symptoms might be caused by the psychotic disorder that may be reemerging as a result of noncompliance with antipsychotics. Medication noncompliance with psychiatric medications is very common among patients with co-occurring disorders, especially when they are actively using substances. If despite this initial treatment the patient shows moderate to severe agitation, then the use of additional pharmacological intervention is indicated.

Pharmacological Intervention

Benzodiazepines
Benzodiazepines (e.g., lorazepam 0.5–2.0 mg orally or intramuscularly every 4–6 hours as needed) are recommended for most patients presenting with agitation and particularly if alcohol withdrawal or stimulant and phencyclidine (PCP) intoxication is considered the leading diagnosis. However, benzodiazepines should not be used during alcohol intoxication or in patients with severe respiratory disorder (i.e., chronic obstructive pulmonary disease).

Antipsychotics
Haloperidol (0.5–5.0 mg orally or intramuscularly every 4–6 hours as needed) is a typical high-potency neuroleptic that has the advantage of being less likely to induce hypotension and bradycardia that are associated with low-potency antipsychotics such as chlorpromazine. However, a high-potency neuroleptic such as haloperidol is associated with dystonic reactions and other extrapyramidal side effects and QT prolongation. Therefore, performing an electrocardiogram when the agitation has subsided is indicated in these cases and particularly if stimulant abuse is considered the cause of this behavior. Also, an anticholinergic medication (e.g., benztropine) may be needed to manage the side effects of these high-potency FGAs.

The following SGAs have been approved for the treatment of acute agitation in schizophrenia and bipolar mania and may have a role in the treatment of substance-induced agitation:

- Ziprasidone (10–20 mg IM/PO every 2–4 hours as needed (maximum = 40 mg/24 hours)
- Olanzapine (10 mg IM/PO every 2–6 hours as needed (maximum = 30 mg/24 hours)
- Aripiprazole (9.75 mg IM/PO every 2–6 hours as needed (maximum = 30 mg/24 hours)

These antipsychotics share the advantage of having an efficacy similar to that of haloperidol but with a better short-term side-effect profile (Citrome 2007). These medications do have serious short- and long-term side effects that must be monitored. It is important to note that SGAs can reduce the seizure threshold and should be used with caution in patients who are prone to seizures. This is especially relevant in patients undergoing alcohol or sedative-hypnotic withdrawal. However, from clinical experience, they appear to have advantages in the acute setting compared with the high-potency FGAs.

Psychomotor Agitation Due to Intoxication

Determining what specific substances the patient has been consuming is important. Urine (or blood) toxicology assessment is very important because the patient may not be a good historian or may not even know what he or she consumed. Specific clinical symptoms and signs are also very helpful. Polydrug use is common and can make the assessment more complicated clinically.

Stimulant Intoxication (Cocaine and Amphetamine)

Patients with stimulant intoxication may show symptoms such as agitation, hyperactivity, hyperthermia, irritability, diaphoresis, mydriasis, hyperpyrexia, flushing, nausea or vomiting, tachycardia, hypertension, arrhythmias, confusion, hallucinations, psychosis, seizures, dyskinesias, dystonias, or coma.

Cocaine is a potent blocker of the presynaptic dopamine transporter (DAT) as well as the transporters for serotonin and norepinephrine. Amphetamines, in addition to blocking the monoamine transporters, increase the release of these neurotransmitters by blocking the vesicular monoamine transporter and preventing their storage in synaptic vesicles.

Patients presenting with stimulant-induced agitation should be carefully evaluated to rule out life-threatening conditions such as severe toxicity that may result in seizure, intracranial hemorrhage, and coronary vasoconstriction. A serious complication of psychomotor agitation is the development of hyperthermia, which is associated with high mortality. Therefore, hyperthermia should be monitored and treated promptly. The general pharmacological approach previously outlined with benzodiazepines should be sufficient to control this syndrome. However, antipsychotic medication also may be used if needed. β-Adrenergic blockers should not be used to treat hypertension or tachycardia because unopposed α-adrenergic stimulation may increase the risk of myocardial ischemia.

Phencyclidine Intoxication

Patients presenting with psychomotor agitation related to PCP may have vertical or horizontal nystagmus, hypertension, tachycardia, numbness or diminished responsiveness to pain, ataxia, dysarthria, muscle rigidity, seizures, coma, and hyperacusis.

PCP is an *N*-methyl-D-aspartate antagonist and at high doses may also block the dopamine and norepinephrine transporters. This latter effect may explain in part the presence of hypertension, tachycardia, and agitation associated with this intoxication.

The treatment of PCP intoxication usually involves observation and close monitoring in a controlled and quiet environment to decrease overstimulation. Treatment with benzodiazepines may be needed, and the use of antipsychotic medications may be added for moderate to severe agitation.

If the patient presents with serious medical complications such as cardiovascular complications, seizures, renal dysfunction, or hyperpyrexia, then the patient should be treated by the medical team.

Alcohol Intoxication

Psychomotor agitation in the context of alcohol intoxication is usually easily diagnosed and confirmed by smelling alcohol on the patient's breath. In addition to disruptive and combative behavior, patients show slurred speech, incoordination, ataxia, nystagmus, and impairment in attention or memory and may develop stupor or coma.

The use of benzodiazepines during psychomotor agitation in the case of acute alcohol intoxication is not recommended because of the synergistic effects of two central nervous system depressants. Management with general supportive measures, fluids, and occasionally isolation or restraints may be considered to control combative and assaultive behavior. The use of antipsychotic medication in these extreme cases of psychomotor agitation is preferable to benzodiazepines. All patients also should receive thiamine and folate as part of their initial treatment. Patients with severe alcohol dependence syndrome may still have relatively high blood alcohol levels by Breathalyzer measure but already present with alcohol withdrawal. In such cases, initiating benzodiazepines as standard treatment for alcohol withdrawal is clearly indicated.

Psychomotor Agitation Due to Withdrawal

Psychomotor agitation is also possible during acute withdrawal from substances, particularly alcohol and other sedatives. Withdrawal comprises two phases: acute and protracted withdrawal. The acute phase varies in length of time depending on the type of substance and its half-life. The protracted phase of withdrawal is more similar across substances and is likely to last 3–6 months. Common symptoms are sleep difficulty, mood difficulties, difficulty concentrating, and persistent cravings triggered by external or internal cues.

Alcohol Withdrawal

Patients with psychomotor agitation in the context of alcohol withdrawal are also likely to have autonomic hyperactivity such as diaphoresis, tachycardia, tremor, insomnia, nausea or vomiting, and anxiety. In severe alcohol withdrawal, hallucinations and seizure also may occur.

Treatment is with general supportive measures, including thiamine 100 mg/day, folate 1 mg/day, multivitamins, and magnesium and potassium replacement as needed. Benzodiazepine treatment may be on a fixed schedule or symptom triggered.

Fixed-schedule treatment

- *Lorazepam:* 1 mg every 6 hours for day 1; 1 mg every 8 hours for day 2; 1 mg every 12 hours for day 3; and for each day thereafter, 1 mg every 2 hours as needed for persistent withdrawal symptoms.
- *Chlordiazepoxide:* 100 mg every 6 hours for day 1; 50 mg every 6 hours for day 2; 25 mg every 6 hours for day 3; and for each day thereafter, 50 mg every 2 hours as needed for persistent withdrawal symptoms.

Symptom-triggered treatment

- *Lorazepam:* 1 mg every 2–4 hours as needed with a Clinical Institute Withdrawal Assessment for Alcohol (CIWA-Ar; Sullivan et al. 1989) score greater than 10.
- *Chlordiazepoxide:* 50 mg every 2–4 hours as needed with a CIWA-Ar score greater than 10.

The use of antipsychotic medication is usually not recommended during alcohol withdrawal. However, if the psychomotor agitation is severe and all other measures have failed, then the use of antipsychotic medication may be weighed against the risk of seizure. The use of antipsychotic medications during delirium tremens is not recommended.

Substance-Associated Psychotic Symptoms and Disorders

General Approach

Psychotic symptoms may emerge in the context of consumption of drugs of abuse. These symptoms can develop in the acute context secondary to intoxication or withdrawal, but they also can develop secondary to chronic use, particularly with cannabis, stimulants, and alcohol. The current diagnostic system (DSM-IV-TR; American Psychiatric Association 2000) has specific criteria for the diagnosis of substance-induced psychotic disorder. The psychotic symptoms should be hallucinations or delusions that emerge during the direct exposure to a specific substance (intoxication) or recent use (withdrawal), and these symptoms may still be present up to 4 weeks after the direct exposure has subsided. The person should not have insight that the hallucinations are related to the use of the substance, or the disorder is better diagnosed as substance intoxication or withdrawal and not substance-induced psychotic disorder. There is evidence from the history, physical examination, or laboratory findings that these psychotic symptoms emerged during or within 4 weeks of intoxication or withdrawal from the suspected substance. The disorder should not be better accounted for by a psychotic disorder that is not substance induced.

In a recent review, Mathias et al. (2008) made meaningful suggestions that further enhance and clarify the current diagnostic criteria for this disorder. The suggestion to change the name of the disorder from substance-induced to substance-associated disorder may stress better the role of substance use as one etiological factor among other factors and not as the sole cause of this disorder. The person may or may not have insight about the relation of substance use and the presence of psychotic symptoms. Psychotic symptoms emerge within a month of intoxication or withdrawal but also during abuse of or dependence on the substance. The evidence that the psychotic symptoms are not better accounted for by another psychotic disorder that is not substance induced should be expanded to include psychotic symptoms that precede the initiation of substance use and symptoms that persist for more than 6 months after cessation of drug use. If the person has a stable preexisting non-substance-related psychotic disorder, the new psychotic episode was likely induced by the suspected substance. In addition to the positive psychotic symptoms, this disorder may include negative symptoms, and the course of the disorder may be brief if the symptoms last less than 4 weeks or persistent if they last more than 4 weeks. The following substances are associated with this disorder:

- Alcohol
- Amphetamine
- Cannabis
- Cocaine
- Hallucinogen
- Inhalant
- Opioid (meperidine)
- PCP
- Sedative, hypnotic, or anxiolytic

Stimulant-Associated Psychosis

Clinical Description and Onset

Most stimulant-induced psychotic symptoms are brief reactions that usually subside rapidly in hours to days; however, symptoms, signs, and course differ between cocaine- and amphetamine-induced psychosis. Treatment is directed to promote abstinence from stimulant use and to administer antipsychotic medication until the psychotic symptoms resolve. In patients presenting with recurrence of psychotic symptoms after relapse to stimulant abuse, a low dose of an FGA or SGA should be given for a longer period (Curran et al. 2004). Evidence indicates that sensitization following high-dose antipsychotic treatment may be related to the upregulation of the dopamine system, which makes the person more prone to develop psychotic symptoms with stimulant-induced increase of dopamine and norepinephrine neurotransmission in the context of cocaine or amphetamine relapse.

The onset of psychotic symptoms after abuse of stimulants has been related to the duration of use, amount of use, and type of substance. For example, one study (Sato 1992) found that these symptoms started from 4 months to more than 4 years after stimulant abuse. Another study found that these symptoms may occur in less than 2 years if multiple daily injections and higher doses of methamphetamine were used (Yui et al. 2002).

Selection of Antipsychotic Medication

A recent meta-analysis (Shoptaw et al. 2008) that searched all reported clinical trials until 2003 showed that the evidence-based treatment for amphetamine psychosis is scarce, according to their study selection criteria, and they concluded that no controlled trials of treatment for amphetamine psychosis were available to be considered. However, a more recent randomized trial of antipsychotic medications for methamphetamine-induced psychosis (Leelahanaj et al. 2005) reported that olanzapine and haloperidol both showed similar efficacy in resolving psychotic symptoms (93% and 79%, respectively), with olanzapine showing significantly greater safety and tolerability than haloperidol as measured by frequency and severity of extrapyramidal symptoms.

Cannabis-Associated Psychosis

Psychotic symptoms associated with cannabis use are usually time-limited, mostly ending with complete improvement after cessation of cannabis consumption. The psychotic symptoms may appear after use of large amounts of cannabis and include a sudden onset of confusion associated with the development of hallucinations, delusions, and emotional lability. This cannabis-associated psychotic syndrome may have a different time course and prognosis that is dependent on the presence or not of history of personality disorder or psychiatric disorder with and without psychosis. Persons without any history tend to have a shorter course, with the symptoms subsiding completely within days. Persons with a history of personality disorder or psychiatric disorder tend to have a longer period of being symptomatic, and their symptoms may improve completely only after several weeks. Patients who have a history of a psychotic episode tend to have a prolonged course and often receive the diagnosis of schizophrenia (Leweke et al. 2004). Whether exposure to cannabis can result in a chronic psychotic state that persists beyond the period of intoxication is unclear (D'Souza 2007).

Cannabis Use as Risk Factor

Clinical Description and Onset

Evidence suggests that cannabis use may be a risk factor for the development of schizophrenia, in association with other risk factors such as genetic predisposition and environmental stress. For example, in one longitudinal study, cannabis was associated with an increased risk of developing schizophrenia in a dose-dependent fashion, with an adjusted odds ratio reaching 6.7 (95% confidence interval=2.1–21.7) for those using cannabis more than 50 times since adolescence (Zammit et al. 2002). Another study (van Os et al. 2002) showed that baseline use of cannabis predicted at 3-year follow-up the presence of psychotic symptoms among those without baseline psychotic symptoms and worsened psychotic symptoms in those who had a baseline psychotic disorder.

Selection of Antipsychotic Medication

The preferred medications for the treatment of cannabis-associated psychosis are the SGAs. Atypical antipsychotics may be more efficacious than the typical antipsychotics for treating the potential "amotivational syndrome" associated with chronic cannabis use, which resembles the negative symptoms of schizophrenia (Leweke et al. 2004).

Co-occurring Disorders

Antipsychotic medications are important treatments for managing symptoms of schizophrenia (see Chapter 2, "Schizophrenia and Schizoaffective Disorder," in this volume) and bipolar disorder (see Chapter 3, "Mood and Anxiety Disorders,"in this volume). Individuals with these disorders also are very likely to abuse substances, including alcohol, cocaine, cannabis, and tobacco. For this population with co-occurring serious mental illness and addiction, there are issues of medication noncompliance, effect on the liver, sedation, seizure risk, and interaction of the medication and the specific substances of abuse. In this section, we review the antipsychotic medications that have been evaluated to reduce psychotic symptoms in the context of substance use.

Schizophrenia

Substance use disorders represent a major challenge in the management of patients with schizophrenia (Ziedonis et al. 2005) and can have a major effect on patients' functional outcomes. Substance use disorders are the most common comorbidity of patients with schizophrenia. Community epidemiological studies, such as the Epidemiologic Catchment Area Study, have reported a prevalence of substance abuse disorder in patients with schizophrenia of nearly 50% in community samples (Regier et al. 1990). Patients with schizophrenia who have comorbid substance abuse are at increased risk for medical complications, suicide, criminal activity, mental status instability, violence, victimization, incarceration, homelessness, and problems in access to care.

Integrative Approach

Management of substance abuse in patients with schizophrenia requires an integrated approach that addresses both the mental illness and the addiction with a multidisciplinary team (Ziedonis 2004). The treatment plan should include pharmacotherapy, psychosocial interventions, substance abuse counseling, and community supports and should be tailored to the needs of the individual patient. Antipsychotic medications are a critical part of the treatment of schizophrenia and substance abuse but should always be administered as part of a treatment plan that addresses the substance abuse and the psychiatric disorder. Consideration of FDA-approved substance abuse treatment medications such as disulfiram, naltrexone, acamprosate, varenicline, nicotine replacement medications, methadone, and buprenorphine can be used successfully in this population.

Address Noncompliance

Medication and treatment participation noncompliance is common in patients with schizophrenia. Some of the many explanations for noncompliance in this population include the patient's fear of the interaction of medications and substances, simply forgetting to take the medication, being told by uninformed peers at Alcoholics Anonymous to stop taking psychotropic medications, and the increasing disorganization, confusion, and disruption that are caused by the substance abuse (Drake 2007). In addition, noncompliance with treatment for substances of abuse (especially stimulants) may exacerbate psychotic symptoms and result in further decompensation of the patient's condition. A focus on the patient's short- and long-term goals can be a useful introduction to increasing motivation to maintain medication compliance and consider substance cessation.

Selection of Antipsychotic Medication

Oral second-generation (atypical) antipsychotic agents
Several open-label studies have compared the effectiveness of a traditional FGA with that of the newer SGAs in patients with schizophrenia. Most of the studies showed a superior efficacy of SGAs in reducing psychopathology and relapse in substance abuse for these patients; however, larger studies are needed in the future. In addition, the longer-term side effects of the newer SGAs may be an issue that remains unstudied in this population. A few studies have suggested that the FGAs may be associated with more substance abuse than the SGAs for a variety of theoretical and practical reasons. Three studies found that clozapine was associated with less tobacco use compared with haloperidol (McEvoy et al. 1995). The hypotheses as to why rates of substance abuse seemed higher with treatment with traditional antipsychotic medications include self-medication of negative symptoms and neuroleptic dysphoria (Voruganti and Awad 2004).

A review of findings of several open-label studies and case reports (Smelson et al. 2008) suggested that clozapine may offer an advantage in this population in reducing the abuse of substances and the psychotic symptoms. Noordsy and Green (2003) pointed out that although clozapine is not a first-line agent for the treatment of these disorders because of its high side-effect profile, it might have a particular role to play in this population. Obviously, clozapine administration requires a commitment from the patient that should be evaluated before starting this agent. Clozapine is also limited in this population because of risks of seizure, sedation, and poor compliance with treatment providers. Olanzapine, risperidone, quetiapine, aripiprazole, and ziprasidone remain good treatment options for these patients with co-occurring disorders; however, more studies are needed to compare these different medications among themselves and with traditional FGAs. We are unaware of any data on the use of paliperidone. The use of antipsychotic medications over the long term requires appropriate monitoring (see Appendixes 4 and 5).

Long-term intramuscular antipsychotics

Because noncompliance is a significant issue in in patients with schizophrenia, clinical experience suggests that intramuscular depot antipsychotics may have advantages in regard to compliance. In the past, the group of depot antipsychotic agents was limited to haloperidol or fluphenazine. The emergence of long-acting intramuscular risperidone provides an option requiring evaluation and is supported by some clinical experience (Rubio et al. 2006). The recommended doses for long-term intramuscular antipsychotics are presented in Table 5–2.

Bipolar Disorder

Individuals with bipolar disorder I have the highest risk for substance use disorders among persons with psychiatric disorders; according to the Epidemiologic Catchment Area Study (Regier et al. 1990), the lifetime prevalence of substance use disorder is as high as 61% in this population, compared with a 48% rate in individuals with bipolar II disorder. Despite these high comorbidity rates, substance use disorders are frequently overlooked in this population, and the use of substances during mania is explained as just a symptom of the bipolar disorder. Sometimes this omission is a result of the expectations of the treatment providers. Patients with bipolar disorder who present with erratic behavior and mood lability are considered to be manifesting symptoms of the psychiatric condition and not of possible substance abuse.

Patients with co-occurring bipolar disorder and substance abuse have a greater risk for medical and psychiatric complications, as well as for violence, incarceration, homelessness, and access to care, than do bipolar pa-

TABLE 5–2. Recommended doses for long-term intramuscular antipsychotics

MEDICATION	ADULT DOSING		
	INITIAL	MAINTENANCE	MAXIMUM DOSE
Haloperidol decanoate 50 mg/mL, 100 mg/mL (IM only)	IM monthly dose is calculated by multiplying previous oral dose by 10 to 20 times. Maximum initial dose should not exceed 100 mg.	Adult dosing usually spans from 50 mg to 200 mg every 4 weeks.	300 mg every 4 weeks
Fluphenazine decanoate 25 mg/mL (IM only)	12.5–25 mg IM	50 mg every 1–4 weeks as needed and tolerated (usually every 2 weeks). Dose should be increased in 12.5-mg increments.	100 mg every 2 weeks
Risperdal Consta 12.5 mg, 25 mg, 37.5 mg, and 50 mg	25 mg IM every 2 weeks	Dose may be increased to 37.5 mg or 50 mg at intervals of at least 4 weeks.	50 mg every 2 weeks

tients who do not abuse substances. Thus, early detection of and screening for substance abuse in this population are important. Because of the high rate of denial, the assessment should include direct clinical observation, laboratory testing, and gathering of collateral information, especially in high-risk patients who have a history of substance abuse and are suspected of relapse. Screening instruments can be a valuable tool in higher-functioning patients, although they might be less sensitive in patients with severe psychiatric disorders.

Integrative Team Approach

The treatment of bipolar disorder with comorbid substance abuse requires an integrative approach. Pharmacotherapy should be combined with individual, group, couples, and family psychotherapy, as well as with social skills learning, other psychosocial interventions, and medical care (Ziedonis 2004). Interventions should be tailored to each patient's needs and clinical condition.

Selection of Medications

There is a dearth of information about medication management for patients with bipolar disorder and comorbid substance abuse. Most studies had a small sample size and were open label. Studies have concentrated mostly on the choice of a mood stabilizer, yielding some evidence that sodium valproate may be preferred over lithium in this population. Salloum and colleagues (2005) reported that valproate therapy decreased heavy drinking in patients with comorbid bipolar disorder and alcohol dependence. In addition, valproate reduces substance abuse while improving psychiatric symptoms in patients with bipolar disorder and primary cocaine dependence (Salloum et al. 2007). On the contrary, Geller and colleagues (1998) showed an improvement in both psychopathology measures and weekly random urine test results when lithium was given to adolescents with comorbid bipolar disorder and substance abuse.

Few studies have been published on the choice of antipsychotic agent in this population. The evidence is only preliminary in nature. As with schizophrenia, these data indicate that SGAs may have a promising role in the treatment of co-occurring disorders. For example, Brown and colleagues (2002) reported that the use of quetiapine was associated with substantial improvement in psychiatric symptoms and cocaine cravings in patients with bipolar disorder with comorbid cocaine abuse. They also reported improvement of psychopathology and drug craving after outpatients with bipolar or schizoaffective disorders and substance abuse switched from their current antipsychotic to aripiprazole (Brown et al. 2005).

Recommendations

As with schizophrenia, the management of co-occurring bipolar disorder and substance abuse is a challenging task. The treatment of these disorders requires an integrative approach, with a plan tailored to the patient's needs. Limited information exists about pharmacological management, but antipsychotic treatment can play an important role. Several studies, mostly open label and with limited sample size, have suggested effectiveness of SGAs. Several studies point to clozapine as the most effective medication in reducing psychopathology and substance abuse. If intramuscular depot preparations are required, risperidone could be an agent to consider over FGAs. In terms of mood stabilizers for bipolar disorder with co-occurring substance abuse, the evidence seems to support the selection of valproate over lithium.

Substance Use Disorders

Antipsychotic medications have been considered candidates for the treatment of substance use disorders (abuse and dependence) primarily because of their effect on the dopaminergic system, which is considered the primary reinforcing and reward pathway for substance abuse. In addition, the SGAs have effects on the serotonergic pathway, which appears to be relevant in the treatment of addictions. There have been limited clinical trials of this approach, perhaps because of the limited efficacy shown in studies, the availability of other FDA-approved medications for some addictions, and the potential for serious side effects with SGAs. The evidence for the use of antipsychotic medications for specific substance use disorders is reviewed in the following subsections.

Alcohol Use Disorders

No evidence suggests that antipsychotic medications are likely to be more effective than the current FDA-approved medications for alcohol use disorders (disulfiram, naltrexone, and acamprosate).

Aripiprazole is an SGA (quinolinone derivative) with partial agonist activity at dopamine D_2 and serotonin $5\text{-}HT_{1A}$ receptors and antagonist activity at $5\text{-}HT_{2A}$ receptors. A recent clinical trial (Anton et al. 2008) evaluating aripiprazole 30 mg/day for alcohol dependence showed decreased treatment retention and more adverse events with aripiprazole than with placebo, with no difference in efficacy between aripiprazole and placebo. The authors considered that the lack of superior efficacy of aripiprazole on days of abstinence and days of heavy drinking was related to the high attrition rate secondary to the high dose of aripiprazole and suggested that a lower dose or dose escalation may improve drinking outcomes.

Quetiapine is an antipsychotic medication that is an antagonist of dopamine D_2 and serotonin 5-HT_2 receptors. In type B (more severe) alcohol-dependent patients, quetiapine 400 mg/day was particularly efficacious in reducing the percentage of drinking days and heavy drinking days compared with placebo (Kampman et al. 2007). A larger trial is warranted to confirm these initial promising results.

Stimulant Use Disorders

Antipsychotic medications do not appear to have a role in cocaine dependence, and no FDA-approved medications exist for cocaine addiction. A review of the literature (Amato et al. 2007) did not support the use of antipsychotic medication for cocaine dependence, although most of the studies had a small sample size and a lack of information on relevant outcomes. Risperidone, olanzapine, and haloperidol have been evaluated in small controlled trials and have not been shown to be useful in reducing cocaine use.

Treatment with quetiapine 300–600 mg/day in cocaine-dependent patients was in general well tolerated and appeared to reduce self-reported cocaine use. At these doses, subjects reported sedation and had significant weight gain (Kennedy et al. 2008). Although the abuse potential of quetiapine is considered low, there have been recent case reports of abuse of quetiapine intranasally and intravenously (Reeves and Brister 2007; Waters and Joshi 2007).

No clinical trials of aripiprazole for stimulant abuse have yet been done, but a series of human laboratory studies support the need for additional studies of this SGA in the treatment of stimulant dependence (Stoops 2006; Stoops et al. 2007).

KEY CLINICAL POINTS

- Antipsychotic medications are used in patients with substance abuse disorders for

  — Psychomotor agitation syndrome during intoxication or withdrawal from different substances.

  — Psychotic syndromes that emerge in the context of substance use usually associated with stimulants and cannabis.

  — Co-occurring primary psychotic disorders such as schizophrenia, schizoaffective disorder, and bipolar disorder.

  — Treatment of primary substance use disorders, particularly stimulant disorders.

- It is important to assess whether the patient is presenting with substance intoxication, substance withdrawal, or simultaneous withdrawal from one substance and intoxication with another.

- Psychotic symptoms (e.g. delusions, hallucinations) may emerge secondary to the consumption of drugs of abuse and may still be present up to 4 weeks after the direct exposure has subsided.

References

Amato L, Minozzi S, Pani PP, et al: Antipsychotic medications for cocaine dependence. Cochrane Database Syst Rev (3):CD006306, 2007

American Psychiatric Association: Diagnostic and Statistical Manual of Mental Disorders, 4th Edition, Text Revision. Washington, DC, American Psychiatric Association, 2000

Anton RF, Kranzler H, Breder C, et al: A randomized, multicenter, double-blind, placebo-controlled study of the efficacy and safety of aripiprazole for the treatment of alcohol dependence. J Clin Psychopharmacol 28:5–12, 2008

Brown ES, Nejtek VA, Perantie DC, et al: Quetiapine in bipolar disorder and cocaine dependence. Bipolar Disord 4:406–411, 2002

Brown ES, Jeffress J, Liggin JD, et al: Switching outpatients with bipolar or schizoaffective disorders and substance abuse from their current antipsychotic to aripiprazole. J Clin Psychiatry 66:756–760, 2005

Citrome L: Comparison of intramuscular ziprasidone, olanzapine, or aripiprazole for agitation: a quantitative review of efficacy and safety. J Clin Psychiatry 68:1876–1885, 2007

Curran C, Byrappa N, McBride A: Stimulant psychosis: systematic review. Br J Psychiatry 185:196–204, 2004

Drake RE: Management of substance use disorder in schizophrenia patients: current guidelines. CNS Spectr 12 (10 suppl 17):27–32, 2007

D'Souza DC: Cannabinoids and psychosis. Int Rev Neurobiol 78:289–326, 2007

Geller B, Cooper TB, Sun K, et al: Double-blind and placebo-controlled study of lithium for adolescent bipolar disorders with secondary substance dependency. J Am Acad Child Adolesc Psychiatry 37:171–178, 1998

Huf G, Alexander J, Allen MH: Haloperidol plus promethazine for psychosis induced aggression. Cochrane Database Syst Rev (1):CD005146, 2005

Kampman KM, Pettinati HM, Lynch KG, et al: A double-blind, placebo-controlled pilot trial of quetiapine for the treatment of Type A and Type B alcoholism. J Clin Psychopharmacol 27:344–351, 2007

Kennedy A, Wood AE, Saxon AJ, et al: Quetiapine for the treatment of cocaine dependence: an open-label trial. J Clin Psychopharmacol 28:221–224, 2008

Leelahanaj T, Kongsakon R, Netrakom P: A 4-week, double-blind comparison of olanzapine with haloperidol in the treatment of amphetamine psychosis. J Med Assoc Thai 88 (suppl 3):S43–S52, 2005

Leweke FM, Gerth CW, Klosterkotter J: Cannabis-associated psychosis: current status of research. CNS Drugs 18:895–910, 2004

Mathias S, Lubman DI, Hides L: Substance-induced psychosis: a diagnostic conundrum. J Clin Psychiatry 69:358–367, 2008

McEvoy JP, Freudenreich O, Levin ED, et al: Haloperidol increases smoking in patients with schizophrenia. Psychopharmacology (Berl) 119:124–126, 1995

Noordsy DL, Green AI: Pharmacotherapy for schizophrenia and co-occurring substance use disorders. Curr Psychiatry Rep 5:340–346, 2003

Reeves RR, Brister JC: Additional evidence of the abuse potential of quetiapine. South Med J 100:834–836, 2007

Regier DA, Farmer ME, Rae DS, et al: Comorbidity of mental disorders with alcohol and other drug abuse: results from the Epidemiologic Catchment Area (ECA) Study. JAMA 264:2511–2518, 1990

Rubio G, Martinez I, Ponce G, et al: Long-acting injectable risperidone compared with zuclopenthixol in the treatment of schizophrenia with substance abuse comorbidity. Can J Psychiatry 51:531–539, 2006

Salloum IM, Cornelius JR, Daley DC, et al: Efficacy of valproate maintenance in patients with bipolar disorder and alcoholism: a double-blind placebo-controlled study. Arch Gen Psychiatry 62:37–45, 2005

Salloum IM, Douaihy A, Cornelius JR, et al: Divalproex utility in bipolar disorder with co-occurring cocaine dependence: a pilot study. Addict Behav 32:410–415, 2007

Sato M: A lasting vulnerability to psychosis in patients with previous methamphetamine psychosis. Ann N Y Acad Sci 654:160–170, 1992

Smelson DA, Dixon L, Craig T, et al: Pharmacological treatment of schizophrenia and co-occurring substance use disorders. CNS Drugs 22:903–916, 2008

Shoptaw SJ, Kao U, Ling WW: Treatment for amphetamine psychosis. Cochrane Database Syst Rev (4):CD003026, 2008

Stoops WW: Aripiprazole as a potential pharmacotherapy for stimulant dependence: human laboratory studies with d-amphetamine. Exp Clin Psychopharmacol 14:413–421, 2006

Stoops WW, Lile JA, Lofwall MR, et al: The safety, tolerability, and subject-rated effects of acute intranasal cocaine administration during aripiprazole maintenance. Am J Drug Alcohol Abuse 33:769–776, 2007

Sullivan JT, Sykora K, Schneiderman J, et al: Assessment of alcohol withdrawal: the revised Clinical Institute Withdrawal Assessment for Alcohol Scale (CIWA-Ar). Br J Addict 84:1353–1357, 1989

van Os J, Bak M, Hanssen M, et al: Cannabis use and psychosis: a longitudinal population-based study. Am J Epidemiol 156:319–327, 2002

Voruganti L, Awad AG: Neuroleptic dysphoria: towards a new synthesis. Psychopharmacology (Berl) 171:121–132, 2004

Waters BM, Joshi KG: Intravenous quetiapine-cocaine use ("Q-ball"). Am J Psychiatry 164:173–174, 2007

Yui K, Ikemoto S, Goto K: Factors for susceptibility to episode recurrence in spontaneous recurrence of methamphetamine psychosis. Ann N Y Acad Sci 965:292–304, 2002

Zammit S, Allebeck P, Andreasson S, et al: Self reported cannabis use as a risk factor for schizophrenia in Swedish conscripts of 1969: historical cohort study. BMJ 325:1199, 2002

Ziedonis DM: Integrated treatment of co-occurring mental illness and addiction: clinical intervention, program, and system perspectives. CNS Spectr 9:892–904, 925, 2004

Ziedonis DM, Smelson D, Rosenthal RN, et al: Improving the care of individuals with schizophrenia and substance use disorders: consensus recommendations. J Psychiatr Pract 11:315–339, 2005

CHAPTER 6

Use of Antipsychotics in Children and Adolescents

Bruce Meltzer, M.D.

ANTIPSYCHOTICS ARE CLASSIFIED into two large groups: the first-generation antipsychotics (FGAs; typical antipsychotics, conventional antipsychotics, or neuroleptics) and the second-generation antipsychotics (SGAs; atypical antipsychotics). Antipsychotic medications are not disease-specific; they provide clinical benefit for a range of syndromes in children, adolescents, and adults. In adults, antipsychotics help in the treatment of the psychotic symptoms of schizophrenia and in both the manic and the depressive phases of bipolar illness. In children and adolescents, they are prescribed for severe tic disorders, explosive aggression, and conduct problems in youths with autism and developmental delay; conduct disorder; psychosis; psychotic depression; and early-onset bipolar disorder.

The estimated number of children and adolescents prescribed antipsychotic medications increased about sixfold from 1993 to 2002. From 2000 to 2002, 92% of the visits that involved prescriptions for an antipsychotic included a second-generation medication. The most frequent mental health diagnoses were disruptive behavior disorders (38%), mood disorders (32%), pervasive developmental disorders or mental retardation (17%), and psychotic disorders (14%).

The sixfold increase in antipsychotic prescriptions for children and adolescents in the past decade is a result of the availability of newer SGAs that are associated with less sedation, fewer extrapyramidal and anticholinergic effects, and a lower risk for tardive dyskinesia. Other contributing factors include a wider range of target behaviors for treatment, declining access to and duration of inpatient psychiatric treatment, a scarcity of empirically supported nonpharmacological treatments, and limited use of psychotherapy.

FGAs have been studied in pediatric psychopharmacology since the 1960s. Now, because of their serious adverse side-effect profile, they are more rarely used and less frequently studied in child psychiatry. With the exception of risperidone, almost all of the methodologically controlled research on SGAs has focused on adults. SGAs have been less well studied in pediatric psychopharmacology. However, clinical trial information is accumulating on the use of SGAs in children and adolescents, especially in those with developmental delay, autism, psychotic conditions, and conduct disorder. Recent empirical studies have documented the efficacy and safety of risperidone for treatment of disruptive symptoms in children with autistic spectrum disorder, disruptive behavior disorder, and mental retardation. In this chapter, I focus on the use of SGAs in pediatric psychopharmacology, with briefer coverage of the FGAs.

The SGAs currently in clinical use in pediatric psychopharmacology are shown in Table 6–1.

Appendixes 1 and 2 contain information about names, strengths, formulations, and pharmacokinetics of the FGAs and SGAs.

Indications and Efficacy

FDA-Approved Pediatric Indications

Two SGAs, risperidone and aripiprazole, are currently approved by the U.S. Food and Drug Administration (FDA) for psychiatric conditions in children and adolescents.

TABLE 6–1. U.S. Food and Drug Administration–approved pediatric indications for antipsychotics

MEDICATION	INDICATION
Second-generation antipsychotics	
Aripiprazole	Acute treatment of schizophrenia in adolescents ages 13–17 years.
	Acute monotherapy for manic and mixed episodes associated with bipolar I disorder with or without psychotic features in pediatric patients ages 10–17 years.
	Adjunctive therapy with either lithium or valproate for the acute treatment of manic and mixed episodes associated with bipolar I disorder with or without psychotic features in pediatric patients ages 10–17 years.
Clozapine	Clozapine has not been approved for use in pediatric patients.
Olanzapine	Olanzapine has not been approved for use in pediatric patients.
Quetiapine	Quetiapine has not been approved for use in pediatric patients.
Risperidone	Autistic disorder irritability in patients ages 5–10 years.
	Short-term monotherapy for manic and mixed episodes associated with bipolar I disorder with or without psychotic features in pediatric patients ages 10–17 years.
	Acute treatment of schizophrenia in adolescents ages 13–17 years.
Ziprasidone	Ziprasidone has not been approved for use in pediatric patients.
First-generation antipsychotics	
Chlorpromazine	Children age 6 months or older with severe behavior problems and/or psychotic conditions.
Thioridazine	Children age 2 years or older who meet diagnostic criteria for schizophrenia and who fail to show an acceptable clinical response to adequate courses of treatment with at least two other antipsychotic medications.

TABLE 6–1. U.S. Food and Drug Administration–approved pediatric indications for antipsychotics *(continued)*

MEDICATION	INDICATION
First-generation antipsychotics *(continued)*	
Haloperidol	Psychotic disorders and Tourette syndrome in children age 3 years or older.
	Explosive aggression in children age 3 years or older only after psychosocial interventions and nonantipsychotic medications have failed to achieve a satisfactory clinical response.
Pimozide	Severe Tourette syndrome in children age 2 years or older in those who have not adequately responded to a trial of a standard medication such as haloperidol.
Fluphenazine	Psychotic disorders in youths age 12 years or older.
Molindone	Psychotic disorders in youths age 12 years or older.
Trifluoperazine	Psychotic disorders in children age 6 years or older.

Aripiprazole

- Bipolar I disorder: adjunctive therapy with lithium or valproate for acute manic or mixed episodes (ages 10–17 years)
- Bipolar I disorder: monotherapy for manic or mixed episodes with or without psychotic features (ages 10–17 years; acute therapy)
- Schizophrenia (ages 13–17 years)

Risperidone

- Autistic disorder: irritability (ages 5–17 years)
- Bipolar I disorder, acute treatment: manic or mixed episodes (ages 10–17 years; oral therapy only)
- Schizophrenia, acute treatment (ages 13–17 years; oral therapy only)

No FDA-approved pediatric indications are available for clozapine, olanzapine, quetiapine, or ziprasidone at this time.

Other Uses of Second-Generation Antipsychotics in Children and Adolescents

Other possible uses of SGAs in children and adolescents include

- Explosive aggression in conduct disorder
- Disruptive behaviors and agitation in youths with developmental delay (mental retardation, autism, or pervasive developmental disorders)
- Tic disorders and Tourette syndrome
- Adolescent-onset bipolar disorders
- Childhood- and adolescent-onset schizophrenia
- Early-onset psychotic depression
- Psychotic symptoms in organic mental disorders
- Disruptive behaviors and agitation in youths with traumatic brain injury

Controlled studies of SGAs in pediatric psychopharmacology are presented in Table 6–2.

Clinical Use

SGAs have been studied in pediatric psychopharmacology and are discussed below.

Clozapine

In an open trial of 11 adolescents (ages 12–17 years) with childhood-onset schizophrenia refractory to other antipsychotic agents, clozapine was started at 12.5–25 mg/day, and the dose was increased every 4 days by one or two times the starting dose to a maximum possible dosage of 900 mg/day. The mean dosage at week 6 of the trial was 370 mg/day. Clozapine appeared effective, with more than half of the subjects improving, and well tolerated. Careful monitoring for hematological side effects was completed during the clinical trial (Frazier et al. 1994).

Remschmidt et al. (1994) reported a retrospective study of 36 adolescent inpatients (ages 14–22 years) with schizophrenia diagnoses who were given clozapine after treatment failures with at least two other antipsychotic drugs. The dosage of clozapine ranged from 50 to 800 mg/day. Symptom improvement was seen in 75% of the patients. Three patients showed no improvement. Six patients developed side effects that required clozapine discontinuation, including leukopenia, hypertension, tachycardia, and electrocardiogram (ECG) abnormalities.

TABLE 6–2. Some controlled studies of second-generation (atypical) antipsychotics in pediatric psychopharmacology

STUDY	DRUG	DISORDER	N	AGE RANGE (YEARS)	DOSAGE	DURATION	OUTCOME
Aman et al. 2002	Risperidone	Mental retardation and disruptive behaviors	118	5–12	0.02–0.06 mg/kg/day	6 weeks	Improvement in conduct problems, aggression, and hyperactivity
Buitelaar et al. 2001	Risperidone	Mental retardation and disruptive behaviors	38	Adolescents	1.5–4 mg/day	6 weeks	Improvement in disruptive behaviors
Delbello et al. 2002	Quetiapine + divalproex	Adolescent bipolar disorder	30	12–18	Divalproex 20 mg/kg + quetiapine up to 450 mg/day	6 weeks	Addition of quetiapine to divalproex significantly improved bipolar symptoms
Findling et al. 2000	Risperidone	Conduct disorder	20	6–14	0.7–1.5 mg/day	10 weeks	Improvement in conduct symptoms

TABLE 6–2. Some controlled studies of second-generation (atypical) antipsychotics in pediatric psychopharmacology *(continued)*

STUDY	DRUG	DISORDER	N	AGE RANGE (YEARS)	DOSAGE	DURATION	OUTCOME
Fleischhaker et al. 2008	Clozapine vs. olanzapine vs. risperidone	Weight gain	33	9–21.3		45 weeks	Olanzapine associated with extreme long-term weight gain more than in adults and more than in study of risperidone and clozapine
Kryzhanovskaya et al. 2009	Olanzapine vs. placebo	Schizophrenia or bipolar I	88	13–17	2.5–20 mg/day	6 weeks	Olanzapine significantly improved symptoms
Kumra et al. 1996	Clozapine vs. haloperidol	Early-onset schizophrenia	21	Average age=14	Clozapine average dosage= 176 mg/day; Haloperidol average dosage= 16 mg/day	6 weeks	Clozapine superior to haloperidol

TABLE 6–2. Some controlled studies of second-generation (atypical) antipsychotics in pediatric psychopharmacology *(continued)*

STUDY	DRUG	DISORDER	N	AGE RANGE (YEARS)	DOSAGE	DURATION	OUTCOME
McCracken et al. 2002	Risperidone	Autism + disruptive behaviors	101	5–17	0.5–3.5 mg/day	8 weeks	Improvement in aggression, tantrums, irritability, and self-injurious behavior
Sallee et al. 2000	Ziprasidone	Tic disorder	28	7–17	40 mg/day	8 weeks	Ziprasidone appears effective
Scahill et al. 2003	Risperidone	Tic disorder	34	6–62	Average dosage = 2.5 mg/day	8 weeks	Risperidone effective
Schimmelmann et al. 2007	Quetiapine	Schizophrenia spectrum disorders	56	12–17.9	200–800 mg/day; average dosage = 584.2 mg/day	12 weeks	Significant improvements occurred
Shaw et al. 2006	Clozapine vs. olanzapine	Childhood-onset schizophrenia	25	7–16		8 weeks with 2-year follow-up	Clozapine more favorable clinical response/more adverse events

TABLE 6–2. Some controlled studies of second-generation (atypical) antipsychotics in pediatric psychopharmacology *(continued)*

Study	Drug	Disorder	N	Age range (years)	Dosage	Duration	Outcome
Sikich et al. 2008	Molindone vs. Risperidone vs. Olanzapine	Early-onset schizophrenia and schizoaffective disorder	116		Molindone 10–140 mg/day Olanzapine 2.5–20 mg/day Risperidone 0.5–6 mg/day	8 weeks	Risperidone and olanzapine did not show superiority over molindone
Tohen et al. 2007b	Olanzapine	Bipolar I	161	13–17	2.5–20 mg/day	3 weeks	Olanzapine effective
Van Bellinghen and de Troch 2001	Risperidone	Mental retardation and disruptive behaviors	13	6–14	Mean dose = 1.2 mg/day	4 weeks	Improvement in disruptive behaviors
Williams et al. 2006	Risperidone	Autism	48	5–16.5	0.5–3.5 mg/day	6 months	Significant improvement in adaptive behavior

Source. Adapted from Connor and Meltzer 2006, p. 150.

The efficacy and adverse effects of clozapine and haloperidol were compared for 21 children and adolescents (14.0±2.3 years) with onset of DSM III-R-defined schizophrenia that began by age 12 years in a 6-week National Institute of Mental Health (NIMH)–funded double-blind parallel comparison of clozapine (mean final dose=176 mg/day) with haloperidol (16 mg/day) (Kumra et al. 1996). All participants had not responded to typical antipsychotics. Clozapine had striking superiority to haloperidol on all measures of psychosis in treatment-refractory childhood-onset schizophrenia. However, neutropenia and seizures were major concerns, and one third of the group discontinued using clozapine. The authors warned that, because of possibly increased toxic effects in this pediatric population, close monitoring for adverse events is essential.

Olanzapine and clozapine were compared in an NIMH-funded 8-week RCT with a 2-year open-label follow-up (Shaw et al. 2006). Children and adolescents, ages 7 to 16 years, who met the unmodified DSM-IV criteria for schizophrenia and had been resistant to treatment with at least two antipsychotics, were randomly assigned after drug washout and a 1- to 3-week antipsychotic-free period to treatment with clozapine ($n=12$) or olanzapine ($n=13$). Clozapine was associated with a significant reduction in all outcome measures, whereas olanzapine showed a less consistent profile of clinical improvement. Clozapine was associated with more overall adverse events. At 2-year follow-up, 15 patients were receiving clozapine and showed evidence of sustained clinical improvement, but additional adverse events emerged, including lipid anomalies ($n=6$) and seizures ($n=1$). While not demonstrating definitively the superiority of clozapine over olanzapine in treatment-refractory childhood-onset schizophrenia, the study suggested that clozapine has a more favorable profile of clinical response, which needs to be balanced against more associated adverse events.

Two recent studies by Kumra (2008a, 2008b) evaluated the effectiveness and safety of clozapine versus "high-dose" olanzapine in adolescents with treatment-refractory schizophrenia. In the initial RCT, children, ages 10–18 years, who met DSM-IV criteria for schizophrenia and who were resistant or intolerant to at least two antipsychotic drugs were randomly assigned to receive 12 weeks of double-blind, flexibly dosed treatment with clozapine ($n=18$) or "high-dose" olanzapine (up to 30 mg/day) ($n=21$). Significantly more clozapine-treated adolescents met the response criteria (66%) compared with olanzapine-treated subjects (33%). Clozapine was superior to olanzapine in terms of reduction of the psychosis cluster scores and negative symptoms from baseline to endpoint. However, both treatments were associated with significant weight gain and related metabolic abnormalities. Kumra et al. (2008a) then conducted a 12-week, open-label follow-up study of 33 youths, of whom 14 received clozapine and 19 olanzapine, to examine changes in lipid and glucose metabolism in youths maintained on clozapine and to determine whether patients who were previously randomly assigned to high-dose olanzapine (up to 30 mg/day) responded to clozapine. Fourteen youths were treated with clozapine for a total of 24 weeks. In addition, the clinical outcomes for 10 of the 19 olanzapine-treated patients who were switched after 12 weeks to clozapine because of treatment nonresponse are included in this report. The incidences of hypertriglyceridemia and of "prediabetes" at week 24 in the clozapine-treated subjects were notable. Seven of 10 patients with schizophrenia (70%) who failed treatment with "high-dose" olanzapine were found to respond to a 12-week, open-label clozapine trial. Clinicians and caregivers need to be aware of potential metabolic adverse events of long-term clozapine treatment. Adolescents with a poor response to olanzapine may do better taking clozapine.

Risperidone

Risperidone was beneficial in children and adolescents with pervasive developmental disorder. Starting doses of 0.25 mg were given twice daily, and the dosage was increased in increments of 0.25 mg/day every 5–7 days (Fisman and Steele 1996). Optimal dosages ranged from 0.75 to 6 mg/day in these patients.

The efficacy of risperidone 0.5–2.5 mg/day or 3–6 mg/day compared with placebo was demonstrated in a 3-week RCT of 169 youths with DSM-IV bipolar disorder who were acutely manic (Pandina et al. 2007). Response was defined as >50% reduction in Young Mania Rating Scale (YMRS) score. Both dose ranges showed significantly higher response rates compared with placebo: 59% for the low-dose group and 63% for the high dose group compared with 26% for the placebo group. Dosages greater than 2.5 mg/day were not associated with increased benefit but were associated with increased rates of adverse events (somnolence, fatigue, agitation) in this study. Weight gain over the 3-week study was 1.9 kg in the low-dose arm, 1.4 kg in the high-dose arm, and 0.7 kg in the placebo arm.

The short-term safety and efficacy of risperidone and olanzapine monotherapy in preschoolers with bipolar disorder was evaluated in a prospective, open-label, 8-week study of 31 children ages 4–6 years (Biederman et al. 2005a). Risperidone was initiated at a dosage of 0.25 mg/day, with the dosage increased weekly according to response and tolerability to a maximum dosage of 2.0 mg/day. Olanzapine was initiated at 1.25 mg/day, and the dosage was increased to no more than 10 mg/day. At study endpoint there was a 18.3 ± 11.9 point reduction in risperidone-treated subjects and a 12.1 ± 10.4 point reduction in olanzapine-treated subjects in YMRS scores that did not differ between groups ($t = 1.4$, $P = 0.2$). Treatment with both risperidone and olanzapine resulted in a rapid reduction of symptoms of mania in preschool children with BPD. Despite this response, substantial residual symptomatology and adverse effects were present.

Pavuluri et al. (2006) assessed the safety and efficacy of risperidone augmentation of lithium in 38 youths ages 4–17 with preschool-onset bipolar disorder, manic or mixed episode, who had insufficiently responded to lithium monotherapy. The children and adolescents were entered into a 12-month trial. All subjects received lithium monotherapy. Those who failed to adequately respond to lithium monotherapy after 8 weeks and those who relapsed after an initial response were given risperidone augmentation for up to 11 months. The YMRS was the primary outcome measure. Response was defined as a ≥50% decrease from baseline. Of the 38 subjects treated with lithium monotherapy, 17 responded, whereas 21 required augmentation with risperidone. The response rate in the youths treated with lithium plus risperidone was 85.7%. Combination treatment of lithium and risperidone was found to be safe and well tolerated. Significant predictors of inadequate response to lithium monotherapy requiring augmentation were attention-deficit/hyperactivity disorder (ADHD), severity at baseline, history of sexual or physical abuse, and preschool age.

A prospective 6-month open trial examined the safety and efficacy of two combination therapies for children and adolescents with manic or mixed episodes associated with type I bipolar disorder (Pavuluri et al. 2004). Thirty-seven youths, ages 5 to 18 years, with DSM IV current mixed or manic episode and YMRS scores >20 were sequentially assigned to receive either divalproex sodium plus risperidone (DVPX+Risp) or lithium plus risperidone (Li+Risp). Response rates (≥50% change from baseline YMRS score at the end of study) were 80% for the DVPX+Risp group and 82.4% for the Li+Risp group. Both combination treatments were well tolerated. There were no significant group differences in safety or tolerability, and no serious adverse events during the 6-month trial.

An 8-week, open-label, prospective study of risperidone monotherapy (1.25±1.5 mg/day) for 30 youths, ages 6–17 years, with bipolar illness (manic, mixed, or hypomanic) evaluated the potential of risperidone as a treatment of pediatric bipolar disorder (Biederman et al. 2005b). Twenty-two of 30 youths completed the study. Risperidone treatment was associated with a significant short-term improvement in symptoms of pediatric bipolar disorder. The response for manic symptoms was 70% at endpoint, indicating mild residual symptoms. Weight increased significantly from baseline (2.1±2.0 kg), and there was a fourfold increase in prolactin levels from baseline.

Olanzapine

A small study of olanzapine pharmacokinetics in children and adolescents with schizophrenia was reported by Grothe et al. (2000). Eight inpatients (ages 10–

18 years) with treatment-resistant childhood-onset schizophrenia received olanzapine (2.5–20 mg/day) over 8 weeks. Blood samples, collected during dose titration and at a steady state, provided pharmacokinetic data. The final evaluation at week 8 included extensive sampling for 36 hours after a 20-mg dose. Results showed that olanzapine concentrations in these eight pediatric patients were of the same magnitude as those for nonsmoking adult patients with schizophrenia but may be as much as twice the typical olanzapine concentration in adult patients with schizophrenia who smoke. Evaluation of olanzapine pharmacokinetics found an apparent mean oral clearance of 9.6 ± 2.4 L/hr and a mean elimination half-life of 37.2 ± 5.1 hours in these young patients.

Kumra et al. (1998) studied olanzapine in eight pediatric patients with treatment-refractory schizophrenia who had developed the disorder by age 12 years. Two different FGA trials had not been successful in each of the subjects. For the eight patients, treatment benefits accrued with olanzapine over and above those found with FGAs over an 8-week open trial.

The efficacy and tolerability of olanzapine were assessed in an RCT up to 6 weeks in 107 inpatient and outpatient adolescents with DSM-IV-TR criteria for schizophrenia treated with flexible doses of olanzapine (2.5–20 mg/day) or placebo (Kryzhanovskaya et al. 2009). Olanzapine-treated adolescents with schizophrenia experienced significant symptom improvement. Significant increases in weight, most liver function tests, and levels of triglycerides, uric acid, and prolactin were observed during olanzapine treatment. More olanzapine-treated versus placebo-treated patients completed the trial.

The efficacy and safety of olanzapine for the treatment of acute manic or mixed episodes associated with bipolar disorder in adolescents were evaluated in a 3-week multicenter RCT (Tohen et al. 2007b). The participants were 161 outpatient and inpatient male and female adolescents 13–17 years of age with an acute manic or mixed episode. Subjects received either olanzapine (2.5–20 mg/day) or placebo. Olanzapine was effective in the treatment of bipolar mania in adolescent patients. Patients treated with olanzapine, however, had significantly greater weight gain and increases in levels of hepatic enzymes, prolactin, fasting glucose, fasting total cholesterol, and uric acid. This same industry-sponsored group continued 146 adolescents in an open-label follow-up study of up to 26 weeks (Tohen et al. 2007a). At the completion of the study, a 50% reduction in YMRS score was achieved. Weight gain over the 29 weeks of study was about 7.5 kg, with 69% of adolescents having a >7% body weight and 40% experiencing elevated prolactin levels.

Quetiapine

Quetiapine therapy was effective in the reduction of motor and phonic tics in pediatric patients with Tourette syndrome (Mukaddes and Abali 2003). In a prospective, open-label study ($N=12$), patients ages 8–16 years (11 boys, 1 girl) with Tourette syndrome received 8 weeks of quetiapine therapy at an initial dosage of 25 mg/day, titrated to a maximum dosage of 75 mg/day (younger than 12 years) or 100 mg/day (12 years and older). The mean dosage of quetiapine was 72.9 mg/day, with a range of 50 to 100 mg/day. The mean total tic score on the Yale Global Tic Severity Scale was significantly reduced from baseline to 4 weeks (61.17 vs. 30.67; $P<0.01$) and from baseline to 8 weeks (61.17 vs. 24.17; $P<0.001$). All 12 patients showed a 30%–100% improvement in tic severity (mean change $=61.91$; 95% confidence interval [CI] $=$ 50.03–73.79 for week 8). Mild, transient sedation was reported in 3 patients; however, extrapyramidal adverse effects and statistically significant weight gain were not observed (Mukaddes and Abali 2003).

An open-label quetiapine trial was completed in psychotic adolescents. Quetiapine was initiated at a dose of 25 mg twice daily and reached 400 mg twice daily by day 20. Quetiapine significantly improved both positive and negative symptoms of schizophrenia, and the medication appeared well tolerated (McConville et al. 2000). In an extension of this trial, all 10 patients continued open-label treatment with quetiapine (initial: 800 mg/day titrated over 2 weeks to optimal dose; mean dosage $=600$ mg/day) for up to 88 weeks. Significant improvements in mean scores from baseline to end point were seen at all time points through week 64 for the Brief Psychiatric Rating Scale (BPRS) and Clinical Global Improvement—Severity of Illness scale (CGI-S) ($P<0.05$). Improvements in mean scores on the Scale for the Assessment of Negative Symptoms (SANS) were significant through week 52 ($P<0.05$). Quetiapine was well tolerated, and adverse events were mild to moderate, with somnolence (60%), headache (50%), and pharyngitis (40%) being reported most frequently. Extrapyramidal symptoms (EPS) were not observed during the trial; however, 30% of the patients reported increases in mean weight and body mass index (BMI) as a "mild" adverse event (McConville et al. 2003).

A 28-day, double-blinded study compared the efficacy and tolerability of quetiapine and divalproex for the treatment of impulsivity and reactive aggression in adolescents with co-occurring bipolar disorder and disruptive behavior disorders (Barzman et al. 2006). The researchers identified 33 adolescents who scored >14 on the Positive and Negative Syndrome Scale (PANSS) Excited Component (EC) and >4 on at least one of the PANSS EC items and who also had a current diagnosis of bipolar I disorder, manic or mixed episode, and a lifetime and/or current diagnosis of a disruptive behavior disorder (conduct disorder or oppositional defiant disorder) were randomly assigned to receive quetiapine (400–600 mg/day) or divalproex (serum level ± 80–120 µg/mL). Quetiapine and divalproex showed similar efficacy and were both useful as monotherapy for the treatment of impulsivity and reactive aggression in adolescents with bipolar and disruptive behavior disorders.

A single-blind, 12-week, prospective study investigated the effectiveness and tolerability of quetiapine for the treatment of adolescents at high risk for developing bipolar I disorder (DelBello et al. 2007). Twenty youths, ages 12–18 years, with mood symptoms that did not meet the DSM-IV-TR criteria for bipolar I disorder and who had at least one first-degree relative with bipolar I disorder participated. Mood disorder diagnoses in the adolescents consisted of bipolar disorder NOS ($n=11$), dysthymia ($n=3$), bipolar II disorder ($n=3$), cyclothymia ($n=2$), and major depressive disorder ($n=1$). The majority of patients ($n=12$, 60%) had not responded to previous trials of psychotropic agents. Fifteen youth completed all study visits. Eighty-seven percent of patients were responders to quetiapine at week 12. The most frequently reported adverse events were somnolence, headache, musculoskeletal pain, and dyspepsia. No subjects discontinued study participation because of adverse events. Quetiapine may be an effective treatment for mood symptoms in adolescents with a familial risk for developing bipolar I disorder.

Despite the general positive trend in studies to date, a pressing need exists to identify additional safe and effective treatments for the management of bipolar illness in this high-risk population.

Aripiprazole

An open-label study of aripiprazole was completed in 23 children and adolescents, ages 6–17 years, with conduct disorder (Findling and McNamara 2004). Aripiprazole dosing was initiated at 1 mg/day for children and 5 mg/day for adolescents. Treatment was associated with improvements in the symptoms of conduct disorder. The most common side effects were dyspepsia, vomiting, somnolence, and lightheadedness.

Recently, Findling et al. (2008) undertook a 6-week, randomized, double-blind study of placebo or 10 or 30 mg/day of aripiprazole in 302 adolescents, ages 13–17 years, with a DSM-IV diagnosis of schizophrenia. Aripiprazole at both dosages (10 and 30 mg/day) was superior to placebo in the acute treatment of adolescents with schizophrenia and was generally well tolerated. Adverse events occurring in more than 5% of either aripiprazole group were extrapyramidal disorder, somnolence, and tremor. Mean body weight changes were –0.8, 0.0, and 0.2 kg for placebo and 10 mg and 30 mg of aripiprazole, respectively. A multiple-center, randomized, double-blind, placebo-controlled study of oral aripiprazole for treatment of adolescents with schizophrenia is under way.

An 8-week open-label trial of aripiprazole in 19 youths with bipolar disorder (Biederman et al. 2007a) found that aripiprazole treatment was associated with clinically and statistically significant improvement in mean YMRS scores. Extrapyramidal symptoms precipitated dropout in two cases. Aripiprazole was well tolerated, with no statistically significant increase in body weight.

A 6-week open trial of aripiprazole in 10 children and adolescents with Bipolar illness with comorbid ADHD (Tramontina et al. 2007) found that aripiprazole significantly improved global functioning scores, manic symptoms, and ADHD symptoms, but remission of neither bipolar disorder nor ADHD symptoms was achieved in most of the cases. Although overall positive tolerability was reported, significant weight gain was observed, This research group followed their open-label study with a 6-week randomized trial of aripiprazole in 43 youths diagnosed with DSM-IV bipolar illness with comorbid ADHD. The group receiving aripiprazole showed a significantly greater reduction in YMRS, Child Mania Rating Scale—Parent Version, and CGI-S scores from baseline to endpoint than the placebo group. In addition, higher rates of response and remission were found for the aripiprazole group. Aripiprazole was effective in reducing manic symptoms, and global functioning improved (Tramontina et al. 2009). No significant between-group differences were found in weight, ADHD symptoms, and depressive symptoms. Adverse events reported significantly more frequently in the aripiprazole group were somnolence and sialorrhea.

A 4-week randomized clinical trial (RCT) of aripirazole in 296 youths ages 10–17 years diagnosed with bipolar I disorder manic or mixed episode who received either 10 or 30 mg/day found significant benefit from both aripiprazole doses compared with placebo (Chang et al. 2007).

Ziprasidone

The effectiveness and tolerability of ziprasidone for treating pediatric mania was assessed in an 8-week, open-label, prospective study of ziprasidone monotherapy (57.3±33.9 mg/day) in 21 bipolar youth, ages 6–17 years, diagnosed with DSM-IV manic, mixed, or bipolar NOS (Biederman et al. 2007b). Ziprasidone treatment was associated with a significant short-term improvement of symptoms of pediatric bipolar disorder.

To characterize the tolerability of ziprasidone, 63 youths, ages 10–17 years, with bipolar mania, schizophrenia, or schizoaffective disorder entered a 3-week fixed-dose (period 1) and a subsequent 24-week flexible-dose (period 2) open-label study. In period 1, youths received ziprasidone 80 or 160 mg/day in two divided doses, with the dosage titrated over 10 days. In period 2, flexible doses (20–160 mg/day) were dispensed (DelBello et al. 2008). Symptom reductions were observed in all patient groups. Adverse events occurred mostly during dose titration and in the high-dose (160 mg/day) group. The most common adverse events were, during period 1, sedation, somnolence, and nausea and, during period 2, sedation, somnolence, and headache. The incidence of movement disorder adverse events was 22% and 16% during periods 1 and 2, respectively. Six percent of study participants discontinued participation due to adverse events during period 1, and 20% discontinued during period 2. Thirty-three percent of subjects gained >7% of their baseline weight. No Fridericia-corrected QT (QTcF) intervals of >450 ms were observed during period 1, and only one occurred during period 2. No QTcF increase >60 ms from baseline was observed. On the basis of the results, a starting dosage of 20 mg/day titrated to between 80 and 160 mg/day over 1–2 weeks appears optimal for most patients.

Four children, ages 7–16 years, with bipolar disorder were switched to ziprasidone from mood stabilizers, anticonvulsants, or other atypical antipsychotics because of poor response, troubling side effects, breakthrough symptoms, or concern over potential toxicity (Barnett 2004). Within 3 days, patients experienced a resolution of hypomania, hallucinations, aggression, irritability, depression, and insomnia. One 16-year-old, who had been switched from carbamazapine, also required adjunctive lorazepam for situational anxiety; the others either responded to, or were ultimately managed with, ziprasidone monotherapy. Side effects were mostly mild and transitory. Patients experiencing sedation or wakefulness at dose escalation were maintained at the previous 20- or 40-mg dose level until side effects resolved.

Versavel (2005) demonstrated the efficacy of multiple doses of ziprasidone in a 3-week study of 46 youths, ages 10–17 years, with bipolar I mixed or manic episode. Ziprasidone 40 mg twice daily was compared with 80 mg twice daily. YMRS scores improved 14.9 points in the low-dose group and 11.1 points in the high-dose group.

Comparison With First-Generation Antipsychotics

SGAs are considered standard treatment for children and adolescents with early-onset schizophrenia and schizoaffective disorder. However, the superiority of SGAs over FGAs had not been demonstrated until recently (Sikich et al. 2004, 2008), and psychiatrists have had a limited evidence base to guide treatment of children and adolescents. Two important NIMH-funded studies are now available to help elucidate this area.

An 8-week pilot RCT compared the acute antipsychotic effect and side-effect profiles of risperidone and olanzapine with those of haloperidol in 50 youths, ages 8–19 years, with prominent positive psychotic symptoms (Sikich et al. 2004). All treatments reduced symptoms significantly. In all, 88% of subjects treated with olanzapine, 74% treated with risperidone, and 53% treated with haloperidol met response criteria. The magnitude of the antipsychotic response with these two atypical agents is comparable to that observed with haloperidol. The primary side effects observed in all patients were mild to moderate sedation, extrapyramidal symptoms, and weight gain. The prevalence and severity of weight gain and extrapyramidal effects in youth treated with risperidone and olanzapine appeared to be greater than those reported in adults.

Sikich et al. (2008) compared the efficacy and safety of olanzapine and risperidone with a first-generation antipsychotic, molindone, in the treatment of 119 youths with early-onset schizophrenia and schizoaffective disorder. Patients were assigned to treatment with either olanzapine (2.5–20 mg/day), risperidone (0.5–6 mg/day), or molindone (10–140 mg/day, plus 1 mg/day of benztropine) for 8 weeks. Risperidone and olanzapine did not demonstrate superior efficacy over molindone, as no significant differences were found among treatment groups in response rates or magnitude of symptom reduction. Adverse effects were frequent but differed among medications. Olanzapine and risperidone were associated with significantly greater weight gain. Olanzapine showed the greatest risk of weight gain and significant increases in fasting cholesterol, low-density lipoprotein, insulin, and liver transaminase levels. Molindone led to more self-reports of akathisia. The results question the nearly exclusive use of SGAs to treat early-onset schizophrenia and schizoaffective disorder. The safety findings related to weight gain and metabolic problems raise important public health concerns, given the widespread use of SGAs in youths for nonpsychotic disorders.

Despite the general positive trend in studies to date, a pressing need exists to identify additional safe and effective treatments for the management of schizophrenia in this high-risk population.

Guidelines for Selection and Use

Only aripiprazole and risperidone are currently approved by the FDA for the treatment of select pediatric neuropsychiatric disorders. Nevertheless, these agents are commonly used for a variety of psychotic disorders, tic disorders, bipolar disorders, and conduct disorders in referred children and adolescents. Risperidone is the best-studied agent in the pediatric age range to date.

Before Initiating Treatment With SGAs

- Complete a baseline physical examination and medical history. An examination within the 6–12 months before the start of medication is generally sufficient in the medically healthy child and adolescent.
- Obtain a careful history in the patient and family of any metabolic disorders and/or diabetes. SGAs are associated with weight gain in children and adolescents that could exacerbate risk for metabolic disorders. It is recommended that the clinician obtain a fasting blood glucose, cholesterol, and lipid panel prior to initiating treatment with an SGA.
- Obtain a baseline height, weight, and BMI.

- Complete a baseline Abnormal Involuntary Movement Scale (AIMS) examination. Although these agents are associated with a low risk of abnormal involuntary movement disorders, they can occur. A baseline examination is necessary for a comparison if the child develops abnormal involuntary movements while taking the medication.

Monitoring During SGA Treatment

- Follow up height and weight monthly.
- Calculate a BMI every 4–6 months during medication administration.
- Complete a follow-up AIMS examination to search for abnormal involuntary movement disorders every 6–12 months during treatment.

Second-Generation Antipsychotics

Specific Agents

Risperidone

Risperidone was approved by the FDA for marketing in the United States in 1993. It has a high affinity for blocking dopamine D_2 receptors and serotonin 5-HT_{2A} receptors. These actions are thought responsible for its antipsychotic action. It also antagonizes α_1- and α_2-adrenergic and histamine H_1 receptors, causing the side effects of hypotension and sedation, respectively.

Available risperidone formulations

- Tablets: 0.25 mg, 0.5 mg, 1 mg, 2 mg, 3 mg, and 4 mg
- Oral solution: 1 mg/mL
- Orally disintegrating tablets: The orally disintegrating tablet formulations are bioequivalent to oral risperidone tablets and available in 0.5-mg, 1-mg, and 2-mg strengths.
- Intramuscular: Risperidone is available as a long-acting depot injection. The recommended dosing is 25 mg IM every 2 weeks for adults with schizophrenia. The safety and efficacy of intramuscular risperidone in the pediatric age range have not been established. For adult patients not responding to a dose of 25 mg IM, the dose may be increased to 37.5 or 50 mg at intervals of at least 4 weeks. The maximum dose for adults should not exceed 50 mg given every 2 weeks. It is recommended that oral medication be continued without taper for the first 8 weeks of intramuscular therapy.

Risperidone dosing suggestions

The safety and effectiveness of risperidone in children and adolescents 5–17 years of age have been established. Risperidone has been studied in numerous controlled clinical trials in children and adolescents.

- For children and adolescents 15 years and younger, risperidone should be started at the lowest possible dose and the dose titrated upward every 3–7 days within a dosage range of 0.25 to 6.0 mg/day.
  - At a total daily dose greater than 6 mg, extrapyramidal side effects may appear out of proportion to benefit.
  - Risperidone dosages greater than 6 mg/day have not been shown to have any increased clinical efficacy compared with lower doses in children and adolescents.
- For prepubertal children, risperidone should be given in two to three divided daily doses.
- For adolescents 16 years or older, risperidone should be initiated at 0.5–1.0 mg/day and the dose titrated upward every 3–7 days within a dosage range of 0.5 to 6.0 mg/day. In postpubertal adolescents, risperidone should be given in two divided daily doses or one dose at bedtime.
- Starting at a lower dose and titrating the dose more slowly are associated with less risk for side effects than initiating treatment at higher doses and titrating the dose upward rapidly.

Olanzapine

Olanzapine was approved by the FDA for marketing to adults in the United States in 1996. In addition to antagonizing dopamine D_2 and serotonin 5-HT_2 receptors, olanzapine blocks acetylcholine receptors and α_1-adrenergic receptors. Olanzapine's actions at dopamine and serotonin receptors are thought responsible for its antipsychotic action. Its action at acetylcholine receptors causes anticholinergic side effects, and its action at adrenergic receptors increases the incidence of hypotension.

Available olanzapine formulations

- Tablets: 2.5 mg, 5 mg, 7.5 mg, 10 mg, and 15 mg
- Zyprexa orally disintegrating tablets: 5 mg, 10 mg, 15 mg, and 20 mg

Olanzapine dosing suggestions

- The safety and efficacy of olanzapine have not been established for children and adolescents age 17 years or younger.

- For adolescents, a single initial dose of 5–10 mg given at bedtime is recommended. Further titration within a dosage range of 5–20 mg/day should occur at weekly intervals to allow steady-state serum concentrations to develop.
- Olanzapine dosages greater than 10 mg/day have not been shown to increase efficacy, and the safety and tolerability of dosages greater than 20 mg/day have not yet been established.
- Starting at a lower dose and titrating the dose more slowly are associated with less risk for side effects than initiating treatment at higher doses and titrating the dose upward rapidly.

Quetiapine

Quetiapine was approved by the FDA for marketing to adults in the United States in 1997. This agent antagonizes D_1, D_2, 5-HT_{1A}, 5-HT_2, and 5-HT_3 receptors. These actions are thought responsible for its antipsychotic action. It also blocks α_1- and α_2-adrenergic receptors and H_1 histamine receptors, which are thought to mediate the side effects of hypotension and sedation, respectively. Quetiapine has no appreciable anticholinergic effects.

Available quetiapine formulations

- Tablets: 25 mg, 50 mg, 100 mg, 200 mg, 300 mg, 400 mg
- Slow-release: 50 mg, 150 mg, 200 mg, 300 mg, 400 mg

Quetiapine dosing suggestions

- The safety and efficacy of quetiapine have not been established for children and adolescents age 17 years or younger.
- For patients 18 years or older with psychotic disorders, quetiapine should be initiated at a dosage of 25 mg twice a day. The dose should be increased every 3–7 days depending on effectiveness and tolerability to a dosage range between 200 and 800 mg given in two divided daily doses. Some symptoms of aggression, anxiety, and sleep disturbance may respond to lower doses.
- Starting at a low dose and titrating the dose more slowly are associated with less risk for side effects, especially sedation, than initiating treatment at higher doses and titrating the dose upward rapidly.

Ziprasidone

Ziprasidone was approved by the FDA for marketing to adults in the United States in 2001. Ziprasidone has high affinity for dopamine D_2 and D_3 receptors and for serotonin 5-HT$_2$ receptors. The antagonism of these receptors is thought responsible for ziprasidone's antipsychotic action. It blocks α_1-adrenergic receptors, which may result in increased risk for hypotension, and has moderate affinity for H$_1$ histamine receptors, which may cause sedation. Ziprasidone has received very little research attention in pediatric psychopharmacology. Little is currently known about its use in children and adolescents. Almost all available data have accrued from studies of adults with psychotic disorders.

Available ziprasidone formulations

- Capsules: 20 mg, 40 mg, 60 mg, and 80 mg
- Intramuscular injection: 20 mg/mL; 1.2 mL of sterile water must be added to each single-dose intramuscular vial and shaken vigorously until all drug is dissolved. The safety and effectiveness of the intramuscular formulation has not been tested in the pediatric age group.

Ziprasidone precautions

- In the adult schizophrenia ziprasidone trials, a dose-dependent lengthening of the ECG QTc interval was found. Lengthening of the QTc interval also was found in a small prospective study of children and adolescents given ziprasidone (Blair et al. 2005). Patients with a cardiac history, and specifically, a history of prolonged QT syndromes, should not be given ziprasidone. Prolonged QT syndromes are clinically identified by a family history of unexplained and recurrent syncope and early sudden cardiac death, with or without a family history of congenital deafness.
- Because of concerns of additive effects on prolongation of the QT interval, ziprasidone should not be given with medications that prolong QTc such as moxifloxacin, chlorpromazine, pentamidine, pimozide, droperidol, quinidine, mefloquine, thioridazine, or mesoridazine.
- The pediatric psychopharmacologist may wish to consider a baseline and on-drug ECG when using ziprasidone (Blair et al. 2005).

Ziprasidone dosing suggestions

- The safety and efficacy of ziprasidone have not been established for children and adolescents age 17 years or younger.
- For patients 18 years or older with psychotic disorders, ziprasidone should be initiated at 20 mg twice a day and the dose titrated upward by 20–40 mg every 3–7 days as needed. For psychotic disorders, the effective dosage range of ziprasidone is 120 mg/day to 160 mg/day, given in two divided doses.

- Starting at a low dose and titrating the dose more slowly are associated with less risk for side effects than initiating treatment at higher doses and titrating the dose upward rapidly.
- Ziprasidone should be taken with food. Taking ziprasidone on an empty stomach decreases absorption and clinical effect by as much as 50%.

Aripiprazole

Aripiprazole was approved by the FDA for marketing in the United States in 2002. Aripiprazole is a novel antipsychotic with partial agonist and antagonist properties and may possess a unique mechanism of action. The efficacy of the drug in adult schizophrenia appears related to partial agonist activity at D_2 and 5-HT_{1A} receptors. Antagonist activity at 5-HT_{2A} receptors also has been speculated. In vitro data have indicated D_2 agonist activity of aripiprazole at presynaptic autoreceptors, with antagonist activity at postsynaptic D_2 receptors. The dual effects of aripiprazole are unlike those of conventional antipsychotic drugs and other atypical agents. It also shows relatively high affinity for dopamine D_3 receptors. Preclinical and clinical data suggest that these actions minimize extrapyramidal and endocrine (e.g., prolactin increases) side effects. Aripiprazole is only just beginning to be studied in pediatric psychopharmacology, and most data are from adults. Data from open-label trials of conduct disorder (Findling and McNamara 2004) and a controlled trial of tic disorders (Sallee et al. 2000) in children and adolescents suggest that the dose range for children might be lower than that published for adults with schizophrenia.

Available aripiprazole formulations

- Tablets: 2 mg, 5 mg, 10 mg, 15 mg, 20 mg, and 30 mg
- Oral solution: 1 mg/mL

Aripiprazole dosing suggestions

- The safety and efficacy of aripiprazole have not been established for children and adolescents ages 10–17 years (see "Indications and Efficacy").
- According to the aripiprazole pediatric trials currently available (Findling and McNamara 2004; Sallee et al. 2000), aripiprazole should be initiated at a dose of 1 mg in children who weigh less than 25 kg, 2 mg in children who weigh 25–49 kg, 5 mg in children who weigh 50–69 kg, and 10 mg in youths who weigh 70 kg or more. The dose should be titrated every 3–7 days to an optimum dose within a dosage range of 1 to 30 mg/day. Steady-state aripiprazole serum concentrations are attained within 14 days of a dose change (Findling and McNamara 2004).

Clozapine

Clozapine was approved by the FDA for marketing to adults in the United States in 1989. Unlike FGAs (neuroleptics), clozapine was the first agent that blocks both dopamine D_1 and D_2 receptors and appears to preferentially block dopamine receptors in central nervous system (CNS) limbic regions more than in striatal regions. This action may account for a very low prevalence of movement disorders reported with clozapine use. Clozapine has effectiveness in treating the negative and positive symptoms of schizophrenia and may have a beneficial effect on tardive dyskinesia in patients with a preexisting antipsychotic-induced abnormal involuntary movement disorder.

A serious adverse event profile limits the use of clozapine in clinical populations. Because of the increased risk for serious and life-threatening hematological side effects and seizures, the use of clozapine is appropriate only for patients with bipolar disorders or schizophrenia who have *not* clinically responded to trials of at least two other antipsychotic medications or who cannot tolerate the side effects of other agents, resulting in subtherapeutic and ineffective doses.

Contraindications to clozapine

- Hypersensitivity to the agent
- Myeloproliferative disorders
- Uncontrolled epilepsy
- A history of clozapine-induced agranulocytosis or severe granulocytopenia
- Concomitant use of agents known to cause agranulocytosis or to suppress bone marrow functioning (e.g., carbamazepine) (Clozapine should not be administered together with these agents.)
- Myocarditis: clozapine is associated with an increased risk of fatal myocarditis, and complaints of chest discomfort or weakness need to be evaluated emergently in clozapine-treated patients. Patients with myocarditis should not be prescribed clozapine.

Available clozapine formulations

- Tablets: 12.5 mg, 25 mg, 50 mg, 100 mg, and 200 mg

Before initiating clozapine treatment

- Patients must have a severe psychotic disorder that has not responded adequately to at least two previous trials of antipsychotic medications.

- A thorough physical examination and medical history must be completed prior to initiating a trial of clozapine.

  - Patients with a history of seizures must be taking an anticonvulsant that does not suppress their bone marrow and results in good seizure control before the initiation of clozapine.
  - Patients with a history of bone marrow disease are not candidates for a clinical trial of clozapine.
  - Patients with a history of myocarditis are not candidates for a clinical trial of clozapine.

- Because of the known propensity of clozapine to induce seizures, the clinician might consider a baseline and on-drug electroencephalogram. Clozapine dose appears to be an important predictor of seizures, with more risk at clozapine dosages above 600 mg/day.
- Baseline pulse and blood pressure should be measured. Clozapine can induce hypotension and tachycardia in patients.
- Baseline height and weight should be measured. Clozapine is associated with weight gain in patients. Increased BMI is associated with increased risk for metabolic disorders and type 2 diabetes. For patients with a history of diabetes or familial metabolic disorders, a baseline fasting glucose and lipid profile must be obtained.
- The patient must be enrolled in a clozapine monitoring protocol. This is mandatory for all patients. Clinicians can obtain details about enrolling patients at the patient's local pharmacy or through the drug manufacturer.
- Because agranulocytosis is reported to occur in association with administration of clozapine in 1%–2% of patients, hematological monitoring is required for prescription dispensation. Baseline (before drug) complete blood count with differential must be obtained. To prescribe clozapine,

  - Baseline white blood cell (WBC) count must be 3,500/mm^3 or higher.
  - Baseline absolute neutrophil count (ANC) must be 1,500/mm^3 or higher.

Medical monitoring during clozapine treatment
See Appendix 5 for guidelines on how to initiate and monitor the patient taking clozapine.

Clozapine dosing suggestions

- Clozapine is not recommended for use in children age 15 years or younger.
- For adolescents age 16 years or older, clozapine should be initiated at a dosage of 12.5 mg once or twice daily. The dose can be increased by 25–

50 mg daily as tolerated, to reach a target dosage of 300–600 mg/day for treatment-resistant psychotic disorders. Subsequent dose increases of a maximum of 100 mg can be made once or twice weekly. The total daily clozapine dose should not exceed 900 mg.

Important clozapine adverse effects

- *Agranulocytosis:* defined as an ANC of 500/mm^3 or less. Agranulocytosis is a medical emergency, and clozapine should be immediately discontinued. Medical care and hematology consultation should be emergently sought. The highest incidence of agranulocytosis occurs within the first 4–10 weeks after initiating clozapine. In the United States, since 1997, 585 cases of agranulocytosis with 19 fatalities out of a total of 150,409 clozapine-treated patients have been described (Physicians' Desk Reference 2003).
- *Seizures:* administration of clozapine is associated with an increased incidence of seizures that is dose dependent (Green 2001).
  - At dosages lower than 300 mg/day, 1%–2% develop seizures.
  - At dosages between 300 and 599 mg/day, 3%–4% develop seizures.
  - At dosages between 600 and 900 mg/day, 5% develop seizures.
- *Myocarditis:* In adults receiving clozapine, an increased association with myocarditis has been reported. Postmarketing surveillance data from the United States of clozapine-treated patients identified 30 reports of myocarditis with 17 fatalities in 205,493 patients. The risk of myocarditis in clozapine-treated pediatric patients appears to be 17–322 times greater than that in the general population (Physicians' Desk Reference 2003). The possibility of myocarditis should be considered in clozapine-treated patients who present with unexplained fatigue, dyspnea, tachypnea, fever, chest pain, and/or ECG abnormalities.

Side Effects and Their Management

Second-generation atypical antipsychotics are frequently used in child and adolescent psychopharmacology. However, they are associated with a wide range of side effects. See Appendixes 7 and 8 for side effects of antipsychotic medications and the management of these side effects.

SGA-induced weight gain may be more problematic for children and adolescents than for adults. Marked weight gain increases risks for insulin resistance and development of type 2 diabetes and the metabolic syndrome. This may be especially true for children who have a family history that is positive for diabetes. Besides weight gain, the most common side effect in youths prescribed SGAs is sedation. Histamine receptor blockade appears to mediate this side effect. Sedation may impair children's and adolescents' daily life and cause them to appear drugged.

Regarding serum level measurement in children, only one small study of therapeutic serum levels is available for clozapine. In six children with schizophrenia, clinical improvement was seen in five of six youths at a clozapine serum level of 289 ng/mL and a norclozapine (an active metabolite) serum level of 410 ng/mL (Frazier et al. 2003).

Management of Drug Overdose

Symptoms of Toxicity

Overdose information with SGAs remains limited, especially in the pediatric age group. Most information is from adult atypical antipsychotic overdose reports. In general, symptoms may include CNS depression, somnolence, slurred speech, ataxia, and dizziness. Acute EPS, including cogwheel rigidity, tremors, trismus, and severe dystonia, have been reported with SGA overdose. Tachycardia and ECG changes may occur, including QTc prolongation, QRS widening, and premature ventricular contractions. With ziprasidone overdose, ECG QTc prolongation must be especially considered. Hepatic toxicity may occur with elevated liver transaminases. Clozapine overdose may result in bone marrow suppression and blood dyscrasias.

General Supportive Measures

Appropriate supportive measures should be instituted. No specific antidote to SGAs is available. The possibility of multiple drug involvement should be considered.

- Serum levels of SGAs are not readily available at most facilities and are not useful for guiding therapy after overdose.
- Respiratory function and vital signs should be monitored after significant overdose.
- Blood pressure should be monitored.
- An ECG should be obtained, and continuous cardiac monitoring should be instituted because of the potential for tachydysrhythmias.
- Liver function tests should be monitored after significant overdose.
- The clinician should monitor for CNS depression, seizures, and extrapyramidal reactions after a toxic ingestion.
- Emesis is not recommended because of the potential for CNS depression and seizures with SGA overdose.
- Pulse oximetry and/or arterial blood gases should be monitored in patients with respiratory depression.

First-Generation Antipsychotics

Although the FGAs continue to be used in pediatric psychopharmacology, their use has decreased with the availability of the newer SGAs. FGAs have many side effects, such as increased risk for EPS, tardive dyskinesia, and anticholinergic effects, that make them difficult to use. Some FGAs such as thioridazine and pimozide cause QTc prolongation on the ECG and increase risk for fatal arrhythmias such as torsades de pointes. See Appendixes 1 and 2 for formulations and pharmacokinetics of the FGAs.

In this section, I briefly review several FGAs that continue to be widely used in children and adolescents, including chlorpromazine, thioridazine, haloperidol, pimozide, fluphenazine, molindone, and trifluoperazine.

Clinical Use

Very few studies have investigated the use of FGAs in youth with psychotic symptoms. Both loxapine and haloperidol, when compared with placebo, were found to be superior to placebo in treating the positive symptoms of psychosis, but neither was significantly different from the other (Poole et al. 1976).

A study (Realmuto et al. 1984) of 21 adolescents with schizophrenia who were receiving thiothixene, an FGA of moderate potency, or thioridazine, an FGA of low potency, found that half of each group experienced significant decrease in positive symptoms. However, many responded poorly or experienced sedation, which requires dose lowering and therefore limits therapeutic response. The authors concluded that for adolescents with schizophrenia, high-potency neuroleptics may be preferable to the more sedating low-potency medications.

A 10-week, crossover RCT assessed the safety and efficacy of haloperidol in hospitalized children with schizophrenia, nine boys and three girls, ages 5.5–11.75 years, diagnosed by DSM-III-R criteria (Spencer et al. 1992). After a 2-week placebo baseline period, the subjects were entered into double-blind treatment for 8 weeks receiving either haloperidol for 4 weeks followed by placebo for 4 weeks, or, alternatively, placebo for 4 weeks followed by haloperidol for 4 weeks. Dosage ranged from 0.5 to 10 mg/day. Haloperidol was superior to placebo for reduction of target symptoms, with the optimal haloperidol dosage ranging from 0.5 to 3.5 mg/day (0.02–0.12 mg/kg/day), but extrapyramidal side effects limited the utility of haloperidol.

Specific Agents

Chlorpromazine

Chlorpromazine is the prototype FGA and is used in children and adolescents for the treatment of psychotic disorders and for severe behavior problems such as explosive aggression. This agent also may have some usefulness in treating severe hyperactivity, impulsivity, and agitation found commonly in youngsters with severe attention-deficit/hyperactivity disorder (ADHD), although it is not as effective as stimulant medications for this purpose. Chlorpromazine also may be used as an antiemetic in the treatment of postoperative nausea and vomiting or following radiation or cytotoxic drugs.

FDA-approved indications for chlorpromazine in pediatric psychopharmacology

- Children age 6 months or older with severe behavior problems and/or psychotic conditions

Possible indications

- Severe ADHD
- Severe agitation, ADHD symptoms, or explosive aggression in children and adolescents with developmental delay and/or autism spectrum conditions

Contraindications to chlorpromazine use

- A history of seizures (Chlorpromazine may lower the CNS threshold for seizures. This agent should not be given to seizure-prone individuals.)
- Hypersensitivity to the agent

Available chlorpromazine formulations

- Tablets: 10 mg, 25 mg, 50 mg, 100 mg, and 200 mg
- Sustained-release spansules: 30 mg, 75 mg, 150 mg
- Syrup: 10 mg/5 mL
- Rectal suppositories: 25 mg and 100 mg
- Concentrate: 30 mg/mL
- Intramuscular injection: 25 mg/1 mL

Chlorpromazine dosing suggestions

- Oral: 25 mg/kg every 4–6 hours as needed. Treatment should be initiated at a dose of 10–25 mg for children and 25–50 mg for adolescents. The dose should be titrated upward by 25–50 mg twice weekly until a dosage range between 50 and 600 mg/day is reached. For severe psychotic or aggressive symptoms, dosages of 200 mg/day or higher may be needed. For young children with rapid metabolic rates, chlorpromazine should be given in three to four divided daily doses. Adolescents should receive one to two daily oral doses.
- Rectal suppositories: 1 mg/kg every 6–8 hours as needed
- Intramuscular injection for children 12 years or younger: 0.5 mg/kg every 6–8 hours as needed. Chlorpromazine is a hypotensive agent. When giving intramuscular injections, the clinician should monitor the blood pressure.
  - For children 5 years or younger, the maximum intramuscular dose is 40 mg/day.
  - For children 6–12 years old, the maximum intramuscular dose is 75 mg/day.
- Intramuscular injections for adolescents 13 years or older: 25 mg every 6–8 hours as needed. Chlorpromazine is a hypotensive agent. When giving intramuscular injections, the clinician should monitor the blood pressure. For these adolescents, the maximum intramuscular dose is 125 mg/day.

Thioridazine

Thioridazine labeling has undergone extensive revisions since 2000. A boxed warning indicating that thioridazine has been shown to prolong the QTc interval in a dose-related manner is now included in the labeling for this agent. Medications with this potential, such as thioridazine, have been associated with fatal cardiac arrhythmias such as torsades de pointes. Consequently, the use of thioridazine for the treatment of childhood severe behavior problems, explosive aggression, ADHD and conduct problems, mood lability, and poor frustration tolerance is no longer approved by the FDA. At present, thioridazine is indicated only for the treatment of schizophrenia in patients whose symptoms have responded insufficiently to adequate clinical medication trials of at least two previous antipsychotics because of lack of efficacy and/or intolerable side effects.

FDA-approved indications for thioridazine in pediatric psychopharmacology

- Children age 2 years or older who meet diagnostic criteria for schizophrenia and who fail to show an acceptable clinical response to adequate courses of treatment with at least two other antipsychotic medications

Contraindications to thioridazine use

- Genetically related reduced levels of cytochrome P450 2D6 activity. This occurs in about 7%–10% of the Caucasian population and results in diminished metabolism of thioridazine and increased risk for QTc lengthening and fatal cardiac arrhythmias.
- Concomitant fluvoxamine, propranolol, fluoxetine, paroxetine, or pindolol use. These agents inhibit the metabolism of thioridazine.
- Congenital long QT syndrome.
- On baseline ECG, a QTc interval greater than 450 ms.
- A history of cardiac arrhythmia.

Available thioridazine formulations

- Tablets: 10 mg, 15 mg, 25 mg, 50 mg, 100 mg, 150 mg, and 200 mg
- Concentrate: 30 mg/mL, 100 mg/mL
- Suspension: 25 mg/5 mL, 100 mg/5 mL

Thioridazine dosing suggestions

- For children 2–12 years old, the usual dosage of thioridazine ranges from 0.5 mg/kg/day to 3 mg/kg/day. Thioridazine should be initiated at a dose between 10 and 25 mg and the total daily dose titrated upward twice weekly by 10–25 mg, depending on tolerability and effect. For prepubertal children, thioridazine should be given in three to four divided daily doses.
- For adolescents 13 years or older, thioridazine should be initiated at a dose between 25 and 50 mg and the total daily dose titrated upward twice weekly by 25–50 mg, depending on tolerability and effect. A maximum thioridazine dosage of 800 mg/day is recommended to minimize the risk of pigmentary retinopathy that is reported to develop at higher thioridazine doses.

Haloperidol

Haloperidol comes in a variety of formulations and continues to be used in pediatric psychopharmacology, frequently for emergent pharmacotherapy in the treatment of aggression or acute behavioral agitation in the context of a psychiatric disorder. Haloperidol is a high-potency FGA and has a side-effect profile characterized by low rates of anticholinergic symptoms and high rates of EPS and long-term risk for tardive dyskinesia. This agent is labeled for use in the treatment of psychotic disorders and Tourette syndrome in children older than 3 years. Haloperidol has been approved for treating severe behavior disorders (e.g., explosive aggression and hyperexcitability, impulsive aggression, severe conduct problems, mood lability, poor frustration tolerance, and difficulty with sustained attention) in children only after psychosocial interventions and non-antipsychotic medications have been tried and have not resulted in a satisfactory clinical response.

FDA-approved indications for haloperidol in pediatric psychopharmacology

- Psychotic disorders and Tourette syndrome in children age 3 years or older.
- Explosive aggression in children age 3 years or older only after psycho-social interventions and nonantipsychotic medications have failed to achieve a satisfactory clinical response.

Available haloperidol formulations

- Tablets: 0.5 mg, 1 mg, 2 mg, 5 mg, 10 mg, and 20 mg
- Concentrate: 2 mg/1 mL
- Intramuscular injection: 5.0 mg/1 mL
- Haloperidol decanoate, a long-acting depot intramuscular preparation: Haldol Decanoate 50 and Haldol Decanoate 100 contain 50 mg and 100 mg of haloperidol, respectively. The safety and efficacy of haloperidol decanoate have not been established in the pediatric age group. The decanoate formulation is used primarily for treating chronic schizophrenia in adults.

Haloperidol dosing suggestions

- For children 3–12 years old and weighing 15–39 kg, haloperidol should be initiated at a dosage of 0.5 mg/day and the dose titrated upward by 0.5-mg increments at weekly intervals. Haloperidol should be given in two to three divided daily doses in younger children.
  - Therapeutic dosage range for nonpsychotic behavior disorders and Tourette syndrome in children: 0.05–0.075 mg/kg/day.
  - Therapeutic dosage range for psychotic disorders in children: 0.05–0.15 mg/kg/day.
- For adolescents age 13 years or older or children weighing 40 kg or more, haloperidol should be initiated at a dosage between 0.5 and 5 mg/day, depending on symptom severity. Haloperidol should be given in one to two daily doses in older adolescents.

Pimozide

Pimozide is an FGA that is labeled for the treatment of motor and vocal tic suppression in patients with Tourette syndrome who have failed to respond to other standard treatments such as haloperidol. This agent is not intended as a treatment of first choice because pimozide increases the risk for QTc prolongation. Sudden, unexpected deaths have occurred in patients taking doses of pimozide greater than 10 mg/day. Pimozide should not be used for behavioral disturbances, aggression, or psychotic disorders in children and adolescents.

FDA-approved indications for pimozide in pediatric psychopharmacology

- Severe Tourette syndrome in children age 2 years or older who have not adequately responded to a trial of a standard medication such as haloperidol.

Contraindications to pimozide use

- Pimozide is contraindicated in the treatment of mild motor and vocal tics because its risk-benefit ratio is unfavorable in all but severe tic symptoms.
- Concomitant use of other drugs that may exacerbate tics such as stimulants or bupropion.
- A history of congenital long QT syndrome, unexplained and recurrent syncope, and a history of cardiac arrhythmias.
- Concomitant use of other medications that prolong the QTc interval, such as thioridazine or ziprasidone.
- Concomitant use of other medications that inhibit pimozide's metabolism (thus increasing pimozide plasma concentrations and increasing risk for QTc prolongation) (These include macrolide antibiotics, azole antifungal agents, protease inhibitors, nefazodone, and zileuton.)
- Uncontrolled seizure disorders (Pimozide may lower the CNS threshold for seizures and should not be given to patients with uncontrolled seizure disorders.)

Available pimozide formulations

- Tablets: 1 mg and 2 mg

Pimozide dosing suggestions

- For children and adolescents ages 2–17 years, pimozide should be initiated at low doses and titrated upward slowly. Treatment should begin with a dose of 0.05 mg/kg/day at bedtime, and the dosage can be increased every 3–5 days by 0.5 mg to a maximum of 0.2 mg/kg/day, not to exceed 10 mg/day. Unexplained deaths and seizures have been reported when the pimozide dosage exceeds 10 mg/day.

Mandatory medical monitoring

- A baseline and on-drug ECG are mandatory for cardiac monitoring during pimozide treatment.

Fluphenazine

Fluphenazine is a high-potency FGA with few anticholinergic effects but increased risk for EPS and long-term tardive dyskinesia. Because it is available in a variety of formulations, it is sometimes used to treat acute aggression and behavioral dyscontrol in children and adolescents with psychiatric disorders. However, it is labeled by the FDA only for the treatment of psychotic disorders in adolescents.

FDA-approved indications for fluphenazine in pediatric psychopharmacology

- Psychotic disorders in youths age 12 years or older.

Available fluphenazine formulations

- Tablets: 1 mg, 2.5 mg, 5 mg, and 10 mg
- Elixir: 0.5 mg/1 mL (or 2.5 mg/5 mL)
- Concentrate: 5 mg/1 mL
- Injectable preparation: 2.5 mg/1 mL
- Decanoate preparations for parenteral administration: fluphenazine enanthate 25 mg/1 mL and fluphenazine decanoate 25 mg/1 mL. The safety and efficacy of fluphenazine enanthate and decanoate preparations have not been established in the pediatric age group. The decanoate formulation is used primarily for treating chronic schizophrenia in adults.

Fluphenazine dosing suggestions

- For adolescents age 12 years or older, fluphenazine should be initiated at a dose of 1–2.5 mg at bedtime and the dose titrated twice weekly to a total daily dose between 2.5 and 10 mg. The dose should be administered in two to three divided daily doses.

Molindone

Molindone is a medium-potency FGA that is one of the few antipsychotics to exert no effects on the ECG QTc interval. It is also one of the few antipsychotics that is weight neutral. In some patients, molindone even promotes weight loss. It is approved for the treatment of psychotic disorder.

FDA-approved indications for molindone in pediatric psychopharmacology

- Psychotic disorders in youths age 12 years or older.

Available molindone formulations

- Tablets: 5 mg, 10 mg, 25 mg, 50 mg, and 100 mg
- Concentrate: 20 mg/1 mL

Molindone dosing suggestions

- For adolescents age 12 years or older, the usual starting dose of molindone for the treatment of early-onset psychotic disorders is between 50 and 75 mg/day. The dose may be titrated every 3–5 days by 25–50 mg up to a maximum dosage of 225 mg/day. Molindone should be given in two to three divided daily doses.

Trifluoperazine

Trifluoperazine is a high-potency FGA with few anticholinergic effects but increased risk for EPS and long-term tardive dyskinesia. It is recommended for the treatment of psychotic disorders in children and adolescents.

FDA-approved indications for trifluoperazine in pediatric psychopharmacology

- Psychotic disorders in children age 6 years or older

Available trifluoperazine formulations

- Tablets: 1 mg, 2 mg, 5 mg, and 10 mg
- Concentrate: 10 mg/1 mL
- Intramuscular injection: 2 mg/1 mL. There is currently little experience in the use of intramuscular trifluoperazine in the pediatric age group.

Trifluoperazine dosing suggestions

- For children 6–12 years old, a starting dose of 1 mg once or twice daily is recommended. The dose may be titrated upward depending on patient tolerability and effectiveness by 1–2 mg twice weekly. Generally, trifluoperazine dosages of 15 mg/day or greater are required for therapeutic benefits to occur in psychotic disorders.

- For adolescents age 13 years or older, trifluoperazine should be initiated at a dosage between 1 and 5 mg once or twice daily. The dosage may be titrated upward by 2–5 mg once or twice weekly. For adolescents, dosages of 15–20 mg/day are generally optimal. Occasionally, the dosage may have to be increased to a maximum recommended total daily dose of 40 mg in adolescents.

Side Effects and Their Management

FGAs have many side effects in children and adolescents. Adverse effects of greatest concern include the effect of sedation on cognition and the effects of EPS. Of particular concern is the development of tardive dyskinesia in youths taking FGAs over a long time during development. Usually, high-potency FGAs cause fewer anticholinergic effects, fewer autonomic nervous system effects, and less sedation than the low-potency FGAs. However, high-potency agents may increase the risk for EPS and tardive dyskinesia compared with low-potency FGAs. Appendix 7 lists FGA treatment-emergent side effects.

For management of the side effects of FGAs, see Appendix 8.

Antipsychotic Treatment of Pediatric Psychiatric Disorders

Pediatric Bipolar Illness

The assessment of children and adolescents with pediatric bipolar illness includes a comprehensive psychiatric evaluation that reviews current and past mood symptoms and comorbid psychiatric disorders. An adequate evaluation obtains information from multiple sources, including the child, parents, and reports on school functioning and interpersonal relationships. Symptoms of bipolar illness must be distinguished from more common childhood mood disorders, conduct disorder, and ADHD and take into account normal developmental excitability. Excitability that is pleasurable, is readily suppressible, and does not interfere with daily functioning is not considered symptomatic of bipolar illness or its disorders. These are in contrast to intense mood episodes that are recurrent, bothersome, and interfere with daily functioning. In those suspected of having bipolar illness, substance use and suicidal ideation should be assessed. Once a diagnosis of bipolar illness is established, symptom severity can be determined with the use of a reliable and valid parent-report measure such as the Young Mania Rating Scale (Gracious et al. 2002).

Research in pediatric psychopharmacology for the treatment of early-onset bipolar illness is not sufficiently advanced to inform clinicians specifically about treatment in children and adolescents. Pediatric clinical practice in this area is largely influenced by the adult literature. Studies of bipolar illness in the pediatric age range are included in Table 6–2. These studies suggest that combination therapy, either with an atypical antipsychotic and a mood stabilizer or with a combination of two mood stabilizers, is more effective for bipolar illness than is monotherapy.

Duration of Treatment for Pediatric Bipolar Illness

- The optimal duration of medication treatment for children and adolescents with bipolar illness is currently unknown.
- Expert consensus suggests 9–18 months of treatment after symptom resolution or stabilization to prevent relapse of the index depressive, manic, or mixed bipolar episode.
- Medications should be discontinued gradually (about 25% every 1–2 months) with careful psychiatric monitoring for any return of bipolar illness.
- Bipolar illness is generally a chronic condition. When bipolar illness medication is discontinued, the child should continue to be monitored periodically for the possible return of bipolar illness.
- The lifetime prevalence of suicide in adults with bipolar illness is high compared with control samples. Adolescents with bipolar illness are also at risk for suicidality. When bipolar illness medication is tapered and discontinued, the physician should carefully monitor the bipolar patient for any suicidal ideation or plan.

Treatment of ADHD in Pediatric Bipolar Illness

ADHD: Given the high rates of comorbidity between ADHD and pediatric bipolar disorder, there exists concern that treatment of ADHD symptoms with stimulants or noradrenergic antidepressants in bipolar youths might destabilize symptoms of bipolar illness. This issue is further complicated because many of the symptoms of ADHD are similar to the symptoms of pediatric bipolar illness. Treating ADHD with medication and not recognizing an underlying comorbid bipolar illness may lead to an exacerbation of manic symptoms in such youths.

- Current recommendations for the treatment of ADHD in the context of bipolar illness emphasize the need to treat bipolar disease first with antipsychotic and/or mood-stabilizing medications.
- If ADHD symptoms persist after successful treatment of bipolar illness, then stimulants can be added to ongoing bipolar medications without destabilizing comorbid bipolar symptoms (G.A. Carlson et al. 2000; P.J. Carlson et al. 2004; Scheffer et al. 2005).

Pediatric Psychosis

Psychotic symptoms occur in a wide variety of neuropsychiatric conditions in children and adolescents and are not pathognomonic for any one disorder. Developmental issues need to be considered in the assessment of childhood psychotic disorders. Psychotic phenomena are relatively uncommon in the elementary school years, and comorbidity is the rule rather than the exception in children who come to the clinician with early-onset psychotic disorders. Illogical thinking and loose associations of ideas are common in nonpsychotic preschoolers. Comorbid conditions may confound accurate diagnosis, affect responses to treatment, and increase the possibility of poorer outcomes in these disorders.

Comorbid Conditions in Pediatric Psychosis

Disruptive behavior disorders

Premorbid and concurrent ADHD, oppositional defiant disorder, and conduct disorder are noted frequently in children and adolescents with bipolar illness, schizophrenia, and other psychotic disorders. In the sample of Biederman and colleagues (2004), children and adolescents with psychoses frequently had comorbid disruptive behavior disorders.

- ADHD: 70%
- Conduct disorder: 30%
- Oppositional defiant disorder: 70%

Mood disorders

Youths with psychotic symptoms often have accompanying mood disorders.

- Major depressive disorder: 40%
- Bipolar disorder: 55%

Anxiety disorders

Youths with psychotic symptoms often have accompanying anxiety disorders.

- Multiple anxiety disorders: 65%
- Obsessive-compulsive disorder: 20%

Substance abuse

Up to 60% of adolescents with psychotic disorders may abuse illicit substances.

Neurological disease

Children with epilepsy can develop psychotic signs and symptoms. Children who experience traumatic brain injury may develop psychotic symptoms. After about age 7 years, psychotic signs and symptoms seen in neurological disease are not so commonly observed in normally developing children (Isohanni et al. 2004). During adolescence, the frequency of psychotic illness increases markedly, and symptomatology becomes generally similar to that in adults.

Summary

Despite the lack of controlled clinical trial evidence, SGAs are thought to play a crucial role in treating the specific symptoms of psychosis. Few controlled studies of antipsychotic medications for pediatric schizophrenia have been done. Most of the available scientific evidence for antipsychotic effectiveness in children and adolescents comes from clinical experience and open case series. Table 6–2 presents some of this evidence. Note that current use of these agents to treat schizophrenia before age 13 years is off label except with risperidone and aripiprazole. However, these agents are frequently prescribed to children and adolescents with psychotic disorders.

Pediatric Anorexia Nervosa

Although the cornerstone of treatment for anorexia nervosa encompasses cognitive and behavioral therapy, pharmacological treatment can be useful in some cases, generally as an adjunct or in treating comorbid diseases that may be associated with anorexia nervosa.

Chlorpromazine

Although no controlled studies have established the efficacy of chlorpromazine to promote weight gain, this agent has been used for decades and was initially believed to improve anxiety and promote weight gain. Chlorpromazine is still used in low doses in patients with anorexia who also present with obsessions or agitation.

Haloperidol

Eleven patients with the restricting subtype of anorexia nervosa were given oral haloperidol at dosages of 1–2 mg/day. Six patients were taking concomitant fluoxetine, 4 were taking sertraline, and 3 were taking amitriptyline but were still not improving. Significant improvements on several rating scales were noted. Within the Eating Disorder Inventory, significant improvement was noted on the Drive for Thinness ($P=0.009$), Interoceptive Awareness

(P=0.001), and Ineffectiveness (P=0.032) subscales. Within the Eating Attitudes Test, improvement occurred on Total Score (P=0.009), Diet (P=0.005), and Bulimia (P=0.01) subscales. Significant improvement occurred in the CGI-S score (P=0.001), and BMI increases with haloperidol use were statistically significant (P=0.03) (Connor and Meltzer 2006).

Olanzapine

A series of four case reports found that adjunctive use of olanzapine in pediatric patients with anorexia nervosa may help to reduce anxiety, compulsive-type behaviors, and poor sleeping. The four patients were between ages 10 and 12 years (three girls and one boy). All had significantly reduced BMIs and showed various degrees of premeal and postmeal anxiety, obsessive-compulsive behaviors, poor sleep patterns, depression, and agitation. Each child began taking olanzapine 2.5 mg/day, and all were hospitalized and given adequate nutrition. On discharge, all four children had BMIs within the expected normal range for their height, and all showed a marked decrease in anxiety and other psychological symptoms. Olanzapine was eventually discontinued in all four patients, with no return of symptoms or loss of BMI (Connor and Meltzer 2006).

Pimozide

Vandereycken and Pierloot (1982) conducted a double-blind, controlled crossover study of pimozide in 18 female patients with anorexia nervosa. The patients received either pimozide 4–6 mg/day or placebo for 3-week periods. Pimozide produced an almost significant enhancement in weight gain during the first two study periods.

Pediatric Autism Spectrum Disorders and Pervasive Developmental Delay

Antipsychotic medications have been used to treat severe behavior problems. Among the FGAs, such as haloperidol, thioridazine, fluphenazine, and chlorpromazine, haloperidol was found in more than one study to be more effective than a placebo in treating serious behavior problems. However, even though haloperidol is helpful for reducing symptoms of aggression, it can also have adverse side effects, such as sedation, muscle stiffness, impaired new learning, and abnormal movements.

Other atypical antipsychotics that have been studied recently with encouraging results are olanzapine, risperidone, and ziprasidone. Of these, only risperidone has an FDA indication for the treatment of autistic disorder irritability in patients age 5 years and older. Ziprasidone has not been associated with significant weight gain.

Pediatric Tourette Syndrome

Quetiapine therapy was effective in the reduction of motor and phonic tics in pediatric patients with Tourette syndrome (Mukaddes and Abali 2003). In a prospective, open-label study with 12 patients ages 8–16 years, 11 boys and 1 girl with Tourette syndrome received 8 weeks of quetiapine therapy at an initial dosage of 25 mg/day, titrated to a maximum dosage of 75 mg/day (younger than 12 years) or 100 mg/day (12 years and older). The mean dosage of quetiapine was 72.9 mg/day (range=50–100 mg/day). The mean total tic score on the Yale Global Tic Severity Scale was significantly reduced from baseline to 4 weeks and from baseline to 8 weeks. All 12 patients had a 30%–100% improvement in tic severity. Mild, transient sedation was reported in 3 patients; however, extrapyramidal adverse effects and statistically significant weight gain were not observed.

Discontinuing Antipsychotic Treatment

Antipsychotic agents should not be abruptly stopped. A variety of withdrawal side effects may occur if patients suddenly discontinue antipsychotics. These may include abnormal involuntary movements called neuroleptic withdrawal dyskinesias. Generally, these abnormal involuntary movements spontaneously remit but may cause distress for the patient and family. Antipsychotics should be tapered by 10%–25% every 5–7 days when treatment is being stopped. The clinician should monitor for the emergence of treatment withdrawal symptoms.

KEY CLINICAL POINTS

- With second-generation antipsychotics, youths gain more weight more quickly than do adults.

- With first-generation antipsychotics, adverse effects of greatest concern include the effect of sedation on cognition and the effects of EPS.

- Risperidone has shown clear effectiveness for irritability seen in autistic disorder and in the treatment of impulsive aggression seen in pervasive developmental disorder spectrum populations.

- No evidence indicates that SGAs are superior to FGAs.

- No evidence suggests that one SGA is better than any other in the treatment of pediatric schizophrenia or bipolar illnesses.

- Neither FGAs (with the possible exception of chlorpromazine) nor SGAs have shown benefit in the treatment of ADHD.

- A pressing need exists for additional information on the long-term efficacy and safety of each SGA during maintenance therapy for the pediatric population.

References

Aman MG, De Smedt G, Derivan A, et al: Double-blind, placebo-controlled study of risperidone for the treatment of disruptive behaviors in children with subaverage intelligence. Am J Psychiatry 159:1337–1346, 2002

Barnett MS: Ziprasidone monotherapy in pediatric bipolar disorder. J Child Adolesc Psychopharmacol 14:471–477, 2004

Biederman J, Petty C, Faraone SV, et al: Phenomenology of childhood psychosis, findings from a large sample of psychiatrically referred youth. J Nerv Ment Dis 192:607–614, 2004

Barzman DH, DelBello MP, Adler CM, et al: The efficacy and tolerability of quetiapine versus divalproex for the treatment of impulsivity and reactive aggression in adolescents with co-occurring bipolar disorder and disruptive behavior disorder(s). J Child Adolesc Psychopharmacol 16:665–670, 2006

Biederman J, Mick E, Hammerness P, et al: Open-label, 8-week trial of olanzapine and risperidone for the treatment of bipolar disorder in preschool-age children. Biol Psychiatry 58:589–594, 2005a

Biederman J, Mick E, Wozniak J, et al: An open-label trial of risperidone in children and adolescents with bipolar disorder. J Child Adolesc Psychopharmacol 15:311–317, 2005b

Biederman J, Mick E, Spencer T, et al: An open-label trial of aripiprazole monotherapy in children and adolescents with bipolar disorder. CNS Spectr 12:683–689, 2007a

Biederman J, Mick E, Spencer T, et al: A prospective open-label treatment trial of ziprasidone monotherapy in children and adolescents with bipolar disorder. Bipolar Disord 9:888–894, 2007b

Blair J, Scahill L, State M, et al: Electrocardiographic changes in children and adolescents treated with ziprasidone: a prospective study. J Am Acad Child Adolesc Psychiatry 44:73–79, 2005

Buitelaar JK, van der Gaag RJ, Cohen-Kettenis P, et al: A randomized controlled trial of risperidone in the treatment of aggression in hospitalized adolescents with subaverage cognitive abilities. J Clin Psychiatry 62:239–248, 2001

Carlson GA, Loney J, Salisbury H, et al: Stimulant treatment in young boys with symptoms suggesting childhood mania: a report from a longitudinal study. J Child Adolesc Psychopharmacol 10:175–184, 2000

Carlson PJ, Merlock MC, Suppes T: Adjunctive stimulant use in patients with bipolar disorder: treatment of residual depression and sedation. Bipolar Disord 6:416–420, 2004

Chang KD, Nyilas M, Aurang C, et al: Efficacy of aripiprazole in children (10–17 years old) with mania. Poster presented at the 54th annual meeting of the American Academy of Child and Adolescent Psychiatry, Boston, MA, October 23–28, 2007

Connor DF, Meltzer BM: Pediatric Psychopharmacology: Fast Facts. New York, WW Norton, 2006

Delbello MP, Schwiers ML, Rosenberg HL, et al. A double-blind, randomized, placebo-controlled study of quetiapine as adjunctive treatment for adolescent mania. J Am Acad Child Adolesc Psychiatry 41:1216–1223, 2002

DelBello MP, Adler CM, Whitsel RM, et al: A 12-week single-blind trial of quetiapine for the treatment of mood symptoms in adolescents at high risk for developing bipolar I disorder. J Clin Psychiatry 68:789–795, 2007

DelBello MP, Versavel M, Ice K, et al: Tolerability of oral ziprasidone in children and adolescents with bipolar mania, schizophrenia, or schizoaffective disorder. J Child Adolesc Psychopharmacol 18:491–499, 2008

Findling RL, McNamara NK: Atypical antipsychotics in the treatment of children and adolescents: clinical applications. J Clin Psychiatry 65 (suppl 6):30–44, 2004

Findling RL, McNamara NK, Branicky LA, et al: A double-blind pilot study of risperidone in the treatment of conduct disorder. J Am Acad Child Adolesc Psychiatry 39:509–561, 2000

Findling RL, Robb A, Nyilas M, et al: A multiple-center, randomized, double-blind, placebo-controlled study of oral aripiprazole for treatment of adolescents with schizophrenia. Am J Psychiatry 165:1432–1441, 2008

Fisman S, Steele M: Use of risperidone in pervasive developmental disorders: a case series. J Child Adolesc Psychopharmacol 6:177–190, 1996

Fleischhaker C, Heiser P, Hennighausen K, et al: Weight gain in children and adolescents during 45 weeks treatment with clozapine, olanzapine and risperidone. Neural Transm 115:1599–1608, 2008

Frazier JA, Gordon CT, McKenna K, et al: An open trial of clozapine in 11 adolescents with childhood-onset schizophrenia. J Am Acad Child Adolesc Psychiatry 33:658–663, 1994

Frazier JA, Cohen LG, Jacobsen L, et al: Clozapine pharmacokinetics in children and adolescents with childhood-onset schizophrenia. J Clin Psychopharmacol 23:87–91, 2003

Gracious BL, Youngstrom EA, Findling RL, et al: Discriminative validity of a parent version of the Young Mania Rating Scale. J Am Acad Child Adolesc Psychiatry 41:1350–1359, 2002

Green WH: Antipsychotic drugs, in Child and Adolescent Clinical Psychopharmacology, 3rd Edition. Edited by Green WH. Philadelphia, PA, Lippincott Williams & Wilkins, 2001, pp 89–149

Grothe DR, Calis KA, Jacobsen L, et al: Olanzapine pharmacokinetics in pediatric and adolescent inpatients with childhood-onset schizophrenia. J Clin Psychopharmacol 20:220–225, 2000

Isohanni M, Isohanni I, Koponen H, et al: Developmental precursors of psychosis. Curr Psychiatry Rep 6:168–175, 2004

Kryzhanovskaya L, Schulz SC, McDougle C, et al: Olanzapine versus placebo in adolescents with schizophrenia: a 6-week, randomized, double-blind, placebo-controlled trial. J Am Acad Child Adolesc Psychiatry 48:60–70, 2009

Kumra S, Frazier JA, Jacobsen LK, et al: Childhood-onset schizophrenia: a double-blind clozapine-haloperidol comparison. Arch Gen Psychiatry 53:1090–1097, 1996

Kumra S, Jacobsen LK, Lenane M, et al: Childhood-onset schizophrenia: an open-label study of olanzapine in adolescents. J Am Acad Child Adolesc Psychiatry 37:377–385, 1998

Kumra S, Kranzler H, Gerbino-Rosen G, et al: A pilot study of risperidone, olanzapine, and haloperidol in psychotic youth: a double-blind, randomized, 8-week trial. J Child Adolesc Psychopharmacol 18:307–316, 2008a

Kumra S, Kranzler H, Gerbino-Rosen G, et al: Clozapine versus "high-dose" olanzapine in refractory early onset schizophrenia: an open-label extension study. Biol Psychiatry 63:524–529., 2008b

McConville BJ, Arvanitis LA, Thyrum PT, et al: Pharmacokinetics, tolerability, and clinical effectiveness of quetiapine fumarate: an open-label trial in adolescents with psychotic disorders. J Clin Psychiatry 61:252–260, 2000

McConville B, Carrero L, Sweitzer D, et al: Long-term safety, tolerability, and clinical efficacy of quetiapine in adolescents: an open-label extension trial. J Child Adolesc Psychopharmacol 13:75–82, 2003

McCracken JT, McGough J, Shah B, et al: Risperidone in children with autism and serious behavioral problems. N Engl J Med 347:314–321, 2002

Mukaddes NM, Abali O: Quetiapine treatment of children and adolescents with Tourette's disorder. J Child Adolesc Psychopharmacol 13:295–299, 2003

Pandina G, DelBello MP, Kushner S, et al: Risperidone for the treatment of acute mania in bipolar youth. Poster presented at the 54th annual meeting of the American Academy of Child and Adolescent Psychiatry, Boston, MA, October 23–28, 2007

Pavuluri MN, Henry DB, Carbray JA, et al: Open-label prospective trial of risperidone in combination with lithium or divalproex sodium in pediatric mania. J Affect Disord 82 (suppl 1):S103–S11, 2004

Pavuluri MN, Henry DB, Carbray JA, et al: A one-year open-label trial of risperidone augmentation in lithium nonresponder youth with preschool-onset bipolar disorder. J Child Adolesc Psychopharmacol 16:336–350, 2006

Physicians' Desk Reference, 57th Edition. Montvale, NJ, Thomson Healthcare, 2003, pp 991–995

Pool D, Bloom W, Mielke DH, et al: A controlled evaluation of loxitane in seventy-five adolescent schizophrenic patients. Curr Ther Res Clin Exp 19:99–104, 1976

Realmuto GM, Erickson WD, Yellin AM, et al: Clinical comparison of thiothixene and thioridazine in schizophrenic adolescents. Am J Psychiatry 141:440–442, 1984

Remschmidt HE, Schulz E, Martin M, et al: Childhood-onset schizophrenia: history of the concept and recent studies. Schizophr Bull 20:727–745, 1994

Sallee FR, Kurlan R, Goetz CG, et al: Ziprasidone treatment of children and adolescents with Tourette's syndrome: a pilot study. J Am Acad Child Adolesc Psychiatry 39:292–299, 2000

Scahill L, Leckman JF, Schultz RT, et al: A placebo-controlled trial of risperidone in Tourette syndrome. Neurology 60:1130–1135, 2003

Scheffer RE, Kowatch RA, Carmody T, et al: Randomized, placebo-controlled trial of mixed amphetamine salts for symptoms of comorbid ADHD in pediatric bipolar disorder after mood stabilization with divalproex sodium. Am J Psychiatry 162:58–64, 2005

Schimmelmann BG, Mehler-Wex C, Lambert M, et al: A prospective 12-week study of quetiapine in adolescents with schizophrenia spectrum disorders. J Child Adolesc Psychopharmacol 17:768–778, 2007

Shaw P, Sporn A, Gogtay N, et al: Clozapine and "high-dose" olanzapine in refractory early onset schizophrenia: a 12-week randomized and double-blind comparison. Arch Gen Psychiatry 63:721–730, 2006

Sikich L, Hamer RM, Bashford RA, et al: Double-blind comparison of first- and second-generation antipsychotics in early onset schizophrenia and schizoaffective disorder: findings from the Treatment of Early-Onset Schizophrenia Spectrum Disorders (TEOSS) study. Neuropsychopharmacology 29:133–145, 2004

Sikich L, Frazier JA, McClellan J, et al: Double-blind comparison of first- and second-generation antipsychotics in early-onset schizophrenia and schizoaffective disorder: findings from the Treatment of Early-Onset Schizophrenia Spectrum Disorders (TEOSS) study. Am J Psychiatry 165:1420–1431, 2008

Spencer EK, Kafantaris V, Padron-Gayol MV, et al: Haloperidol in schizophrenic children: early findings from a study in progress. Psychopharmacol Bull 28:183–186, 1992

Tohen M, Kryzhanovskaya L, Carlson G, et al: Olanzapine in the treatment of adolescents with bipolar mania: 26-week open-label extension. Poster presented at the 47th annual meeting of the New Clinical Drug Evaluation Unit (NCDEU), Boca Raton, FL, June 13, 2007a

Tohen M, Kryzhanovskaya L, Carlson G: Olanzapine versus placebo in the treatment of adolescents with bipolar mania. Am J Psychiatry 164:1547–1556, 2007b

Tramontina S, Zeni CP, Pheula GF, et al: Aripiprazole in juvenile bipolar disorder comorbid with attention-deficit/hyperactivity disorder: an open clinical trial. CNS Spectr 12:758–762, 2007

Tramontina S, Zeni CP, Ketzer CR, et al: Aripiprazole in children and adolescents with bipolar disorder comorbid with attention-deficit/hyperactivity disorder: a pilot randomized clinical trial. J Clin Psychiatry 70:756–764, 2009

Van Bellinghen M, de Troch C: Risperidone in the treatment of behavioral disturbances in children and adolescents with borderline intellectual functioning: a double-blind, placebo-controlled pilot trial. J Child Adolesc Psychopharmacology 11:5–13, 2001

Vandereycken W, Pierloot R: Pimozide combined with behavior therapy in the short-term treatment of anorexia nervosa: a double-blind placebo-controlled cross-over study. Acta Psychiatr Scand 66:445–450, 1982

Versavel M, DelBello MP, Ice K, et al: Ziprasidone dosing study in pediatric patients with bipolar disorder in pediatric patients with bipolar disorder, schizophrenia, and schizoaffective disorder. Neuropsychopharmacology 30 (suppl 1):S122–S213, 2005

Williams SK, Scahill L, Vitiello B, et al: Risperidone and adaptive behavior in children with autism. J Am Acad Child Adolesc Psychiatry 45:431–439, 2006

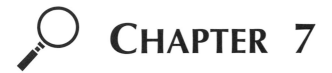

CHAPTER 7

Use of Antipsychotics in Geriatric Patients

Ellen M. Whyte, M.D.
Charles Madeira

ANTIPSYCHOTIC MEDICATIONS have a unique role in geriatric psychiatry. In addition to being prescribed for patients whose psychiatric illness started earlier in life, this class of medication is commonly used to manage psychosis and behavioral disturbances in the setting of common late-life disorders such as dementia. However, few medications, and none of the antipsychotic medications, have received specific U.S. Food and Drug Administration (FDA) approval for use in the geriatric population, and no medications are specifically FDA approved for the psychiatric consequences of dementia, a condition that mainly affects the elderly. Nevertheless, antipsychotic medications can be an important part of the pharmacological armamentarium available to treat psychiatric illness in late life, whether it be for a patient whose illness started earlier in life (e.g., schizophrenia) or for a patient with a late-onset illness (e.g., dementia). However, clinicians need to be particularly mindful about the risks when prescribing medications for non-FDA-approved indications and need to document carefully that the patient (and their families) understands the potential risks and benefits and agrees to proceed with the medication trial.

In addition, late life presents numerous challenges in pharmacotherapy management. Elderly patients are at increased risk for aberrant drug responses and adverse drug events because of the physiological changes caused by both age and disease, the high prevalence of polypharmacy (e.g., drug-drug interactions), and the prevalence of malnutrition syndromes common in late life. These factors, in addition to the individual's genetic constitution, increase the variability of response and tolerability to medications in late life when compared with midlife patients.

General Principles of Medication Management

"Start low and go slow," the mantra of pharmacotherapy in geriatrics, applies to the use of antipsychotic medications as well. By starting the medication at a low dose, the clinician is able to monitor for and minimize initial potential side effects. By titrating up slowly, the clinician is able to find the optimal dose for the particular patient that balances the risks of side effects with the benefits of treatment. However, elderly patients may still require "full doses" to achieve symptomatic improvement. Hence as long as the patient remains symptomatic and is tolerating the medication, the dose can be increased to "adult" doses in an attempt to capture a clinical response. The typical starting doses of antipsychotic medications in late life are shown in Table 7–1.

TABLE 7–1. Typical starting doses of antipsychotic medications commonly used in late life

DRUG	STARTING DOSAGE (MG/DAY)
Haloperidol	0.25–2.5
Risperidone	0.25–1
Clozapine	12.5
Olanzapine	1.25–5.0
Quetiapine	12.5–50
Aripiprazole	5

Source.   Based on Alexopoulos et al. 2004.

Age-Specific Issues Related to Side Effects

Older patients are generally at risk for the same side effects as those in younger patients. However, the relative rates of some side effects vary with age (see Table 7–2). In addition, some potential side effects become more common and more clinically meaningful in late life because of the elderly patient's decreased ability to compensate physiologically for the side effect. For example, some antipsychotic medications can cause orthostatic hypotension. An older patient may become dizzy and fall given a particular decline in blood pressure on standing, whereas a younger patient experiencing the same decline in blood pressure may be asymptomatic.

TABLE 7–2. Side-effect profile of antipsychotic medications in older patients compared with younger patients

SIDE EFFECT	INCIDENCE IN OLDER VS. YOUNGER PATIENTS
Extrapyramidal symptoms	
Tardive dyskinesia	↑↑↑
Akathisia	↔
Acute dystonia	↓↓↓
Antipsychotic-induced parkinsonism	↑↑
Neuroleptic malignant syndrome	↑?
Hyperprolactinemia	↔?
Anticholinergic effects	↑↑
Metabolic	
Weight gain	↓?
Glucose intolerance	↓?
Hyperlipidemia	↓?
Cardiovascular	
Orthostatic hypotension	↑↑
QTc prolongation	↑

Note.   Compared with younger adults, the incidence of specific side effects may be increased (↑), decreased (↓), or unchanged (↔) in older adults. Uncertainty in the relative incidence of side effects is indicated by a "?".
Source.   Based on Alexopoulos et al. 2004; Jeste et al. 2008.

In general, the primary strategy for managing adverse drug events is dose reduction. Clearly, dose reduction may not always be feasible. Switching to an agent with a more beneficial side-effect profile (for that particular patient) is also an option. Adding an augmenting agent to address side effects (such as adding benztropine to manage extrapyramidal symptoms [EPS]) is a less desirable strategy in the elderly because the second medication adds potential new side effects and increases the risk for drug-drug interactions. Nevertheless, using an augmentation strategy may be an appropriate option for an individual patient, depending on his or her unique risk-benefit profile. The discussion in the following sections highlights differences in side-effect profile between older and younger patients and is not meant to be an all-inclusive list of possible side effects of antipsychotic medications.

Cardiovascular Effects

Orthostatic Hypotension

Antipsychotic medications, through α_1 antagonism, can cause orthostatic hypotension. Older individuals may be particularly prone to developing orthostatic hypotension in response to antipsychotic exposure as a result of both concurrent medical illness and diminished ability to compensate physiologically for the α_1 blockage. Orthostatic hypotension, defined as a decrease in systolic pressure of more than 20 mm Hg, a decline in diastolic pressure of more than 10 mm Hg, or an increase in heart rate greater than 20 beats per minute on standing from a sitting or lying position, can result in fatigue, dizziness, falls, syncope, myocardial infarction, and cerebral ischemia. Orthostatic hypotension is especially common with the low-potency first-generation, or typical, antipsychotics (FGAs) chlorpromazine and thioridazine as well as with the second-generation, or atypical, antipsychotics (SGAs) clozapine and olanzapine. Expert guidelines suggest that risperidone and quetiapine are the drugs of choice in the setting of orthostatic hypotension (Alexopoulos et al. 2004). Clinicians should monitor orthostatic blood pressure both before and after initiating treatment with an antipsychotic and should avoid antipsychotic medications with the strongest potential for inducing orthostasis when treating individuals who already have mild positional blood pressure changes pretreatment (Jacobson et al. 2007).

QTc Prolongation

QTc prolongation is a known side effect of antipsychotic medications, which may lead to *torsades de pointes*, an arrhythmia that can cause syncope, ventricular fibrillation, and death. Older adults may be at increased risk for QTc prolongation because several other risk factors associated with QTc prolongation—including heart disease and hepatic and renal impairment—are common in the elderly. A pretreatment QTc value of 500 ms or a posttreatment increase in QTc of 60 ms or greater is considered an indication that a patient is at significant risk for torsades de pointes and other arrhythmias (Haddad and Sharma 2007). Studies involving younger patients suggest that thioridazine and ziprasidone have the greatest potential to prolong QTc interval (Pfizer Inc. 2000). Unfortunately, few specific data in late life are available. In late life, it would be reasonable to obtain an electrocardiogram (ECG) prior to initiating antipsychotic therapy, especially if a patient is receiving other medications that may prolong QTc or has underlying cardiac disease. Expert consensus guidelines suggest that risperidone, quetiapine, and olanzapine are the drugs of choice in the setting of preexisting QTc prolongation. If therapy with ziprasidone is being considered, then a pretreatment ECG must be obtained, and electrolytes need to be assessed. Ziprasidone is contraindicated in patients with a QTc interval greater than 500 ms, history of prolonged QTc syndrome or cardiac arrhythmia, recent myocardial infarction, or uncompensated congestive heart failure. If ziprasidone therapy is initiated, clinicians should assess patients for palpitations, dizziness, or syncope because these may indicate cardiac arrhythmias and also should monitor electrolytes for those patients at risk for electrolyte disturbances (e.g., due to diuretic use). The utility of repeated ECGs is unclear because the natural variability of QTc interval makes serial assessment difficult.

Extrapyramidal Symptoms

Antipsychotic-induced EPS include several different movement disorders, such as a parkinsonian-like disorder, tardive dyskinesia (TD), akathisia, and acute dystonia. These drug-induced movement disorders can be disturbing and uncomfortable for patients; may contribute to nonadherence with therapy; may cause disability; and, especially in the elderly, may increase the risk of falls and injury.

Antipsychotic-Induced Parkinsonism

Antipsychotic-induced parkinsonism is characterized by psychomotor slowing, tremor, rigidity, and shuffling gait. Antipsychotic-induced parkinsonism can significantly impair a person's ability to carry out basic activities of daily living. Older patients and those receiving FGAs are at particular risk for developing antipsychotic-induced parkinsonism. An estimated 30%–60% of older patients taking a FGA develop antipsychotic-induced parkinsonism; in contrast, fewer than 10% of older patients taking an SGA will do so (Caligiuri et al. 2000). However, many SGAs have a dose-response relation whereby the risk of EPS significantly increases with dose increase. For example, risperidone does not cause antipsychotic-induced parkinsonism (compared with placebo) at dosages of 1 mg/day or less but can cause significant antipsychotic-induced parkinsonism at dosages of 2 mg/day (Herrmann and Lanctot 2006). Overall, among the SGAs, risperidone and olanzapine are associated with the highest risk of antipsychotic-induced parkinsonism, whereas clozapine, quetiapine, and aripiprazole have the least risk (Haddad and Sharma 2007; Schneider et al. 2006b).

Patients with preexisting parkinsonian symptoms, including those with Parkinson's disease, are at particular risk for developing antipsychotic-induced parkinsonism. Patients with dementia with Lewy bodies (DLB) are at risk for a very severe form of antipsychotic-induced parkinsonism, which is associated with sedation, confusion, and death (Aarsland et al. 2005).

Antipsychotic-induced parkinsonism is generally aggressively managed in late life because of the assumption that antipsychotic-induced parkinsonism puts patients at greater risk for falls and injury. The primary management strategy is dose reduction. If that is not successful, switching to an SGA with less potential to cause antipsychotic-induced parkinsonism is recommended. If antipsychotic-induced parkinsonism continues to be bothersome, use of a low-dose anticholinergic medication, such as benztropine, may be considered. Clinicians must monitor for side effects of anticholinergic medication, including cognitive impairment, blurred vision, urinary retention, and constipation, which can be especially prominent in the elderly (Dayalu and Chou 2008).

Tardive Dyskinesia

Tardive dyskinesia consists of a variety of involuntary, repetitive movements caused by exposure to antipsychotic medications. Characteristically, TD involves involuntary movements of the muscles of the face, mouth, and tongue but can involve other muscle groups, including the fingers, hands, toes, or trunk. TD can lead to impaired balance, falls, difficulty swallowing and eating with resultant weight loss, social embarrassment, and depression.

Older patients have a five to six times higher risk of developing TD compared with younger patients. In addition, older patients may develop TD after much shorter period of antipsychotic medication exposure compared with younger patients, for whom TD may develop after months to years of antipsychotic medication treatment. The cumulative incidence of TD after 1, 2, and 3 years of treatment with a conventional antipsychotic medication is 29%, 50%, and 63%, respectively, for adults older than 65; the comparative rates for younger adults are 5%, 10%, and 15%, respectively. An older patient has a significantly lower risk of developing TD with SGAs.

Even though SGAs have a much lower incidence of TD, clinicians still need to use the lowest effective dose to reduce the risk of emergent TD. Treatment of

TD consists of switching from a conventional antipsychotic to an SGA, gradual dose reduction, or discontinuation if possible. Initially, symptoms of TD may worsen or even emerge for the first time on drug discontinuation, but these symptoms usually fade over time. Use of antiparkinsonian medications may actually worsen the TD syndrome and is not recommended (Jeste 2004).

Akathisia

Akathisia is an uncontrollable desire to move with or without inner restlessness. It usually occurs within the first 2 weeks of treatment and may take the form of pacing, fidgeting, or inability to sit for more than a few minutes. Akathisia is as common or slightly less common in older patients than in younger patients. Unfortunately, older patients may be at increased risk for developing chronic akathisia. Risk factors for akathisia include higher drug dose, use of FGAs (especially high-potency drugs), and the development of concurrent antipsychotic-induced parkinsonism. Use of SGAs is associated with a reduced incidence of akathisia.

In treating dementia and agitation in elderly patients, clinicians may misinterpret akathisia as a worsening of agitation. The diagnosis of akathisia can be informed by asking the patient whether he or she is experiencing a new uncontrollable and irresistible urge to move. The primary treatment of akathisia in late life is to lower the dose of the antipsychotic medication. Switching to another antipsychotic, if necessary, may decrease the akathisia symptoms. Mitigation of akathitic symptoms with β-blockers is an option that must be used cautiously in patients with significant medical illness because β-blockers can worsen asthma and can cause bradycardia, hypotension, conduction block, and fatigue. Use of benzodiazepines to manage akathisia is also an option that must be used with caution in the elderly because benzodiazepines can lead to confusion, sedation, incoordination, and falls (Dayalu and Chou 2008).

Acute Dystonia

Acute dystonia is characterized by muscle spasms, typically of the muscles of the head and neck, which can present as abnormal neck positioning, a clenched jaw, difficulty speaking and swallowing, eye deviation, or odd positioning of the extremities or trunk. Most cases of acute dystonia occur within the first 4 days of treatment (Dayalu and Chou 2008). Acute dystonia is significantly less common in older adults compared with younger adults. The incidence of acute dystonia is 5% in late-life patients. Given the low incidence of acute dystonia and the potential adverse effects of anticholinergic medication in the elderly, the clinician should not prophylactically prescribe anticholinergic agents for older patients.

Mild dystonic reactions may be left untreated if not bothersome to the patient. Treatment of acute dystonia includes the use of oral diphenhydramine 25–50 mg or benztropine 1–2 mg. Intravenous diphenhydramine or benztropine may be considered for treatment of severe reactions. After the acute crisis is over, the physician needs to weigh the risks and benefits of continued antipsychotic treatment, with or without anticholinergic medication, for that individual patient.

Falls

It is unclear whether the use of antipsychotic medications increases the risk of falling for elderly patients. A recent meta-analysis of 11 randomized placebo-controlled trials involving more than 3,500 subjects did not find an increased risk of injury or falls with SGAs in the elderly (Schneider et al. 2006a). In contrast, a recent case-control study of nursing home residents found an approximately 1.3 times increased risk of fall-related fractures with both FGAs and SGAs (Liperoti et al. 2007). Nevertheless, the prudent clinician needs to be mindful of such a potential risk and monitor for antipsychotic medication side effects, such as EPS, confusion, and sedation, that may contribute to the risk of falls.

Neuroleptic Malignant Syndrome

Neuroleptic malignant syndrome (NMS) is a life-threatening complication of antipsychotic treatment characterized by fever, muscle rigidity, autonomic hyperreactivity (e.g., brady- or tachycardia, hyper- or hypotension), and mental status changes. NMS results in death in about 10% of cases. Although age is not an independent risk factor for the development of NMS, other factors correlated with increased incidence of NMS are more likely to develop in the elderly. These include agitation, dehydration, use of restraints, parkinsonian symptoms, and iron deficiency. All antipsychotic agents have been associated with NMS, but high-potency conventional antipsychotic medications carry the greatest risk.

Prompt recognition of this syndrome is essential. Muscle rigidity may be less prominent in NMS associated with use of an SGA or in the presence of preexisting parkinsonian features. A diagnosis of NMS must be considered in any older patient receiving an antipsychotic medication who experiences a change in mental status, instability of vital signs, or fever. Laboratory tests that may help with diagnosis include elevations in creatine kinase or myoglobin, and/or myoglobinuria. If NMS is considered, the antipsychotic medication needs to be discontinued, and supportive medical therapy should be implemented to address volume depletion, electrolyte abnormalities, and hyperthermia, with monitoring for cardiac, respiratory, renal, or infectious complications. If NMS does not reverse with cessation of antipsychotic medication, treatment with a benzodiazepine or a dopamine agonist (bromo-criptine, amantadine) may be indicated. Dantrolene may be used to reverse hyperthermia and rigidity in severe cases, but this agent is associated with hepatic toxicity (Strawn et al. 2007).

Anticholinergic Side Effects

Many medications, including antipsychotic drugs, have significant anticholinergic activity, which results from blockade of muscarinic receptors either centrally or peripherally (Chew et al. 2008). Peripheral effects may include tachycardia, urinary retention, constipation, increased intraocular pressure (with resultant glaucoma exacerbation), dry mouth, and constipation. These peripheral effects are bothersome and potentially dangerous to elderly patients. For example, an elderly man with significant prostatic hypertrophy can develop urinary retention in response to an anticholinergic medication. Central anticholinergic effects include cognitive slowing, delirium, and sedation. These side effects may be particularly prominent in patients with preexisting cognitive impairment and may lead to dangerous behaviors and accidental injury. Low-potency FGAs, as well as clozapine and olanzapine, are considered the most strongly anticholinergic drugs.

Metabolic Abnormalities

Antipsychotic medications, particularly the SGAs, have been reported to be associated with metabolic abnormalities, which include hyperlipidemia, weight gain, and diabetes mellitus. The risk of SGA–induced metabolic abnormalities has not been well studied in older adults. However, evidence suggests that older patients may be less susceptible to the metabolic side effects of SGAs (especially weight gain and glucose intolerance) than are younger patients (Etminan et al. 2003). Nevertheless, the clinician needs to monitor for metabolic side effects. In addition, clozapine, olanzapine, and conventional antipsychotic medications (especially low- and mid-potency agents) should be avoided or the dose minimized in older patients with preexisting dyslipidemias, obesity, or diabetes mellitus. Clinicians should routinely discuss diet, nutrition, and exercise while regularly monitoring weight, waist circumference, blood pressure, fasting glucose, and lipids (see Appendixes 4 and 5).

Hyperprolactinemia

Use of antipsychotic medications can lead to elevated prolactin levels. Clinicians caring for older patients who have had long-term exposure to antipsychotic medications should be watchful for osteopenia and an increase in the risk for breast and endometrial cancer—both long-term effects of prolactin elevation—and encourage patients to receive appropriate screening tests. Older men and women also may experience poor libido, gynecomastia, and galactorrhea as acute side effects. Management of acute side effects can include an attempt to lower the dose. Risperidone is the SGA most likely to induce elevated prolactin levels (Henderson and Doraiswamy 2008).

Monitoring for Side Effects

Late life presents numerous challenges when managing pharmacotherapy. Elderly patients are at increased risk for aberrant drug responses and adverse drug events because of the physiological changes caused by both age and disease, the high prevalence of polypharmacy (e.g., drug-drug interactions), and the prevalence of malnutrition syndromes common in late life. These factors, in addition to the individual's genetic constitution, increase the variability of response and tolerability to medications in late life when compared with midlife patients. Patients should be monitored closely for EPS, including antipsychotic-induced parkinsonism and TD; metabolic side effects such as glucose intolerance, elevated lipids, and weight gain; orthostatic blood pressure changes; and other side effects. General recommendations for monitoring older patients receiving antipsychotic medication are summarized in Table 7–3. The individual patient's medical situation will dictate how often safety surveillance should occur and whether additional assessments are needed.

Risks Unique to
Patients With Dementia

Risk of Death

The FDA has issued a black-box warning regarding an increased risk of death when FGAs or SGAs are prescribed for elderly patients with dementia. The FDA initially issued this black-box warning in April 2005 for all SGAs after a meta-analysis of 17 placebo-controlled trials found that subjects taking an SGA over the course of 8–12 weeks had a 4.5% risk of dying compared with a 2.6% risk for placebo-treated subjects. The cause of death was primarily attributed to cardiac causes or infections. Subsequently, in June 2008, the FDA extended this black-box warning to FGAs after two large retrospective observational epidemiological studies found that conventional antipsychotic medications also were associated with an increased risk of death (Gill et al. 2007; Schneeweiss et al. 2007).

TABLE 7–3. General recommendations for side-effect monitoring in older patients receiving antipsychotic medication

PARAMETER OR SIDE EFFECT	FREQUENCY OF ASSESSMENT	COMMENT
Vital signs; weight and height	Baseline and every 3 months	Includes pulse, blood pressure, and orthostatic blood pressure
Metabolic laboratory evaluation	Baseline, months 3 and 6, and then every 6 months thereafter	Includes fasting blood glucose (or hemoglobin A1c) and fasting lipid panel
QTc prolongation	Baseline. Consider repeat electrocardiogram for patients with cardiac disease or after addition of other medications affecting QTc interval.	Normal QTc is <430 ms for men and <450 ms for women. Pretreatment electrocardiogram (and electrolyte assessment) needed prior to treatment with ziprasidone.
Extrapyramidal symptoms, including antipsychotic-induced parkinsonism and tardive dyskinesia	Baseline and every 3 months	Clinical assessment of abnormal involuntary movements. Ask about occurrence of falls.
Side effects due to anticholinergic burden or hyperprolactinemia	Review every 3 months.	Screening for osteopenia and gynecological cancers appropriate for patients receiving long-term antipsychotic treatment.

Source. Based on Alexopoulos et al. 2004; Jeste et al. 2008.

It is important to note that the black-box warning does not represent a contraindication to using these agents in elderly patients with dementia who have psychosis or dangerous or distressing agitation. Indeed, both pharmacological and nonpharmacological interventions for dementia-related behavioral disturbances and psychosis are limited. Antipsychotic medication remains an appropriate tool in managing behaviors that in and of themselves may put the patient at risk for injury or death. However, these black-box warnings force the clinician to seriously consider the risk-benefit ratio of using this class of medications for a non-FDA-approved indication. In addition, these warnings should guide clinicians when discussing the risk-benefit ratio with patients' families.

Cerebrovascular Events

The use of SGAs and FGAs is associated with an increased risk of cerebrovascular events (e.g., transient ischemic attack, stroke) in elderly patients with dementia. A recent meta-analysis of 16 placebo-controlled trials found that subjects taking an SGA over the course of 10–12 weeks had a 1.9% risk of a cerebrovascular event compared with a 0.9% risk for placebo-treated subjects (Schneider et al. 2006a). The risk of cerebrovascular events is also elevated with FGAs and is likely equivalent to the risk posed by SGAs. Although only risperidone, olanzapine, and aripiprazole have the increased risk of cerebrovascular events noted in their FDA-approved labeling, clinicians should assume that the same risk of cerebrovascular events exists for all medications within this class.

Use of Antipsychotic Medications in Long-Term-Care Facilities

The Omnibus Budget Reconciliation Act (OBRA) of 1987 placed restrictions on the use of psychotropic medications in long-term-care facilities. The goal of these guidelines is to reduce both the number of patients needlessly prescribed antipsychotic medications and the total exposure (e.g., dose and duration) of each individual patient to these drugs. The OBRA rules place limitations on who can receive an antipsychotic medication and mandate an attempt to discontinue these medications once prescribed. These guidelines reflect good clinical practice and do not limit a physician's ability to provide high-quality care to patients. However, adherence to these guidelines requires careful documentation of the rationale for using antipsychotic medications when treating patients in long-term-care settings.

The OBRA Guidelines (U.S. Code of Federal Regulations: 42 CFR §483.25; further elaborated in CMS-Pub. 60AB) state: "When an antipsychotic drug has not been used in the past, it is not given unless antipsychotic drug therapy is necessary to treat a specific condition as diagnosed and documented in the clinical record." Antipsychotic drug use should be limited to the primary psychotic disorders (e.g., schizophrenia), psychotic mood disorders, Tourette syndrome, Huntington's disease, and the short-term symptomatic treatment of hiccups, nausea, vomiting, or pruritus.

Antipsychotic medications may be used in the management of psychotic and agitated behaviors associated with delirium, dementia, or other cognitive disorders in a long-term-care setting only if the psychotic symptoms and agitated behaviors have been quantitatively and objectively documented; are persistent; are not due to a preventable cause (e.g., excessive noise, pain, constipation); cause the patient to be a danger to self or others, to continuously scream, yell, or pace; or result in distress or impairment of functional capacity. However, antipsychotic drugs are not indicated for certain common neuropsychiatric symptoms of delirium, dementia, and other cognitive disorders, including wandering, restlessness, poor self-care, impaired memory, depression, anxiety, insomnia, or unsociability or indifference.

OBRA guidelines mandate gradual dose reduction of the antipsychotic medication, under close clinical supervision, to determine the lowest possible dose that can control target symptoms. Of course, if possible, the medication should be discontinued. Patients who could not tolerate a gradual dose reduction on two occasions over 1 year may continue taking the lowest effective dose with appropriate documentation as to the reason for this decision. However, this mandated gradual dose reduction does not need to be undertaken if the patient has a primary psychotic disorder, a mood disorder with psychotic features, Tourette syndrome, or Huntington's disease and has been stable on a maintenance dose of antipsychotic medications without significant side effects. In addition, physicians can defer mandated gradual dose reductions if they have another compelling clinical reason to do so, as long as an adequate justification of continuation treatment is documented.

Medication Management for Patients With Psychiatric and Neuropsychiatric Disorders

Schizophrenia

Limited data have examined the use of antipsychotic medications in older individuals with schizophrenia, even though 23% of patients with schizophrenia develop it after age 40 and 4% after age 60 (Broadway and Mintzer 2007). The current standard of care for late-life schizophrenia is almost identical to that for nonelderly adults—antipsychotic medications are the treatment of choice for schizophrenia (see Chapter 2, "Schizophrenia and Schizoaffective Disorder," in this volume). Unlike other late-life conditions such as dementia or delirium, the maintenance doses of antipsychotic medications prescribed for older patients with schizophrenia are generally in the same range as those prescribed for younger patients. Nevertheless, compared with younger patients, older patients may need their antipsychotic treatment to be started at a lower dose and be gradually titrated according to both response and side effects. Atypical agents are preferred in the management of schizophrenia in the older patient because of the more generally favorable side-effect profile and the need for long-term treatment. Typical maintenance doses for the preferred SGAs, derived from expert consensus guidelines (Alexopoulos et al. 2004), include

- Risperidone 1.25–3.5 mg/day
- Quetiapine 100–300 mg/day
- Olanzapine 7.5–15 mg/day
- Aripiprazole 15–30 mg/day

Major Depressive Disorder

Major Depression Without Psychosis

The role of antipsychotic medication in nonpsychotic major depression is limited. First-line treatment for nonpsychotic major depression in older patients is antidepressant therapy. However, many patients do not achieve remission of depression with antidepressant monotherapy. A patient whose symptoms do not respond to one or more trials of an antidepressant, of adequate dose and duration, is considered to have treatment-resistant depression. The clinician needs to distinguish true treatment resistance from inadequate treatment (e.g., short treatment duration preventing late responders from achieving remission) and misdiagnosis (e.g., failing to recognize dementia, psychosis, or bipolar disorder). Strategies for managing treatment-resistant depression in adults include combining two antidepressants, augmenting antidepressant monotherapy with lithium, or using electroconvulsive therapy (ECT). Recently, augmentation of antidepressant therapy with aripiprazole (5–15 mg/day) has received an FDA indication for treatment-resistant depression (see Chapter 3, "Mood and Anxiety Disorders," in this volume). This approval is based on pivotal studies that did not include geriatric patients. However, two small studies suggested that aripiprazole may be helpful in geriatric treatment-resistant depression (Rutherford et al. 2007; Sheffrin et al. 2009).

Psychotic Depression

Major depression with psychosis is the second most common cause of psychosis in the elderly. Among older patients hospitalized with depression, approximately 40% have psychosis. Although this diagnosis is associated with significant morbidity and mortality, high-quality evidence to inform treatment of psychotic depression in elderly patients is lacking. Therefore, treatment recommendations are based on those for adult patients in general (see Chapter 3). Specifically, the first-line pharmacotherapy treatment is an antipsychotic medication combined with an antidepressant. The doses of antipsychotic medication required are in the same range as those prescribed for younger patients (Meyers et al. 2009). Nevertheless, compared with younger patients, antipsychotic treatment may need to start at a lower dose and be gradually titrated according to both response and side effects in the older patient. The optimal duration of pharmacological treatment in psychotic depression is unknown. However, gradual discontinuation of the antipsychotic medication after a sustained period of wellness should be considered. Expert consensus guidelines recommend that the clinician initiate a taper no earlier than 6 months after remission. ECT is also appropriate as either a first- or a second-line therapy; however, patients may be less likely to choose this therapy because of availability and stigma (Alexopoulos et al. 2004).

Bipolar Disorder

In adult patients, antipsychotic medications are used in the management of bipolar disorder (see Chapter 3). Unfortunately, the evidence supporting the use of antipsychotic medication in elderly patients with bipolar disorder is limited to case reports and open-label studies. Generally, evidence is suggestive that antipsychotic medications may be beneficial in bipolar disorder in late life. Expert consensus guidelines for the treatment of geriatric mania recommend mood stabilizer monotherapy as first-line therapy. The use of an antipsychotic medication, alone or in combination with a mood stabilizer, should be reserved for cases of severe mania, the presence of psychosis, or cases not responding to first-line therapy. ECT is also a second-line treatment option for geriatric mania. Antipsychotic augmentation may be appropriate for patients with bipolar depression that does not respond to the addition of an antidepressant to the mood stabilizer. There is no evidence informing the use of maintenance antipsychotic medication in geriatric bipolar disorder. Hence an attempt at tapering and discontinuing the antipsychotic medication is appropriate, but such a decision should be based on each patient's unique situation. Expert consensus guidelines suggest that an attempt to taper and discontinue the antipsychotic medication should occur 2–3 months after euthymia is achieved (Alexopoulos et al. 2004; Aziz et al. 2006).

Dementia With Behavioral Disturbances and Psychosis

The most common cause of dementia in the United States is Alzheimer's disease (AD) with or without cerebrovascular disease. The following subsections on dementia with behavioral disturbances and psychosis are primarily based on data derived from studies of AD patients. Management of the neuropsychiatric complications of dementia due to Parkinson's disease, DLB, and frontotemporal dementia (FTD) is discussed separately.

Definitions

Behavioral Disturbance

Behavioral disturbances can be defined as specific patient behaviors that upset and/or jeopardize the safety of the patient or others. Behavioral disturbances are very common in dementia, tend to become more common as the underlying dementia progresses, and are a leading cause of institutionalization. More than 50% of patients with AD have behavioral disturbances at some point in their illness, and 93% of nursing home patients with dementia experience at least weekly behavioral disturbances.

Behavioral disturbances can include, but are not limited to, pacing, attempts at elopement, wandering, day-night confusion, sundowning (e.g., increased nondescript agitation that emerges in late afternoon or early evening), hoarding, picking (at one's own skin), refusal of care, disruptive vocalizations (e.g., screaming), swearing or other verbal abusive behavior, and threatening behavior (including threatening physical gestures, throwing objects, and assault). Aggression in AD is manifested in 5%–20% of patients.

Psychosis

Psychosis is common in the setting of dementia. Approximately 30% of patients with AD experience delusions, and approximately 10% experience hallucinations. Unlike behavioral disturbances, the prevalence of psychosis appears to be stable as the underlying dementia progresses. It is important to note that psychosis in the setting of dementia does not always lead to behavioral disturbance—patients may quietly suffer with their psychosis (Devanand et al. 1997).

Management of Behavioral Disturbances and Psychosis

The first step in managing new-onset or worsening behavioral disturbances or psychosis is to thoroughly investigate and mitigate any potential causes

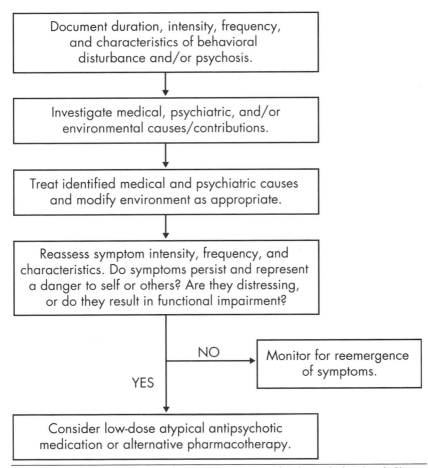

FIGURE 7–1. Algorithm for evaluating psychosis or behavioral disturbances of dementia.

(see Figure 7–1). Behavioral disturbances in the setting of dementia may be a result of the dementia itself, but an underlying medical, psychiatric, or environmental reason may cause or contribute to the disturbance. Although almost any medical problem can trigger behavioral disturbances in dementia, the clinician should be particularly tuned in to those disorders associated with delirium (such as infections, electrolyte disturbances, or medication effects). In addition, pain (either acute or chronic) or sensory alterations (e.g., hearing or vision loss) can lead to behavioral disturbances. Psychiatric causes of behavioral disturbances include delirium, depression, and psychosis. Environmental causes of behavioral disturbances can include any change in environment (e.g., change in room assignment, change in primary caregiver), a mismatch between a patient's level of need and level of care available (e.g., the patient is required to perform tasks that he or she is no longer capable of doing), an immediate environment that is either overstimulating or understimulating, or other interpersonal and social issues. Similarly, psychosis may be due to the dementia or may represent delirium in the setting of dementia. A careful cognitive evaluation to examine for acute worsening of cognition and a thoughtful medical evaluation are needed to rule out a medical cause of the psychosis.

Once a likely underlying cause is identified, first-line treatment is aimed at ameliorating that cause. Preferred first-line treatments include nonpharmacological interventions that address environmental causes (e.g., an understimulated patient is provided more structured activities) or pharmacological interventions that address an underlying medical or psychiatric cause (e.g., a patient with recurrent constipation is prescribed a bowel regimen, or a depressed patient is prescribed an antidepressant).

Patients who do not respond to first-line treatment are candidates for a more targeted psychopharmacological intervention only if their behavioral disturbance or psychosis is persistent and represents a danger to self or others, is distressing, or results in functional impairment. Not initiating a pharmacological treatment is an appropriate option for patients with mild symptoms given the risk of medication side effects and the fact that no class of medication has an FDA-approved indication for the management of dementia with behavioral disturbance or psychosis. Other classes of medications may be beneficial, including citalopram and the acetylcholinesterase inhibitors, for behavioral disturbances and psychosis (Miller 2007; Pollock et al. 2007). Importantly, not all behavioral disturbances will benefit from a trial of an antipsychotic medication. Wandering behaviors and restlessness are generally not responsive to antipsychotic medication, and in the long-term-care setting, OBRA regulations prevent the use of antipsychotic medications for these behaviors (see subsection "Use of Antipsychotic Medications in Long-Term-Care Facilities" earlier in this chapter).

Nevertheless, antipsychotic medications are the best-studied class of medications in the management of dementia-associated behavioral disturbances or psychosis, producing small, but meaningful, changes in behavior (Ballard and Waite 2006; Lanctot et al. 1998; Sultzer et al. 2008). Evidence suggests that FGAs and SGAs are equally effective (Jeste et al. 2008; Lonergan et al. 2002). Both FGAs and SGAs are associated with an increased incidence of death and stroke or transient ischemic attack in the dementia population. However, use of FGAs is associated with greater incidence of EPS and sedation; hence SGAs are preferred for this indication.

Before prescribing an antipsychotic medication to a patient with dementia, the clinician must communicate to the patient (at a level that the person

TABLE 7–4. Dosing of antipsychotic medications for dementia with behavioral disturbance or psychosis

DRUG	STARTING DOSAGE (MG/DAY)	TYPICAL THERAPEUTIC DOSAGE (MG/DAY)
Haloperidol	0.25–0.5	0.25–2
Risperidone	0.25–0.5	0.5–2.0
Clozapine	12.5	50–100
Olanzapine	1.25–5.0	5–10
Quetiapine	12.5–50	50–200
Aripiprazole	2.5–5	2.5–15

Source. Based on Alexopoulos et al. 2004; Jeste et al. 2008.

can understand) and to his or her family or guardian that this indication has no FDA approval, discuss the risks and benefits of antipsychotic treatment (including the risk of death and stroke or transient ischemic attack), and review alternatives. Documentation of this discussion and the family's or guardian's approval is important for medicolegal purposes. Typical starting doses of the most commonly used antipsychotic medications for dementia with behavioral disturbance or psychosis are listed in Table 7–4. Expert consensus guidelines suggest that the clinician should wait 5–7 days before considering a dose adjustment. Breakthrough agitation can be treated with as-needed medications during that period (see the following subsection). After achieving an adequate level of symptom management, expert consensus guidelines recommend waiting 3 months before attempting a dose reduction (Alexopoulos et al. 2004).

Acutely Dangerous Agitation and Aggression in Dementia

At times, the behavioral disturbance encountered in dementia presents an imminent danger to the patient or others. Usually, this occurs in the setting of ongoing behavioral disturbances for which the patient already may be receiving pharmacotherapy. The clinical approach to the acutely and severely agitated patient should include nonpharmacological interventions, such as attempts to redirect or distract the patient. Although as-needed medications generally should be avoided, as-needed antipsychotics and benzodiazepines are commonly used when the patient's behavior is hazardous. Typically, a patient whose behavior is dangerous would not receive treatment as an outpatient but rather at either a psychiatric inpatient unit or a dementia specialty care unit at a nursing home. Ideally, the family or guardian of the patient would have been informed of and consented to the potential risks (stroke, mortality) in anticipation of the need for as-needed antipsychotics. Possible as-needed medication regimens include olanzapine 2.5–5 mg orally or 5 mg intramuscularly; risperidone 0.5–1 mg orally; haloperidol 0.25–2 mg orally or intramuscularly; or lorazepam 0.5–1 mg orally or intramuscularly. Oral disintegrating forms are preferred over tablet form; intramuscular injections should be given only if the patient refused oral medication. After receiving an as-needed dose, the patient should be closely monitored for side effects and for symptom resolution.

Parkinson's Disease

Antipsychotic medications can be used in Parkinson's disease to manage psychosis and to manage disorders of impulse control.

Psychosis

Psychosis in Parkinson's disease patients who are not taking medications is a rare occurrence. However, in the setting of treatment of motor symptoms with dopaminergic agents, the prevalence of illusions or hallucinations jumps to 15%–40%. Although all medications used to manage the motor symptoms of Parkinson's disease have been implicated (L-dopa, dopamine agonists, monoamine oxidase inhibitors, anticholinergic medications, amantadine) in causing psychosis, dopamine agonists and L-dopa account for most cases (Weintraub and Hurtig 2007).

The presence of psychosis does not necessarily indicate a need for antipsychotic treatment. Often patients with Parkinson's disease experience visual perceptual changes or hallucinations, usually of formed animal or human figures, and retain insight into the unreal nature of these symptoms. If patients with Parkinson's disease are not bothered by these symptoms, they probably do not require treatment. However, use of antipsychotic medication is indicated when the patient is clearly distressed by the psychosis or when the psychosis makes the patient a danger to self or others or impairs the patient's functional abilities.

The first step in the management of Parkinson's disease psychosis is to reduce or discontinue antiparkinsonian medications, if possible. Generally, dopamine agonists are the first medication class targeted for reduction or discontinuation, followed by anticholinergic medications, amantadine, and monoamine oxidase inhibitors. L-Dopa is reduced only if other medication adjustments fail to reduce the psychosis.

Second-line treatment would involve initiating an SGA. FGAs are avoided because of the risk of worsening motor symptoms. Clozapine has the strongest evidence supporting its use for treatment of psychosis in Parkinson's disease and does not worsen motor symptoms or cognition. However, clozapine must be used with caution. In addition to the concern regarding agranulocytosis and the increased risk of death when SGAs are prescribed to elderly patients with dementia, approximately 25% of older patients who receive clozapine experience orthostatic hypotension and tachycardia. In addition, the elderly may be particularly susceptible to problematic anticholinergic side effects. Ziprasidone's efficacy has been suggested by small case reports; it does not seem to worsen motor symptoms. Quetiapine is commonly used and frequently listed as a first-line choice in expert consensus guidelines; however, two placebo-controlled trials have not shown benefit with quetiapine. Olanzapine and aripiprazole also have failed to show efficacy for psychosis in Parkinson's disease and often worsen motor symptoms. Some evidence suggests that cholinesterase inhibitors may treat psychosis in patients with Parkinson's disease without exacerbating motor symptoms (Weintraub and Hurtig 2007).

Impulse-Control Disorders

There is growing recognition of impulse-control disorders occurring in the setting of Parkinson's disease, which may be the result of dopamine-stimulating drugs. The impaired impulse control may manifest itself as a gambling addiction or hypersexuality. Gambling addiction afflicts 0.5%–5% of patients with Parkinson's disease. Treatment of pathological gambling involves discontinuation or reduction of dopamine-stimulating drugs, if possible, in addition to addiction counseling. No data support the use of antipsychotic medication for gambling addiction.

Hypersexuality may manifest itself as constant desire for sexual intercourse, excessive viewing of pornography, frequenting prostitutes, partaking in Internet sex chats, or paraphilias. Treatment strategies include reduction or discontinuation of dopaminergic agonists in addition to counseling offered to the patient and his or her family. Case reports suggest that antipsychotic medications may be useful in reducing inappropriate sexual behavior (Stamey and Jankovic 2008).

Dementia With Lewy Bodies

Dementia with Lewy bodies is clinically characterized by the presence of significant cognitive decline, parkinsonian motor features, fluctuations in cognition, and recurrent visual hallucinations. Approximately 75% of patients with DLB experience hallucinations, which are typically colorful images of people or animals. Approximately 50% of DLB patients experience delusions (Weintraub and Hurtig 2007). Many DLB patients are sensitive to antipsychotic medications and experience worsening parkinsonism or drowsiness on exposure to either FGAs or SGAs. DLB patients also can have a severe reaction to antipsychotic medications (typical or atypical), which can involve abrupt cognitive decline, acute worsening of parkinsonian symptoms, drowsiness, NMS, and death (Ballard et al. 1998). Some small studies suggest that olanzapine and quetiapine may be effective in improving psychosis without significantly worsening motor symptoms. However, given the risk of a severe reaction to antipsychotic medications, these agents are rarely used in this condition. Cholinesterase inhibitors are first-line therapy for the treatment of psychosis and behavioral disturbance in DLB (Weintraub and Hurtig 2007).

Frontotemporal Dementia

Frontotemporal dementia is a neurodegenerative dementia that accounts for 2%–5% of all dementias. FTD typically presents in patients 40–60 years old. FTD is subtyped on the basis of whether the initial presentation involves predominantly behavioral impairment with concomitant impaired executive function or prominent language impairment. Patients with the behavioral impairment can show poor impulse control, sexual inappropriateness, stereotyped behaviors, compulsions, disinhibition, and mood instability. Selective serotonin reuptake inhibitors and trazodone are considered first-line agents for the behavioral symptoms of FTD. SGAs are used only when first-line treatments fail, because patients with FTD are at risk for significant EPS (Boxer and Boeve 2007).

KEY CLINICAL POINTS

- "Start low and go slow" when initiating an antipsychotic medication to find the optimal dose that balances risks and benefits for the individual patient.

- Antipsychotic doses used to treat psychosis and agitation occurring as part of dementia are typically much lower than the doses used to treat primary psychotic disorders in late life.

- Both SGAs and FGAs are associated with an increased risk of death and stroke or transient ischemic attack among elderly patients with dementia.

- Patients with Parkinson's disease and DLB are extremely sensitive to antipsychotic medications.

- Older patients are at increased risk for antipsychotic-induced parkinsonism and for TD but are at reduced risk for acute dystonia. Akathisia is as common or slightly less common in older patients than in younger patients, but older patients may be at increased risk for developing chronic akathisia.

- Older patients may be more sensitive to the anticholinergic and α_1 blockade side effects of antipsychotic medications, including dry mouth, constipation, urinary retention, confusion, and orthostatic hypotension.

References

Aarsland D, Perry R, Larsen JP, et al: Neuroleptic sensitivity in Parkinson's disease and parkinsonian dementias. J Clin Psychiatry 66:633–637, 2005

Alexopoulos GS, Streim J, Carpenter D, et al: Expert Consensus Guideline Series: Using antipsychotic agents in older patients. J Clin Psychiatry 65 (suppl 2):5–105, 2004

Aziz R, Lorbeg B, Tampi RR. Treatments for late-life bipolar disorder. Am J Geriatr Pharmacother 4:347–364, 2006

Ballard C, Waite J: The effectiveness of atypical antipsychotics for the treatment of aggression and psychosis in Alzheimer's disease. Cochrane Database Syst Rev (1):CD003476, 2006

Ballard C, Grace J, McKeith I, et al: Neuroleptic sensitivity in dementia with Lewy bodies and Alzheimer's disease. Lancet 351:1032–1033, 1998

Boxer AL, Boeve BF: Frontotemporal dementia treatment: current symptomatic therapies and implications of recent genetic, biochemical, and neuroimaging studies. Alzheimer Dis Assoc Disord 21:S79–S87, 2007

Broadway J, Mintzer J: The many faces of psychosis in the elderly. Curr Opin Psychiatry 20:551–558, 2007

Caligiuri MR, Jeste DV, Lacro JP: Antipsychotic-induced movement disorders in the elderly: epidemiology and treatment recommendations. Drugs Aging 17:363–384, 2000

Chew ML, Mulsant BH, Pollock BG, et al: Anticholinergic activity of 107 medications commonly used by older adults. J Am Geriatr Soc 56:1333–1341, 2008

Dayalu P, Chou KL: Antipsychotic-induced extrapyramidal symptoms and their management. Expert Opin Pharmacother 9:1451–1462, 2008

Devanand DP, Jacobs DM, Tang MX, et al: The course of psychopathologic features in mild to moderate Alzheimer disease. Arch Gen Psychiatry 54:257–263, 1997

Etminan M, Streiner DL, Rochon PA: Exploring the association between atypical neuroleptic agents and diabetes mellitus in older adults. Pharmacotherapy 23:1411–1415, 2003

Gill SS, Bronskill SE, Normand SL, et al: Antipsychotic drug use and mortality in older adults with dementia. Ann Intern Med 146:775–786, 2007

Haddad PM, Sharma SG: Adverse effects of atypical antipsychotics: differential risk and clinical implications. CNS Drugs 21:911–936, 2007

Henderson DC, Doraiswamy PM: Prolactin-related and metabolic adverse effects of atypical antipsychotic agents. J Clin Psychiatry 69 (suppl 1):32–44, 2008

Herrmann N, Lanctot KL: Atypical antipsychotics for neuropsychiatric symptoms of dementia: malignant or maligned? Drug Saf 29:833–843, 2006

Jacobson SA, Pies RW, Katz IR (eds): Clinical Manual of Geriatric Psychopharmacology. Washington, DC, American Psychiatric Publishing, 2007

Jeste DV: Tardive dyskinesia rates with atypical antipsychotics in older adults. J Clin Psychiatry 65 (suppl 9):21–24, 2004

Jeste DV, Blazer D, Casey D, et al: ACNP White Paper: update on use of antipsychotic drugs in elderly persons with dementia. Neuropsychopharmacology 33:957–970, 2008

Lanctot KL, Best TS, Mittmann N, et al: Efficacy and safety of neuroleptics in behavioral disorders associated with dementia. J Clin Psychiatry 59:550–561, 1998

Liperoti R, Onder G, Lapane KL, et al: Conventional or atypical antipsychotics and the risk of femur fracture among elderly patients: results of a case-control study. J Clin Psychiatry 68:929–934, 2007

Lonergan E, Luxenberg J, Colford J: Haloperidol for agitation in dementia. Cochrane Database Syst Rev (2):CD002852, 2002

Meyers BS, Flint AJ, Rothschild AJ, et al; STOP-PD Group: A double-blind randomized controlled trial of olanzapine plus sertraline vs olanzapine plus placebo for psychotic depression: the Study of Pharmacotherapy of Psychotic Depression (STOP-PD). Arch Gen Psychiatry 66:838–847, 2009

Miller LJ: The use of cognitive enhancers in behavioral disturbances of Alzheimer's disease. Consult Pharm 22:754–762, 2007

Pfizer Inc: FDA Psychopharmacological Drugs Advisory Committee: Briefing Document for Zeldox Capsules (Ziprasidone HCl). July 19, 2000. Available at: http://www.fda.gov/ohrms/dockets/ac/00/backgrd/3619b1a.pdf. Accessed September 12, 2009.

Pollock BG, Mulsant BH, Rosen J, et al: A double-blind comparison of citalopram and risperidone for the treatment of behavioral and psychotic symptoms associated with dementia. Am J Geriatr Psychiatry 15:942–952, 2007

Rutherford B, Sneed J, Miyazaki M, et al: An open trial of aripiprazole augmentation for SSRI non-remitters with late-life depression. Int J Geriatr Psychiatry 22:986–991, 2007

Schneeweiss S, Setoguchi S, Brookhart A, et al: Risk of death associated with the use of conventional versus atypical antipsychotic drugs among elderly patients (published erratum appears in CMAJ 176:1613, 2007). CMAJ 176:627–632, 2007

Schneider LS, Dagerman K, Insel PS: Efficacy and adverse effects of atypical antipsychotics for dementia: meta-analysis of randomized, placebo-controlled trials. Am J Geriatr Psychiatry 14:191–210, 2006a

Schneider LS, Tariot PN, Dagerman KS, et al: Effectiveness of atypical antipsychotic drugs in patients with Alzheimer's disease. N Engl J Med 355:1525–1538, 2006b

Sheffrin M, Driscoll HC, Lenze EJ, et al: Pilot study of augmentation with aripiprazole for incomplete response in late-life depression: getting to remission. J Clin Psychiatry 70:208–213, 2009

Stamey W, Jankovic J: Impulse control disorders and pathological gambling in patients with Parkinson disease. Neurologist 14:89–99, 2008

Strawn JR, Keck PE Jr, Caroff SN: Neuroleptic malignant syndrome. Am J Psychiatry 164:870–876, 2007

Sultzer DL, Davis SM, Tariot PN, et al, for the CATIE-AD Study Group: Clinical symptom responses to atypical antipsychotic medications in Alzheimer's disease: phase 1 outcomes from the CATIE-AD effectiveness trial. Am J Psychiatry 165:844–854, 2008

Weintraub D, Hurtig HI: Presentation and management of psychosis in Parkinson's disease and dementia with Lewy bodies. Am J Psychiatry 164:1491–1498, 2007

CHAPTER 8

Use of Antipsychotics in Medically Ill Patients

Marcus W. Tjia, M.D.
David F. Gitlin, M.D.

PATIENTS WITH MEDICAL ILLNESSES occasionally require treatment with antipsychotic medications. Compared with patients with primary psychiatric illnesses, a different approach to the use of antipsychotics is needed. In this population, the use of antipsychotic medications may have some role in essentially three general situations:

1. Patients with medical illnesses may have secondary psychiatric illnesses or neuropsychiatric sequelae due to underlying medical conditions.
2. These patients may have comorbid psychiatric illnesses that may require an alternative approach to management in the medical situation.
3. Some patients will present with acute mental status changes in which it is unclear whether their presentation is a result of a primary psychiatric illness, medical illness, or some combination of both.

In all of these situations, antipsychotic medications may play some role but require a unique approach to their use.

Medical Considerations in the Use of Antipsychotics

Drug-Drug Interactions

Most patients with serious medical illnesses are being prescribed a wide range of medications, with polypharmacy being the rule rather than the exception. Hospitalized medical patients may be taking 10 or more medications each day, thus increasing the potential for significant drug-drug interactions. It is often difficult to predict the interaction between even two medications for a given individual. For patients taking multiple medications, it may be virtually impossible to anticipate all of the potential interactions accurately. Therefore, the addition or dosage change of an antipsychotic medication in medically ill patients should be done more cautiously than in patients taking few other medications.

Pharmacokinetics

The effects of medical illness on medication absorption, serum distribution, metabolism, and elimination can be significant. Patients with infectious diseases, low-flow cardiac conditions, or gastrointestinal disorders, including postoperative ileus, may have impaired absorption. Illnesses affecting the liver, including cirrhosis, hepatic carcinoma, and hepatitis, may markedly change both "first-pass" hepatic effects and overall metabolism of virtually all antipsychotic agents. Chronically medically ill patients typically have reduced protein binding, lower albumin levels, a decreased volume of distribution, and decreased perfusion of both the liver and the kidneys, all of which result in changes in antipsychotic distribution.

Routes of Administration

Patients hospitalized in acute medical settings may not be able to take their medications by mouth. Patients who are recovering from gastrointestinal surgery, intubated in the intensive care unit, and in comatose states will require alternative routes of administration of medications. Several of the antipsychotics are available in intramuscular form. Haloperidol and chlorpromazine are available as intravenous preparations and, although this route of administration is not approved by the U.S. Food and Drug Administration (FDA), are widely used. See Table 8–1 for available routes of administration of commonly used antipsychotic medications.

TABLE 8–1. Routes of administration of antipsychotic medications

MEDICATION	ORAL	INTRAMUSCULAR	INTRAVENOUS
Haloperidol	+	+	+
Chlorpromazine	+	+	+
Aripiprazole	+	+	−
Clozapine	+	−	−
Olanzapine	+	+	−
Quetiapine	+	−	−
Risperidone[a]	+	−	−
Ziprasidone	+	+	−

[a]Risperidone available in intramuscular depot preparation but not available for acute treatment.

Metabolic Disorder

Many of the second-generation, or atypical, antipsychotics (SGAs) are associated with hypercholesterolemia, hyperglycemia, and weight gain. For medical patients with these preexisting conditions, use of these agents may result in further dysregulation of glucose and lipid levels. Antipsychotics thus should be used with caution in patients with obesity, coronary artery disease, and diabetes. Although few controlled data regarding the use of SGAs exist in medical populations, agents that are less likely to affect weight and glucose or lipid metabolism should be preferentially used. Clozapine and olanzapine probably should be avoided in these patients because they are most strongly associated with hyperglycemia, hyperlipidemia, and weight gain and may have a greater propensity for the development of type 2 diabetes mellitus. Quetiapine and risperidone also have been associated with hyperglycemia and weight gain. First-generation, or typical, antipsychotics (FGAs) associated with weight gain and hyperglycemia include haloperidol, thioridazine, and chlorpromazine. Agents such as aripiprazole and ziprasidone are associated with a significantly lower risk of these metabolic complications and may be better options in medically at-risk populations.

Sedation

Patients with medical illnesses, particularly those in acute medical settings, commonly experience insomnia and derangements of the sleep-wake cycle. This may be the result of their underlying medical illness, increased pain, or effects from the myriad of medications they are taking. Sleep disturbances often may simply be caused by the commotion of the acute medical setting where endless disturbances (e.g., lights, vital signs checks, blood draws) make regulated sleep nearly impossible. Sedation is a common side effect of most antipsychotic agents. Excess sedation may complicate the treatment plan but may be used effectively in those patients for whom sedation is a desirable effect. Low-potency first-generation antipsychotics are more likely to be sedating. Among the SGAs, olanzapine and quetiapine are the most sedating, and aripiprazole and ziprasidone are the least sedating.

Extrapyramidal Symptoms

In medical settings, antipsychotic agents are commonly used to treat agitated and aggressive states, especially delirium (see the subsection "Delirium" later in this chapter). The potential development of acute extrapyramidal symptoms (EPS) can greatly complicate the care of these patients. An antipsychotic agent may be recommended to manage agitation or delirium, but some patients then may experience a worsening in their psychomotor excitation. The consulting psychiatrist is then faced with a dilemma. Is the increase in agitation a result of a progression of the underlying condition, or is it a result of antipsychotic-induced akathisia, dystonia, or dyskinesia? Patients with underlying medical conditions with indirect central nervous system (CNS) effects, as well as those with primary brain diseases (e.g., dementia, stroke, traumatic brain injury [TBI]), may be exquisitely sensitive to the dopaminergic blockage of antipsychotic agents. SGAs may offer some advantages in this context. Patients who initially received high-potency neuroleptics such as haloperidol can be switched to an SGA if concerns are raised about potential EPS. In particular, quetiapine and aripiprazole, as well as clozapine if necessary, may be least likely to cause EPS.

General Conditions

Delirium

One of the most common but difficult-to-manage conditions seen in acute medical settings is *delirium,* a neuropsychiatric syndrome caused by an acute and global derangement of brain function. The hallmark feature of this brain dysfunction is an impairment of attention and a "waxing and waning" level of consciousness. Other common symptoms include cognitive deficits, psychomotor agitation or retardation, disturbance of the sleep-wake cycle, disorganization of thought, and perceptual abnormalities. It is typically acute in onset, occurring over hours to days with symptoms often worse at night.

Delirium is not a discrete disease but rather a syndrome of characteristic symptoms, reflective of an underlying medical illness. The etiologies of delirium cover the gamut of physiological disturbances including metabolic, neoplastic, infectious, cardiovascular, cerebrovascular, autoimmune, hypoxic, traumatic, and toxic. Common etiologies are drug and medication intoxication and withdrawal states, pneumonia, urinary tract infection, stroke, head injury, hepatic and uremic encephalopathy, and intracerebral lesions. Patients with preexisting brain disease such as dementia, brain injury, and HIV infection, as well as the elderly in general, are particularly at risk for the development of delirium.

The prevalence of delirium varies in different settings but appears to be directly related to the severity of comorbid medical illness. Medically hospitalized inpatients typically have a prevalence rate of 15%–25% (Trzepacz and Meagher 2005), although an extensive review revealed a range from 3% to 42% (Fann 2000). Rates of delirium may be as high as 82% (Trzepacz and Meagher 2005) in high-risk populations such as postoperative, intensive care unit, and organ transplant patients. Most, but not all, studies indicate that delirium is associated with an increased mortality in hospitalized patients, ranging from 4% to 65% (Trzepacz and Meagher 2005). Posthospital follow-up studies suggest increased mortality at 3 months following discharge (Kelly et al. 2001). Increased mortality risk has been associated with comorbid dementia and increased severity of comorbid medical conditions. Thus, delirium is a marker of serious underlying medical illness, which, if not identified and treated, may result in increased morbidity and mortality.

The primary goal in the management of delirium is the treatment of the underlying etiology. However, the etiology is not always readily identifiable, and management of the symptoms of delirium may be necessary during the workup for the primary etiology. Initial approach to management should be focused on supportive and environmental interventions. Consistent efforts should be made to reorient the patient to place, time, and circumstances. Environmental cues such as clocks and calendars can be helpful. High-stimulus environments such as emergency departments and intensive care units can contribute to confusion and disorientation, and excessive stimuli should be minimized when possible. Conversely, excessively low-stimulus environments may not provide adequate orienting cues and thus may worsen delirium. This may explain, in part, why symptoms of delirium appear to be worse at night. Sensory impairments may be a factor, and the addition of hearing and visual aids can significantly reduce delirious symptoms.

When symptoms of delirium place the patient or staff at risk, pharmacotherapy is usually indicated. Most often, this is necessary when patients have hyperactive symptoms, including agitation, aggression, psychosis, and paranoia. The evidence for medication efficacy in the treatment of hyperactive symptoms is greatest with antipsychotic agents. Haloperidol is considered the mainstay of pharmacotherapy treatment for delirium. According to the American Psychiatric Association "Practice Guidelines for the Treatment of Patients With Delirium," the recommended starting dose of haloperidol is 1–2 mg every 2–4 hours as needed (Trzepacz et al. 2002). Most patients typically respond at 5–10 mg/24 hours. For severe agitation, much higher doses may be necessary, and the titration interval may be decreased to as little as every 30–60 minutes. Doses as high as 25 mg/hour up to 1,000 mg/day are well described, usually given as continuous intravenous infusion. This ultrahigh dose approach is considered controversial, is probably associated with more ventricular dysrhythmias, and should be used only in intensive care settings.

The experience of using haloperidol for the management of delirium is quite extensive, even though the FDA has not approved its use for this condition. Haloperidol can be given orally, intramuscularly, or parenterally. Intravenous haloperidol is also commonly used in the treatment of agitated delirium, although this administration route lacks FDA approval for any condition. Evidence indicates that intravenous administration may be associated with fewer EPS than is oral administration. However, this route is likely associated with an increased risk of QT prolongation. Careful electrocardiogram (ECG) monitoring is necessary when intravenous antipsychotics are used, and additional or alternative interventions are indicated when the QTc is greater than 450 ms (see the subsection "Cardiovascular Disease" later in this chapter).

Second-generation antipsychotics are being used with increased regularity in the treatment of delirium. A few smaller studies have reported efficacy with risperidone and olanzapine equal to that of haloperidol. Case reports regarding the use of ziprasidone, quetiapine, and aripiprazole also have shown these agents to be effective. Dosage ranges for the SGAs tend to be lower as compared with doses used for the treatment of psychosis, but again, higher doses may be needed in more refractory cases of delirium. The daily dosages and routes of administration for first- and second-generation antipsychotics used in the treatment of delirium are summarized in Table 8–2.

Most of the SGAs have been associated with QT prolongation. Olanzapine may be less likely to cause this effect, whereas ziprasidone may have a greater association. Early data suggest that aripiprazole may not be associated with QT prolongation, but further studies are needed to determine whether this may be a useful alternative in delirious patients at risk for ventricular dysrhythmias.

Several of the SGAs are available in intramuscular preparations, which may be of particularly utility in delirious patients. Olanzapine, ziprasidone, and aripiprazole can be given in either oral or intramuscular routes of administration.

TABLE 8–2. Pharmacotherapy for delirium

| | ROUTE OF ADMINISTRATION | | | | MAXIMUM DAILY |
MEDICATION	PO	IM	IV	DAILY DOSAGE	DOSE (MG)
First-generation antipsychotics					
Chlorpromazine	+	+	+	12.5–200 mg q 2–8 hours	2,000
Haloperidol[a]	+	+	+	0.5–5 mg q 1–12 hours	50[a]
Second-generation antipsychotics					
Aripiprazole	+	+	–	2–30 mg q 12–24 hours	30
Olanzapine	+	+	–	2.5–20 mg q 6–24 hours	30
Quetiapine	+	–	–	12.5–200 mg q 6–24 hours	800
Risperidone	+	–	–	0.5–3 mg q 6–24 hours	12
Ziprasidone	+	+	–	10–80 mg q 12–24 hours	160

Note. IM=intramuscular; IV=intravenous; PO=oral.
[a]Protocols exist for ultra-high-dose use of haloperidol IV up to 100 mg/hour continuous bolus.
Source. Adapted from Blumenfield and Strain 2006.

Agitation and Aggressive Behavior in Medical Patients

Agitation and aggression in the medical setting are relatively uncommon. Most medical patients with these symptoms have delirium and/or dementia. Management of agitation and aggression in delirium is described in the previous subsection. Patients with dementia often have chronic, intermittent agitation or aggressiveness, which may be symptoms of their dementing disorder. Long-term management is described by Whyte and Madeira in Chapter 7 ("Use of Antipsychotics in Geriatric Patients") in this volume, and the treatment of acute symptoms in dementia is described later in this chapter.

Occasionally, medically ill patients will show aggressive behavior for other reasons. Patients with personality disorders may require medical treatment but may not tolerate the rules and expectations of the hospital setting.

222 THE EVIDENCE-BASED GUIDE TO ANTIPSYCHOTIC MEDICATIONS

This may result in conflicts with hospital staff that may escalate to aggressiveness. Early recognition of personality styles in which aggressiveness is possible may help hospital staff minimize this risk as well as allow them to maintain their safety. Training staff in de-escalation techniques is important and often allows staff to interact with difficult patients in a less adversarial manner. Early intervention with pharmacotherapy sometimes can be useful, and patients should be offered oral medication. When aggressive behaviors do occur, physical restraint may be necessary. Whenever possible, hospital security staff trained in restraint techniques should be used.

When pharmacotherapy is necessary, benzodiazepines are the most commonly used treatment. However, antipsychotic agents also may be of benefit, particularly in combination with a benzodiazepine. Haloperidol is most commonly used and can be highly effective. Typically, patients may receive 2–5 mg either orally or intramuscularly, but smaller doses should be used in the elderly and in patients with CNS disease. Risperidone and olanzapine also can be used. Olanzapine is also available in intramuscular form.

Medical Disorders

Cardiovascular Disease

Antipsychotic medications can be safely and effectively used in patients with cardiovascular disease. Although antipsychotics are commonly used in patients with primary psychiatric disorders and concurrent cardiovascular disease, these medications are also extremely effective in the treatment of delirium in the context of acute cardiac illness such as congestive heart failure, arrhythmias, or after cardiac surgery (see the subsection "Delirium" earlier in this chapter for the treatment of general delirium). Cardiac side effects of neuroleptics are primarily caused by antagonism at α_1-adrenergic receptors as well as potential prolongation of the QT interval.

α_1-Adrenergic blockade may cause several clinical problems, particularly in patients with preexisting cardiovascular disease. Orthostatic hypotension and dizziness, which may be independent of or secondary to orthostasis, may lead to neurocardiogenic syncope or falls. In addition, the decline in blood pressure that may occur with α-adrenergic and cholinergic blockade may increase cardiac workload, potentially leading to angina in predisposed patients.

Of the antipsychotics, the low-potency FGAs, such as chlorpromazine, are most commonly associated with orthostatic hypotension. The high-potency agents, such as haloperidol, largely avoid any α blockade and any resulting complications. The SGAs cause only minimal α blockade with the exception of clozapine, which is capable of inducing significant hypotension and dizziness. Quetiapine and, to a lesser extent, olanzapine and risperidone are also associated with orthostasis and dizziness.

In patients who may be particularly vulnerable to the side effects of α blockade, such as the elderly and patients with autonomic dysfunction, antipsychotics should be initiated at low doses with slow titration and close monitoring of vital signs.

One of the most frequent topics of discussion in administering antipsychotics to medically ill patients is the potential for QT interval prolongation. The QT interval represents the time of repolarization of the myocardium, and the QTc interval represents the QT adjusted for heart rate. A QTc interval of 450 ms is considered to be the upper limit of normal, whereas an interval of 500 ms or greater is associated with an increased risk of developing the polymorphic ventricular arrhythmia torsades de pointes. Although sometimes self-limiting, torsades de pointes may degenerate into ventricular fibrillation and sudden cardiac death. Other risk factors for torsades de pointes include hypokalemia, hypomagnesemia, hypocalcemia, family history of sudden death, and low ejection fraction. In addition, several other medications such as tricyclic antidepressants, fluoroquinolones, methadone, and several class IA and III antiarrhythmics are known to prolong the QTc interval (Mackin 2008).

Among the antipsychotics, thioridazine is well known to induce the greatest increase in QTc, has been associated with numerous cases of torsades de pointes and sudden death, and was given a black-box warning by the FDA for this reason. Haloperidol also has been associated with prolonged QTc and several reported cases of torsades de pointes (Glassman and Bigger 2001). However, a study by Harrigan et al. (2004) for the FDA evaluated the effects of six antipsychotic drugs on the QTc interval and found haloperidol to have the lowest mean increase in QTc among the six studied drugs (see Table 8–3). Despite its apparent predilection to prolong QTc, ziprasidone's association with torsades de pointes and sudden death is unclear. Data on aripiprazole's effect on QTc are scarce, but aripiprazole thus far appears to have limited cardiotoxicity.

It is recommended that a baseline ECG be obtained in all medically ill patients receiving antipsychotics. Electrolytes should be fully repleted, specifically potassium and magnesium, and other potential QTc-prolonging medications identified. Once antipsychotic treatment has been initiated, a QTc interval greater than 440 ms or an increased QTc interval 25% above baseline warrants close monitoring and elimination of any unnecessary QTc-prolonging factors, including other medications. An interval of 500 ms or more may indicate the need for either cardiology consultation or transition to an alternative psychotropic medication, including nonantipsychotics.

Clozapine warrants special consideration in cardiac disease, as in numerous other medical conditions. Aside from its significant risk of agranulocyto-

TABLE 8–3. Effect of antipsychotic drugs on QTc interval

MEDICATION	MEAN INCREASE IN QTC FROM BASELINE AT STEADY STATE (MS)
Haloperidol	4.7
Olanzapine	6.8
Quetiapine	14.5
Risperidone	11.6
Thioridazine	35.6
Ziprasidone	20.3

Source.   Adapted from Harrigan et al. 2004. Other antipsychotic medications were not included in the study.

sis, clozapine may cause dose-related tachycardia and orthostasis secondary to its considerable anticholinergic load. In addition, it carries an increased risk of myocarditis and cardiomyopathy, with several reported cases of fatal cardiac conditions precipitated by its use (Mackin 2008). In patients with significant cardiac disease, clozapine should be used with extreme caution.

Renal Disease

Despite the complex physiological changes that occur in renal insufficiency, most antipsychotic medications are minimally excreted in urine and require little dose adjustment in patients with renal failure. However, patients with chronic renal failure may have heightened sensitivity to medication side effects and often have comorbid illnesses and symptoms, such as diabetes and hypotension, that require consideration in medication administration. In general, clinicians should consider abiding by the "rule of two-thirds" in dosing most psychotropics in renal failure—use only two-thirds of the dose used for patients with normal renal function (Levenson 2005).

In regard to dialysis, all antipsychotics are lipophilic compounds and are thus not dialyzable. However, the dramatic fluid shifts that may occur around dialysis make these patients even more vulnerable to side effects such as hypotension and sedation. Low-potency FGAs such as chlorpromazine should be used with extreme caution in patients with renal failure, and specifically those receiving dialysis, because of the increased risk of orthostasis, urinary retention, and sedation.

Renal failure has only a minimal effect on the pharmacokinetics of most FGAs, as well as olanzapine, quetiapine, aripiprazole, and clozapine (Cohen et al. 2004). These medications can be used safely in renal insufficiency.

Risperidone is the only antipsychotic that requires definitive dose adjustment in renal insufficiency as recommended by its manufacturer. Clearance of the drug and its active metabolite is decreased by 60% in renal failure (Wyszynski and Wyszynski 2005). It is recommended that initial doses be no more than 0.5 mg twice a day, with individual dose increases of no more than 0.5 mg twice a day (Janssen 2002). Increased doses beyond 1.5 mg twice a day should be made no more often than once per week. If once-a-day dosing is preferred in the elderly or frail, the manufacturer recommends beginning with twice-a-day dosing before switching to a cumulative single daily dose.

The pharmacokinetics of ziprasidone are not significantly affected by renal failure. However, the electrolyte shifts that may occur in renal insufficiency, and specifically in patients reliant on dialysis, may increase the risk of fatal cardiac arrhythmias related to QT prolongation (Cohen et al. 2004). Ziprasidone is therefore a less desirable option in these patients. Electrolytes, specifically potassium, calcium, and magnesium, should be closely monitored when using ziprasidone in patients with renal failure.

Hepatic Insufficiency

All antipsychotics, both typical and atypical, are metabolized primarily by the liver through phase I and phase II metabolism. Phase I metabolism consists of oxidation (via the cytochrome P450 [CYP] isoenzyme family), reduction, or hydrolysis of the drug compound. Phase II metabolism produces mostly inactive compounds via several conjugation and acetylation pathways. Hepatic insufficiency, whether due to alcoholic cirrhosis, acute hepatitis, or other causes, can therefore affect the clearance of all antipsychotic drugs.

The classic adage "start low, go slow" best describes the recommended approach in dosing antipsychotics in patients with significant hepatic failure, with the expectation that clearance may be decreased, resulting in plasma drug levels higher than what might be expected in a healthy individual. Nevertheless, for mild to moderate hepatic insufficiency, haloperidol has been known to be well tolerated without significant dose adjustment. Among the SGAs, respective drug manufacturers recommend no dose changes for olanzapine, aripiprazole, or ziprasidone (Crone et al. 2006; Levenson 2005). Risperidone should be started at a reduced dose of 0.5 mg twice a day (Levenson 2005). Quetiapine should be initiated at a dosage of 25 mg/day, with increases of no more than 50 mg/day (Levenson 2005).

The Child-Pugh score is a measure frequently used by hepatologists to categorize the severity of liver dysfunction. As a standardized measure generalizable to all patients with hepatic failure regardless of etiology, it can be a useful guideline in determining appropriate antipsychotic dosing in patients with severe liver dysfunction. It has been suggested that patients with class

A liver failure may tolerate and respond to 75%–100% of a normal starting dose. Class B patients should be started at 50%–75% of a standard dose (Crone et al. 2006). Hepatic encephalopathy is often present in patients with class C disease, and antipsychotics should be dosed cautiously, avoiding any agents that may worsen delirium such as low-potency phenothiazines.

All antipsychotics may be associated with transient asymptomatic increases in liver aminotransferase levels. Several agents, including quetiapine, olanzapine, risperidone, clozapine, and the phenothiazines, have been implicated in rare cases of acute hepatotoxicity and cholestasis (Wright and Vandenberg 2007). Clearly, when an antipsychotic appears to be playing a role in worsening hepatic functioning, prompt discontinuation of that medication is warranted. Among the SGAs, clozapine may be the most likely to cause hepatotoxicity and should be used warily in those who already have hepatic failure (Wright and Vandenberg 2007). Phenothiazines have been found frequently to exacerbate hepatotoxicity or induce cholestasis and are contraindicated in patients with significant liver disease (Wyszynski and Wyszynski 2005).

Pulmonary Disease

Antipsychotics can be useful tools in the treatment of patients with pulmonary disease. Delirium is a frequent occurrence in pulmonary patients in the intensive care unit setting (see the subsection "Delirium" earlier in this chapter for information on the general treatment of delirium). Antipsychotics also may be extremely helpful in the treatment of patients who struggle with both anxiety and dyspnea, which often exacerbate each other. Although benzodiazepines are often the most effective agents in the treatment of these comorbid symptoms, the risk of respiratory depression may be a significant concern in particular patients. Antipsychotics may be extremely helpful in these situations, particularly in the weaning of anxious patients from mechanical ventilation. Evidence for this practice is limited to anecdotal data and case reports in the literature. Quetiapine at dosages of up to 100 mg three times a day was shown to facilitate quickly and successfully the weaning of an anxious, nondelirious patient from mechanical ventilation who had extreme anxiety not responsive to trials of lorazepam and clonazepam (Rosenthal et al. 2007).

None of the FGAs or SGAs cause respiratory depression and thus can be used safely in patients who have shown evidence of respiratory depression with benzodiazepines. Although extremely rare, the high-potency antipsychotics carry the risk of laryngeal dystonia and tardive dyskinesia with respiratory musculature involvement. EPS should be monitored closely in these patients. The anticholinergic effects of the low-potency FGAs may affect the pulmonary system by drying secretions. Clozapine has been associated with allergic rhinitis and respiratory depression, particularly when used in conjunction with benzodiazepines. Close monitoring is advised when clozapine is used in patients with respiratory failure.

Pregnancy and Breast-Feeding

The use of antipsychotics in pregnancy and breast-feeding requires both a thoughtful clinician and a well-informed patient (see Appendix 9 for detailed information). An extremely limited amount of data supporting their use in the pregnant or lactating female, coupled with the potential adverse effects to not only the patient but also an unborn fetus or newborn infant, requires the clinician to do a careful risk-benefit analysis when using antipsychotic medications in this population. Adding to this calculation is the fact that untreated serious psychiatric disorders may lead to poor prenatal care, increased risk to the fetus and child, and impairment in the patient's parenting ability (Hales et al. 2008). In fact, schizophrenia, independent of medication exposure, has been shown to increase the risk of congenital malformations and fetal demise (Altshuler et al. 1996).

The use of low-potency phenothiazines during the first trimester has been shown to increase the baseline risk of congenital anomalies by a relatively small 0.4% (Wyszynski and Wyszynski 2005). In contrast, the high-potency FGAs have not been associated with an increased rate of congenital malformations. Animal studies have shown evidence of neurobehavioral teratogenicity with the use of FGAs, although no data suggest that this also occurs in humans. Case studies have reported a low incidence of perinatal side effects in newborns, including sedation, tachycardia, irritability, restlessness, impaired feeding, and jaundice, with the use of FGAs, specifically the low-potency medications.

The data on SGAs in pregnancy are limited to a single prospective comparative study and several case reports. In the comparative study (McKenna et al. 2005), none of the studied drugs (olanzapine, risperidone, quetiapine, and clozapine) were associated with a significantly increased risk of major congenital malformations, although they were associated with lower birth weight and an increased rate of therapeutic abortions. Case reports have supported the impression that risperidone, olanzapine, and quetiapine are potentially safe in pregnant women. No information supports or discourages the use of aripiprazole and ziprasidone in pregnancy. Note that all of the SGAs may be capable of causing the same perinatal effects associated with the FGAs detailed earlier. A concern specific to the use of SGAs is the potential for hyperglycemia and impaired glucose metabolism, which may put a pregnant female at risk for gestational diabetes.

Trihexyphenidyl and benztropine, two anticholinergic medications often used to treat EPS caused by antipsychotics, have been associated with minor congenital malformations, urinary retention, and functional bowel obstruction in newborns (Hales et al. 2008). Diphenhydramine, however, has been shown to be relatively safe in pregnant women and is therefore the treatment of choice for EPS in this population.

In summary, few data are available to inform the clinician in the treatment of psychotic symptoms during pregnancy. A minimal amount of information exists on the use of SGAs in pregnancy. FGAs, specifically the high-potency agents such as haloperidol, are therefore recommended as the first line of treatment in this patient population. Women attempting to conceive should be transitioned from atypical to typical agents before conception. SGAs should be reserved for patients who have not responded to FGAs or are at high risk for relapse if transitioned off their SGA. In general, antipsychotics should be used during pregnancy only when needed; a single agent should be used at the lowest doses possible and for the shortest amount of time necessary to control symptoms adequately.

All antipsychotics are expressed in the breast milk, but little is known about their effects on developing infants. A single controlled trial has been done in a small group of infants exposed to FGAs through breast milk, and a minority showed developmental delays up to age 18 months (Yoshida et al. 1998). Many of the FGAs have long half-lives, which would make a nursing infant vulnerable to drug accumulation and subsequent sedation along with other side effects. No studies have examined the effects of SGAs on breast-feeding infants. Given the lack of knowledge regarding antipsychotics and breast-feeding, it is recommended that women being treated with any antipsychotic avoid breast-feeding if possible. If these medications are used during breast-feeding, infants should be closely monitored for sedation and motor abnormalities such as rigidity and tremor.

Dementia

Agitation, aggression, delusions, and hallucinations are unfortunately common in patients with dementia. In the acute medical setting, the psychiatric consultant is frequently asked to help manage such behaviors and symptoms in these often confused and frightened patients. In addition to the cognitive impairment caused by their primary dementing illness, these patients are prone to delirium with even slight changes in their medical status, often resulting in the emergence or worsening of behavioral issues or psychotic symptoms. The first step in the treatment of agitation and psychosis in dementia is to address any reversible and treatable processes such as infection, metabolic disturbances, or pain.

The use of antipsychotics in the elderly with dementia is discussed in detail by Whyte and Madeira in Chapter 7. No FDA-approved antipsychotics are currently designated for the treatment of dementia-related agitation or psychosis. A few studies have shown that FGAs and SGAs may be effective in the treatment of specific symptoms related to dementia (Schneider et al. 2006; Sultzer et al. 2008). However, both classes of drugs also have been associated with an increased risk of stroke and death in this population, and neither has shown efficacy in improving long-term functioning or quality of life (Rochon et al. 2008; Schneider et al. 2006). The risk of stroke may be greater with the use of atypical as compared with typical agents. It is important to note that studies thus far have focused on outpatient populations rather than medically hospitalized patients with dementia.

Nevertheless, when agitation or psychotic symptoms become severely distressing or dangerous, and when nonpharmacological treatments have failed, the use of antipsychotics may be necessary. Patients with dementia may be more prone to EPS and the anticholinergic and cardiovascular side effects of these medications. The low-potency FGAs are therefore less attractive options. Haloperidol is the most extensively used agent in this population, and the availability of intravenous administration provides a reasonable option in the extremely agitated and noncompliant patient. SGAs are becoming increasingly common in the treatment of dementia despite the identified risks mentioned earlier.

Given the physical and neurocognitive impairments of these patients as well as the potential decreased renal clearance and slowed hepatic metabolism that come with aging, any antipsychotic should be started at one-quarter to one-half of the standard starting dose, with dose increases carried out slowly. The need for ongoing use of these medications should be constantly reassessed, and medications should be discontinued as soon as possible. Most importantly, physicians should thoroughly discuss the risks and benefits of these drugs with caregivers and family before prescribing antipsychotics to patients with dementia.

Parkinson's Disease

The use of antipsychotic medications in Parkinson's disease is a challenging, yet often necessary, endeavor. Psychosis, agitation, and delirium are common in patients with Parkinson's disease. The first step in the assessment of any mental status change in these patients is a thorough review of their antiparkinsonian medications. Dose reduction or discontinuation of these medications, specifically dopamine agonists, may significantly improve distressing neuropsychiatric symptoms. When decreases in the dosages of antiparkinsonian agents are not possible, antipsychotics may be extremely helpful in the management of both acute and chronic symptoms. Unfortunately, dopaminergic blockade, the primary mechanism of action of antipsychotics, may significantly worsen parkinsonian symptoms. This unfortunate conundrum places significant limitations on the clinician's choice of antipsychotic medications.

FGAs, specifically the high-potency agents, are well known to worsen the motor symptoms of Parkinson's disease and are therefore not recommended in these patients. Several studies have found significant worsening of Parkinson's motor symptoms without improvement in psychosis with the use of olanzapine and risperidone. Neither of these agents can be recommended in this population. Originally thought to be a potential savior in the treatment of psychosis associated with Parkinson's disease because of its partial agonism at dopamine D_2 receptors, aripiprazole showed a lack of antipsychotic efficacy along with actual worsening of motor symptoms in two small studies. Ziprasidone has not been formally studied in this patient group, although a small case series suggested an improvement in neuropsychiatric symptoms without worsening of parkinsonism (Weintraub and Hurtig 2007).

Clozapine has been the most studied antipsychotic in the treatment of psychosis associated with Parkinson's disease. Low-dose clozapine has been found to be significantly more efficacious than placebo without worsening motor symptoms or overall cognitive functioning. Anecdotal evidence, however, has suggested that quetiapine can be effective as an antipsychotic agent in these patients. Quetiapine has been studied in two placebo-controlled trials. Although quetiapine did not clearly show efficacy in the treatment of psychotic symptoms, it did not worsen the symptoms of Parkinson's disease.

In summary, clozapine is the only antipsychotic that has shown efficacy in the treatment of psychosis associated with Parkinson's disease (Weintraub and Hurtig 2007). However, the need for frequent blood tests because of the risk of agranulocytosis, along with the potential for sedation and even delirium, make it a less than ideal choice in this often tenuous disease. Quetiapine is now considered by some as a first-line agent in the treatment of psychosis and agitation associated with Parkinson's disease. Starting dosages of quetiapine should be 12.5–25 mg/day with titration carried out in a slow and deliberate manner while closely monitoring for potential side effects, including sedation, orthostasis, or worsening parkinsonism. Clozapine should be reserved for those patients who have not responded to or are unable to tolerate quetiapine.

How long Parkinson's disease patients should continue taking antipsychotics once psychotic symptoms remit remains unclear. In a single case series, most psychiatrically stable patients tapered off antipsychotics experienced a relatively quick recurrence of psychosis, some with symptoms worse than during their initial psychotic episode (Weintraub and Hurtig 2007). Many patients may require maintenance antipsychotic treatment with the goal of tapering medications to the lowest necessary doses.

Traumatic Brain Injury

Although the use of antipsychotics in TBI is not without controversy, they remain an important tool in the treatment of the various neuropsychiatric sequelae of TBI. Animal studies have shown a negative effect on neuronal recovery in TBI with the use of these drugs. In the human literature, a small amount of evidence suggests negative effects on stroke and TBI recovery (Elovic et al. 2003). However, these studies examined only FGAs. To date, little evidence indicates that SGAs negatively affect the rehabilitation of patients with TBI.

Although all antipsychotics are known to be efficacious in the treatment of psychosis in TBI, evidence also supports their use in other symptoms of head injury, including acute delirium, mania, anxiety, tic disorders, persistent aggression, and mood instability. Case studies of quetiapine, olanzapine, risperidone, and clozapine have highlighted their effectiveness in this population (Kim and Bijlani 2006; Levenson 2005; Oster et al. 2007).

The use of antipsychotics to treat aggression associated with TBI-induced psychosis is well supported. However, the use of antipsychotics in nonpsychotic aggression due to TBI is more controversial. Some have argued that these medications are overused in these instances, and the benefits of their use lie in their sedative side effects rather than any antiaggression properties. However, a pilot study of quetiapine in the treatment of TBI-related aggression reported significant efficacy at doses of 25–300 mg/day, with only short-term sedation and no emergent cognitive impairments (Kim and Bijlani 2006).

Patients with TBI are potentially more sensitive to the side effects of antipsychotics, specifically anticholinergic effects and EPS. The use of antipsychotics is also complicated by the potential increased seizure risk in these brain-injured patients, and particular caution must be taken, especially when using clozapine. The risk of increased seizures with various antipsychotics is discussed in the subsection "Epilepsy" later in this chapter.

Because of the increased risk of EPS, as well as the question of impaired recovery with FGAs, SGAs are recommended in the treatment of TBI-related symptoms. Only a short duration of treatment may be needed in the acute postinjury stage, but chronic treatment with antipsychotics may be indicated to address the potentially persistent neuropsychiatric sequelae of TBI such as mood instability, aggression, and psychosis.

HIV Disease

Few controlled trials are available in the literature to guide the clinician in the use of antipsychotics in HIV-infected individuals. Psychiatric symptoms in patients with HIV may be the result of a primary psychiatric process or a multitude of HIV-related illnesses such as HIV-associated dementia; CNS lymphoma; or delirium due to CNS infection with toxoplasmosis, cytomegalovirus (CMV), or *Cryptococcus neoformans*. Regardless of etiology, the clinician faces significant challenges in treating neuropsychiatric symptoms in these often seriously ill patients.

Although patients with HIV may respond to lower-than-standard doses of antipsychotics, they also have been shown to be more sensitive to the side effects of these medications, particularly EPS. Degeneration of the basal ganglia and the related loss of CNS dopaminergic neurons found in HIV infection may explain this finding (Levenson 2005). In one study, patients with HIV or AIDS treated with FGAs, even at low doses, were more than twice as likely to develop EPS or tardive dyskinesia as were patients without AIDS (Dolder et al. 2004). In contrast, several studies have reported the successful use of SGAs at low doses without significantly increased rates of EPS. The most frequently examined SGAs thus far have been risperidone, olanzapine, and clozapine (Wyszynski and Wyszynski 2005).

Unfortunately, one possible side effect of SGAs is the metabolic syndrome, which is also a potential side effect of the drugs used in highly active antiretroviral therapy (HAART), specifically protease inhibitors. The risks of dyslipidemia and impaired glucose metabolism are potentially compounded in patients receiving both SGAs and antiretrovirals. Monitoring of patients' metabolic profiles is critical in the continued use of these agents.

Little is known about the direct interactions between antipsychotics and antiretrovirals. All protease inhibitors and non-nucleoside reverse transcriptase inhibitors are metabolized by the CYP system, and all possess either enzyme-inhibiting or enzyme-inducing properties that can affect plasma levels of many antipsychotics (Thompson et al. 2006). It is not clear how frequently antipsychotics affect antiretroviral plasma levels. Ritonavir, a protease inhibitor, was shown to decrease plasma levels of olanzapine significantly as a result of the induction of the CYP1A2 liver enzyme (Repetto and Pettito 2008). Higher doses of olanzapine may be required when used in conjunction with ritonavir. In contrast, ritonavir has been shown to increase the concentrations of clozapine and pimozide, which may lead to toxicity with either agent (Thompson et al. 2006).

Note that even though clozapine has been shown to be efficacious in treating psychosis in HIV-infected patients, it is generally contraindicated in patients with HIV and AIDS because of the risk of agranulocytosis in these already immunocompromised patients.

In summary, SGAs may represent an improved treatment option over FGAs in patients with HIV because of the decreased risk of EPS. However, the possible risk of metabolic syndrome and potential interactions with antiretroviral agents make close monitoring of side effects imperative in the use of SGAs. HIV-infected patients may respond to antipsychotic medications at lower-than-standard doses but also may be more sensitive to side effects. Low starting doses and the slow titration of any antipsychotic medication are recommended.

Epilepsy

The assessment and treatment of psychiatric symptoms in the context of epilepsy are complicated by several issues. The epileptic syndrome may include many neuropsychiatric signs and symptoms, both intrinsic and extrinsic to the primary neurological disease. In addition, all antipsychotics may alter the seizure threshold, and many may interact with antiepileptic drugs. Psychotic symptoms may occur throughout the various stages of the epileptic syndrome. Identifying the stage in which such symptoms occur in a particular patient helps dictate whether treatment with an antipsychotic is indicated.

Postictal psychiatric disturbances occur in approximately 8%–10% of seizure patients, with psychosis being the most common symptom (Stern et al. 2004). Postictal psychosis is often mild and transient and usually can be contained by appropriate adjustment of antiepileptic drugs and regulation of sleep. Interictal psychosis is defined as psychotic symptoms not directly linked to ictal events. Interictal psychosis is sometimes brief and recurrent but more commonly follows a chronic course and often shares features with schizophrenia. Paranoid delusions and visual and auditory hallucinations are common. Because interictal psychiatric symptoms are more frequent in the context of poorly controlled seizures, appropriate antiepileptic drug therapy remains the first line of treatment for interictal psychosis.

A paucity of evidence-based literature is available to guide the clinician in the systematic use of antipsychotics for epilepsy-related psychoses. However, anecdotal information and clinical experience have provided some generally accepted guidelines. For severe acute psychosis and agitation, such that may occur in postictal states or during antiepileptic drug withdrawal, a high-potency neuroleptic, such as haloperidol, may be indicated. The more persistent symptoms of interictal psychosis may be treated successfully with SGAs to minimize potential side effects such as EPS. Higher doses of risperidone may be needed because of hepatic enzyme induction and subsequent increased metabolism by some antiepileptic drugs (Koch-Stoecker 2002). Metabolism of quetiapine takes place via the CYP3A4 enzyme, which also may lead to potential interactions with several antiepileptic drugs.

The probability of drug-induced increased seizure frequency varies among antipsychotic drugs and appears to be dose related. Determining the seizure risk of an individual drug is difficult because of the paucity of standardized data. Chlorpromazine appears to carry the highest risk of seizure among the FGAs, whereas haloperidol is thought to be less seizure-provoking. Among the SGAs, quetiapine, risperidone, and olanzapine appear to have a low to negligible risk of inducing seizures (Koch-Stoecker 2002). Nevertheless, starting at low doses and carefully titrating upward is prudent, with the goal of using the lowest possible dose.

Clozapine is undoubtedly the SGA with the highest risk for increased seizure frequency. In addition, the risk of agranulocytosis with its use can be increased in combination with some antiepileptic drugs, particularly carbamazepine. For these reasons, the use of clozapine is generally warranted only in nonresponders to all other antipsychotic drugs. Patients should be fully educated about the risks associated with clozapine. When used, it should be introduced slowly with frequent electroencephalogram monitoring for increased seizure activity.

The use of antipsychotics in epilepsy has been proved to be safe and efficacious when carried out in a thoughtful and appropriate manner. Treatment in conjunction with a patient's neurologist and frequent reassessment of the need for antipsychotic treatment are imperative in this disorder in which psychiatric symptoms are often closely linked to the particular stage of neurological illness.

Rheumatologic Disorders

The efficacy of antipsychotics in the treatment of psychiatric symptoms related to rheumatologic disorders is supported by several case reports. Acute psychosis has been documented in cases of Behçet's disease, polyarteritis nodosa, scleroderma, and, most frequently, systemic lupus erythematosus (SLE). Such symptoms can be caused not only by the primary illness process but also by secondary etiologies such as medications, infections, and metabolic derangements resulting in delirium.

When psychotic symptoms are due to CNS involvement of the primary rheumatologic disease, treatment with antipsychotics in conjunction with appropriate steroid and immunosuppressant regimens has been shown to be effective. Because of the elevated risk of EPS with FGAs, SGAs may be the preferred treatment in these complicated illnesses. Olanzapine and risperidone have been reported to be effective at moderate doses in the treatment of psychosis in SLE (Pinto et al. 2006).

Patients with SLE also may be at increased risk for agranulocytosis with the use of antipsychotics, thus making the use of clozapine in these patients particularly problematic. Agranulocytosis also has been reported in lupus patients taking olanzapine (Su et al. 2007).

Antipsychotics, particularly phenothiazines, have been linked to the development of positive antinuclear and antiphospholipid antibodies. Drug-induced lupus has been identified in patients who received chlorpromazine, promethazine, clozapine, and ziprasidone and who previously did not have SLE (Pinto et al. 2006; Wolfe et al. 2004).

It has been estimated that two-thirds of neuropsychiatric symptoms in SLE may be due to secondary causes as opposed to the primary illness (Lesser et al. 1997). Corticosteroids are the most infamous culprit, capable of causing affective instability as well as florid mania and psychosis. The use of antipsychotics in steroid-induced psychiatric symptoms is discussed in the following subsection.

Steroid-Induced Psychiatric Symptoms

A vast number of medications are known to precipitate psychiatric symptoms, but the most notorious are corticosteroids. Used in the treatment of a myriad of medical illnesses, steroids can induce a variety of psychiatric states ranging from mild depressed mood and irritability to full-blown mania and psychosis.

The single most important predictive risk factor of steroid-induced psychiatric symptoms is steroid dose, specifically greater than 60 mg of prednisone or its equivalent. Surprisingly, neither psychiatric history nor previous steroid-induced complications, or the lack thereof, reliably predict future steroid-related psychiatric decompensation (Warrington and Bostwick 2006).

The initial treatment of steroid-induced psychiatric complications is discontinuation or reduction of steroid dosage, if possible. When continued steroid administration is necessary, or when psychiatric symptoms continue even with the discontinuation or reduction of steroids, use of psychotropic medications may be indicated. Both typical and atypical antipsychotics have been shown to reduce the severity of several psychiatric symptoms related to steroids and to shorten the duration of such episodes.

The FGAs have been well documented as efficacious in the treatment of steroid-induced mood instability and frank psychosis; chlorpromazine, thioridazine, and haloperidol are most frequently cited (Wyszynski and Wyszynski 2005). The use of both low- and high-potency agents has been described, but high-potency agents such as haloperidol are generally preferred because of their side-effect profile.

The development of SGAs has resulted in multiple relatively new options in the treatment of steroid-induced psychiatric disturbances. Thus far, olanzapine has been most frequently reported in the literature as being useful in this context and specifically in patients with manic or psychotic symptoms. Case reports also have supported the use of risperidone. A recent open-label trial found that olanzapine at moderate doses was effective in treating both mixed and manic symptoms in a small cohort of patients taking corticosteroids (Brown et al. 2004). Additionally, olanzapine was well tolerated with no significant changes in metabolic parameters such as weight or blood glucose levels. However, the risk of hyperglycemia and lipid abnormalities with SGAs may be compounded with the concomitant use of steroids, and close monitoring is indicated.

Both typical and atypical antipsychotics have shown efficacy in the treatment of steroid-induced mood and psychotic symptoms. Metabolic parameters such as weight, lipid levels, and especially glucose levels should be closely monitored when using SGAs and steroids simultaneously. Mood disturbances may require only low to moderate doses of neuroleptics, whereas florid psychosis and agitation may respond only to higher doses.

Burns and Trauma

Although literature on the use of antipsychotics in burn and trauma patients is limited, these medications can be valuable tools in the treatment of these often critically ill patients. The tranquilizing effects of neuroleptics may be useful in addressing agitation, anxiety, delirium, and insomnia in trauma patients. In burn patients, 10%–30% may experience delirium, often in the initial stages after injury (Stern et al. 2004). (See the subsection "Delirium" earlier in this chapter for specific recommendations in the treatment of delirium.)

Because of its high potency and availability in intravenous form, haloperidol has historically been the most commonly used antipsychotic in agitated, anxious, or delirious burn and trauma patients as well as for symptoms of acute stress or posttraumatic stress disorder. Phenothiazines also can be used and may be more sedating, although they are often avoided because of their tendency to cause hypotension and potentially worsen delirium as a result of their anticholinergic properties. SGAs are increasingly being used in burn and trauma patients. Risperidone, specifically, has been shown to be helpful in adult and pediatric burn patients with acute stress disorder (Meighen et al. 2007; Stanovic et al. 2001).

Pain

The question of whether antipsychotic medications possess analgesic properties has been a controversial issue. However, a 1994 review evaluated the available literature with regard to FGAs and pain management and concluded that only methotrimeprazine, a phenothiazine not available in the United States, had efficacy as an analgesic agent (Patt et al. 1994).

A 2004 review investigated the potential analgesic effects of SGAs (Fishbain et al. 2004). Several small controlled trials found tiapride, an SGA not available in the United States, to be an effective analgesic agent in cancer

TABLE 8–4. Use of antipsychotic medications in medical conditions

MEDICAL CONDITION	TREATMENT	TARGETED SYMPTOMS
Intractable hiccups	Chlorpromazine, haloperidol	Hiccups
Nausea and vomiting	Haloperidol, prochlorperazine, chlorpromazine, olanzapine	Nausea
Tourette syndrome	Fluphenazine, pimozide, haloperidol, ziprasidone	Tics
Acute intermittent porphyria	Chlorpromazine	Agitation, abdominal pain
Chronic pain	Olanzapine	Pain
Migraine headache	Quetiapine, chlorpromazine	Headache
Huntington's disease	Haloperidol, risperidone, quetiapine	Chorea
Autistic spectrum disorders	Risperidone	Agitation, irritability
Tetanus	Chlorpromazine	Rigidity, muscle spasm

pain. Two small studies suggested that olanzapine was effective in the treatment of cancer pain, chronic daily headache, and fibromyalgia. A single descriptive study found that quetiapine may be helpful for migraine prophylaxis.

Although antipsychotics are known to be effective in the treatment of conditions that often accompany pain such as delirium and agitation, it remains unclear whether either the typical or the atypical agents have direct analgesic properties.

Other Medical Disorders

Antipsychotic medications have been used to treat a wide variety of somatic symptoms and medical disorders unrelated to their antipsychotic property (see Table 8–4).

Chlorpromazine is considered a primary treatment for intractable hiccups. Nausea and vomiting, especially in the context of chemotherapy treatment, can be well managed by haloperidol and various other dopaminergic agents. Prochlorperazine, a typical neuroleptic, is commonly used to control nausea and vomiting. Tics seen in Tourette syndrome have responded to several different antipsychotics. Chlorpromazine has been used to treat both abdominal pain and delirium seen in acute intermittent porphyria. Chronic pain and migraines may respond to some neuroleptics. Abnormal movements seen in progressive Huntington's disease, including chorea and ballismus, may improve with haloperidol, risperidone, or quetiapine. Muscle spasms and rigidity found in severe tetanus may be responsive to chlorpromazine.

KEY CLINICAL POINTS

- Patients with medical illness occasionally require antipsychotic medication.

- Because medically ill patients are often prescribed several medications, the potential for drug-drug interactions requires a more careful dosing of the antipsychotic medication.

- At times, intramuscular or intravenous preparations of the antipsychotic medication need to be used because patients may not be able to take oral medication.

- Preexisting medical conditions may complicate the use of antipsychotic medications; thus, careful selection and dosing of the antipsychotic are necessary following an individualized assessment of the patient's medical problems and potential side effects of the antipsychotic medication.

References

Altshuler LL, Cohen L, Szuba MP, et al: Pharmacologic management of psychiatric illness during pregnancy: dilemmas and guidelines. Am J Psychiatry 153:592–606, 1996

Blumenfield M, Strain JJ (eds): Psychosomatic Medicine. Philadelphia, PA, Lippincott Williams & Wilkins, 2006

Brown ES, Chamberlain W, Dhanani N, et al: An open-label trial of olanzapine for corticosteroid-induced mood symptoms. J Affect Disord 83:277–281, 2004

Cohen L, Tessier E, Germain M, et al: Update on psychotropic medication use in renal disease. Psychosomatics 45:34–48, 2004

Crone CC, Gabriel GM, Dimartini A: An overview of psychiatric issues in liver disease for the consultation–liaison psychiatrist. Psychosomatics 47:188–205, 2006

Dolder C, Patterson T, Jeste D: HIV, psychosis and aging: past, present and future. AIDS 18 (suppl 1):S35–S42, 2004

Elovic E, Lansang R, Li Y, et al: The use of atypical antipsychotics in traumatic brain injury. J Head Trauma Rehabil 18:177–195, 2003

Fann JR: Epideniology of delirium: a review of studies and methodological issues. Semin Clin Neuropsychiatry 5:86–92, 2000

Fishbain DA, Cutler RB, Lewis J, et al: Do the second-generation "atypical neuroleptics" have analgesic properties? A structured evidence-based review. Pain Med 5:359–365, 2004

Glassman AH, Bigger JT: Antipsychotic drugs: prolonged QTc interval, torsades de pointes, and sudden death. Am J Psychiatry 158:1774–1782, 2001

Hales RE, Yudofsky SC, Gabbard GO (eds): The American Psychiatric Publishing Textbook of Psychiatry, 5th Edition. Washington, DC, American Psychiatric Publishing, 2008

Harrigan EP, Miceli JJ, Anziano R, et al: A randomized evaluation of the effects of six antipsychotic agents on QTc in the absence and presence of metabolic inhibition. J Clin Psychopharmacol 24:62–69, 2004

Janssen: Risperidone Product Information, 2002

Kelly KG, Zisselman M, Cutillo T, et al: Severity and course of delirium in medically hospitalized nursing facility residents. Am J Geriatr Psychiatry 9:72–77, 2001

Kim E, Bijlani M: A pilot study of quetiapine treatment of aggression due to traumatic brain injury. J Neuropsychiatry Clin Neurosci 18:547–549, 2006

Koch-Stoecker S: Antipsychotic drugs and epilepsy: indications and treatment guidelines. Epilepsia 43 (suppl 2):19–24, 2002

Lesser RS, Walters JL, Pebenito R, et al: Improvement of neuropsychiatric lupus with addition of SSRI antidepressant/antipsychotic therapy. J Clin Rheumatol 3:294–298, 1997

Levenson JL (ed): Textbook of Psychosomatic Medicine. Washington, DC, American Psychiatric Publishing, 2005

Mackin P: Cardiac side effects of psychiatric drugs. Hum Psychopharmacol Clin Exp 23:3–14, 2008

McKenna K, Koren G, Tetelbaum M, et al: Pregnancy outcome of women using atypical antipsychotic drugs: a prospective comparative study. J Clin Psychiatry 66:444–449, 2005

Meighen KG, Hines LA, Lagges AM: Risperidone treatment of preschool children with thermal burns and acute stress disorder. J Child Adolesc Psychopharmacol 17:223–232, 2007

Oster TJ, Anderson CA, Filley CM, et al: Quetiapine for mania due to traumatic brain injury. CNS Spectr 12:764–769, 2007

Patt RB, Proper G, Reddy S: The neuroleptics as adjuvant analgesics. J Pain Symptom Manage 9:446–453, 1994

Pfizer Inc.: Study Report of Ziprasidone Clinical Pharmacology Protocol 2000. Rockville, MD, U.S. Food and Drug Administration, Center for Drug Evaluation and Research, Division of Cardiorenal Drug Products Consultation, 2000

Pinto JP, Morais SL, Hallack JEC, et al: Effectiveness of olanzapine for systemic lupus erythematosus-related psychosis (letter). Prim Care Companion J Clin Psychiatry 8:377–378, 2006

Repetto M, Petitto J: Psychopharmacology in HIV-infected patients. Psychosom Med 70:585–592, 2008

Rochon PA, Normand SL, Gomes T, et al: Antipsychotic therapy and short-term serious events in older adults with dementia. Arch Intern Med 168:1090–1096, 2008

Rosenthal LJ, Kim V, Kim D: Weaning from prolonged mechanical ventilation using an antipsychotic agent in a patient with acute stress disorder. Crit Care Med 35:2417–2419, 2007

Schneider LS, Dagerman K, Insel PS: Efficacy and adverse effects of atypical antipsychotics for dementia: meta-analysis of randomized, placebo-controlled trials. Am J Geriatr Psychiatry 14:191–210, 2006

Stanovic JK, James KA, Vandevere CA: The effectiveness of risperidone on acute stress symptoms in adult burn patients: a preliminary retrospective pilot study. J Burn Care Rehabil 22:210–213, 2001

Stern TA, Fricchione GL, Cassem NH, et al (eds): Massachusetts General Hospital Handbook of General Psychiatry, 5th Edition. Philadelphia, PA, Elsevier, 2004

Su JA, Wu CH, Tsang HY: Olanzapine-induced agranulocytosis in systemic lupus erythematosus: a case report. Gen Hosp Psychiatry 29:75–77, 2007

Sultzer DL, Davis SM, Tariot PN, et al: Clinical symptom responses to atypical antipsychotic medications in Alzheimer's disease: Phase 1 outcomes from the CATIE-AD Effectiveness Trial. Am J Psychiatry 165:844–854, 2008

Thompson A, Silverman B, Dzeng L: Psychotropic medications and HIV. HIV/AIDS 42:1305–1310, 2006

Trzepacz PT, Meagher DJ: Delirium, in The American Psychiatric Publishing Textbook of Psychosomatic Medicine. Edited by Levenson JL. Washington, DC, American Psychiatric Publishing, 2005, pp 91–130

Trzepacz P, Breitbart W, Franklin J, et al: Practice guidelines for the treatment of patients with delirium, in American Psychiatric Association Practice Guidelines for the Treatment of Psychiatric Disorders. Washington, DC, American Psychiatric Association, 2002

Warrington TP, Bostwick JM: Psychiatric adverse effects of corticosteroids. Mayo Clin Proc 81:1361–1367, 2006

Weintraub D, Hurtig HI: Presentation and management of psychosis in Parkinson's disease and dementia with Lewy bodies. Am J Psychiatry 164:1491–1498, 2007

Wolfe J, Sartorius A, Alm B, et al: Clozapine-induced lupus erythematosus. J Clin Psychopharmacol 24:236–238, 2004

Wright TM, Vandenberg AM: Risperidone- and quetiapine-induced cholestasis. Ann Pharmacother 41:1518–1523, 2007

Wyszynski AA, Wyszynski BW (eds): Manual of Psychiatric Care for the Medically Ill. Washington, DC, American Psychiatric Publishing, 2005

Yoshida K, Smith B, Craggs M, et al: Neuroleptic drugs in breast-milk: a study of pharmacokinetics and of possible adverse effects in breast-fed infants. Psychol Med 28:81–91, 1998

APPENDIX 1

Names, Strengths, and Formulations of First- and Second-Generation Antipsychotics

First-Generation Antipsychotics

Medication (Brand Name)	Oral Formulations	Oral Solution	Oral Disintegrating Tablets	Intramuscular Injection	Intravenous Injection	Suppository Per Rectum
Chlorpromazine (Thorazine)	Tablets: 10 mg, 25 mg, 50 mg, 100 mg, 200 mg Sustained-release spansules: 30 mg, 75 mg, 150 mg	Concentrate: 30 mg/mL Syrup: 10 mg/5 mL	—	25 mg/mL	25 mg/mL after dilution	25 mg, 100 mg
Thioridazine (Mellaril)	10 mg, 15 mg, 25 mg, 50 mg, 100 mg, 150 mg, 200 mg	Concentrate: 30 mg/mL, 100 mg/mL Suspension: 5 mg/mL, 20 mg/mL	—	—	—	—
Fluphenazine (Prolixin)	1 mg, 2.5 mg, 5 mg, 10 mg	Concentrate: 5 mg/mL Elixir: 0.5 mg/mL	—	2.5 mg/mL	—	—

FIRST-GENERATION ANTIPSYCHOTICS (*CONTINUED*)

MEDICATION (BRAND NAME)	ORAL FORMULATIONS	ORAL SOLUTION	ORAL DISINTEGRATING TABLETS	INTRAMUSCULAR INJECTION	INTRAVENOUS INJECTION	SUPPOSITORY PER RECTUM
Fluphenazine enanthate (Prolixin Enanthate)	—	—	—	25 mg/mL	—	—
Fluphenazine decanoate (Prolixin Decanoate)	—	—	—	25 mg/mL	—	—
Perphenazine (Trilafon)	2 mg, 4 mg, 8 mg, 16 mg	Concentrate: 16 mg/5 mL	—	—	—	—
Trifluoperazine (Stelazine)	1 mg, 2 mg, 5 mg, 10 mg	Concentrate: 10 mg/mL	—	2 mg/mL	—	—
Prochlorperazine (Compazine)	5 mg, 10 mg	—	—	—	—	—

FIRST-GENERATION ANTIPSYCHOTICS (*CONTINUED*)

MEDICATION (BRAND NAME)	ORAL FORMULATIONS	ORAL SOLUTION	ORAL DISINTEGRATING TABLETS	INTRAMUSCULAR INJECTION	INTRAVENOUS INJECTION	SUPPOSITORY PER RECTUM
Haloperidol (Haldol)	0.5 mg, 1 mg, 2 mg, 5 mg, 10 mg, 20 mg	Concentrate: 2 mg/mL	—	5 mg/mL	0.5–100 mg/ 50–100 mL (dextrose 5% in water)	—
Haloperidol decanoate (Haldol Decanoate)	—	—	—	50 mg/mL, 100 mg/mL	—	—
Loxapine (Loxitane)	5 mg, 10 mg, 25 mg, 50 mg	—	—	—	—	—
Molindone (Moban)	5 mg, 10 mg, 25 mg, 50 mg, 100 mg	Concentrate: 20 mg/mL	—	—	—	—
Pimozide (Orap)	1 mg, 2 mg	—	—	—	—	—
Thiothixene (Navane)	1 mg, 2 mg, 5 mg, 10 mg	5 mg/mL	—	—	—	—

SECOND-GENERATION ANTIPSYCHOTICS

MEDICATION (BRAND NAME)	ORAL FORMULATIONS	ORAL SOLUTION	ORAL DISINTEGRATING TABLETS	INTRAMUSCULAR INJECTION	INTRAVENOUS INJECTION	SUPPOSITORY PER RECTUM
Clozapine (Clozaril)	12.5 mg, 25 mg, 50 mg, 100 mg, 200 mg	—	12.5 mg, 25 mg, 100 mg	—	—	—
Risperidone (Risperdal)	0.25 mg, 0.5 mg, 1 mg, 2 mg, 3 mg, 4 mg	1 mg/mL	0.5 mg, 1 mg, 2 mg, 3 mg, 4 mg	—	—	—
Risperidone long-acting injectable (Risperdal Consta)	—	—	—	12.5 mg, 25 mg, 37.5 mg, 50 mg	—	—
Olanzapine (Zyprexa)	2.5 mg, 5 mg, 7.5 mg, 10 mg, 15 mg, 20 mg	—	5 mg, 10 mg, 15 mg, 20 mg	10 mg/mL	—	—
Quetiapine (Seroquel)	25 mg, 50 mg, 100 mg, 200 mg, 300 mg, 400 mg	—	—	—	—	—
Quetiapine slow release (Seroquel XR)	50 mg, 150 mg, 200 mg, 300 mg, 400 mg	—	—	—	—	—

SECOND-GENERATION ANTIPSYCHOTICS (CONTINUED)

Medication (brand name)	Oral formulations	Oral solution	Oral disintegrating tablets	Intramuscular injection	Intravenous injection	Suppository per rectum
Ziprasidone (Geodon)	20 mg, 40 mg, 60 mg, 80 mg	—	—	20 mg/mL	—	—
Aripiprazole (Abilify)	2 mg, 5 mg, 10 mg, 15 mg, 20 mg, 30 mg	1 mg/mL	10 mg, 15 mg	7.5 mg/mL	—	—
Paliperidone (Invega)	Extended-release tablets: 3 mg, 6 mg, 9 mg	—	—	—	—	—
Paliperidone palmitate extended-release injectable suspension (Invega Sustenna)	—	—	—	Pre-filled syringes containing 39 mg, 78 mg, 117 mg, 156 mg, or 234 mg	—	—
Iloperidone (Fanapt)	1 mg, 2 mg, 4 mg, 6 mg, 8 mg, 10 mg, 12 mg	—	—	—	—	—
Asenapine (Saphris)	—	—	5 mg, 10 mg	—	—	—

References

Abilify [package insert]. Tokyo, Otsuka Pharmaceutical Company, 2009

DailyMed (Web site). Available at: http://dailymed.nlm.nih.gov. Accessed December 2008.

DrugDex Evaluations Database Web site. Available at: http://www.thomsonhc.com. ezproxy.umassmed.edu/hcs/librarian. Accessed December 2008.

Geodon [package insert]. New York, Pfizer, 2008

Iloperidone [package insert]. Rockville, MD, Vanda, 2009

Invega [package insert]. Titusville, NJ, Janssen, 2009

Invega Sustenna [package insert]. Titusville, NJ, Janssen, 2009

Micromedex Healthcare Series Web site. Available at: http://www.thomsonhc.com/ hcs/librarian. Accessed December 2008.

Physicians' Desk Reference, 62nd Edition. Montvale, NJ, Thomson Healthcare, 2008

Risperdal [package insert]. Titusville, NJ, Janssen, 2009

Saphris [package insert]. Kenilworth, NJ, Schering-Plough, 2009

APPENDIX 2

Pharmacokinetics of
First- and Second-Generation
Antipsychotics

FIRST-GENERATION ANTIPSYCHOTICS

MEDICATION (BRAND NAME)	CHEMICAL CLASS	CHLORPROMAZINE EQUIVALENCE	METABOLISM AND PLASMA HALF-LIFE ($T_{1/2}$)	ACTIVE METABOLITES	TIME TO PEAK PLASMA CONCENTRATION	DISTRIBUTION
Chlorpromazine (Thorazine)	Phenothiazine (aliphatic)	100 mg	Considerable first-pass metabolism in gut, some enterohepatic recycling; $t_{1/2}=30$ hours but longer for active metabolites	Nor-2-chlorpromazine, nor-2-chlorpromazine sulfate, and 3-hydroxy-chlorpromazine	2–4 hours; wide intersubject variation in concentration	95%–98% protein bound, wide bodily distribution with higher concentration in brain compared with plasma
Thioridazine (Mellaril)	Phenothiazine (piperidine)	100 mg	Extensive hepatic metabolism; $t_{1/2}=21$–24 hours	Mesoridazine is a metabolite of thioridazine that is twice as potent as thioridazine; sulforidazine is another active metabolite		>95% protein bound
Fluphenazine (Prolixin)	Phenothiazine (piperazine)	2 mg	$t_{1/2}=14.7$ hours	Metabolites exist; activities not reported	2.8 hours	

FIRST-GENERATION ANTIPSYCHOTICS *(CONTINUED)*

Medication (Brand Name)	Chemical Class	Chlorpromazine Equivalence	Metabolism and Plasma Half-Life ($T_{1/2}$)	Active Metabolites	Time to Peak Plasma Concentration	Distribution
Fluphenazine enanthate (Prolixin Enanthate)	Phenothiazine (piperazine)	0.22 cc/mo	$t_{1/2}$=6–9 days			
Fluphenazine decanoate (Prolixin Decanoate)	Phenothiazine (piperazine)	0.22 cc/mo	$t_{1/2}$=6–9 days			
Perphenazine (Trilafon)	Phenothiazine (piperazine)	6–10 mg	Extensive hepatic metabolism with marked first-pass effect and likely enterohepatic cycling; $t_{1/2}$=9.5 hours	Perphenazine sulfoxide and 7-hydroxyper-phenazine, both with unknown activity	1–3 hours	Widely distributed
Trifluoperazine (Stelazine)	Phenothiazine (piperazine)	3–5 mg	Hepatic metabolism; multiphasic; $t_{1/2}$=24 hours	*N*-oxide derivative is active; the sulfoxide and 7-hydroxy derivatives' metabolic activity is unknown	2–4 hours	90%–99% protein bound; highly lipophilic with CNS concentrations > plasma concentrations

FIRST-GENERATION ANTIPSYCHOTICS (CONTINUED)

MEDICATION (BRAND NAME)	CHEMICAL CLASS	CHLORPROMAZINE EQUIVALENCE	METABOLISM AND PLASMA HALF-LIFE ($T_{1/2}$)	ACTIVE METABOLITES	TIME TO PEAK PLASMA CONCENTRATION	DISTRIBUTION
Prochlorperazine (Compazine)	Phenothiazine (piperazine)	15 mg	Biphasic, possibly triphasic with $t_{1/2}$=6–9 hours and 18 hours; hepatic and other	N-desmethylprochlorperazine is active	2–4 hours	
Haloperidol (Haldol)	Butyrophenone	2 mg	Hepatic and possibly extrahepatic; $t_{1/2}$=10–38 hours	Hydroxymetabolite is active	2–6 hours after ingestion; 20 minutes after intramuscular injection; wide intersubject variation in plasma concentrations	>90% protein bound
Haloperidol decanoate (Haldol Decanoate)	Butyrophenone	20 mg/mo	Hepatic and possibly extrahepatic; $t_{1/2}$=3 weeks		6 days	
Loxapine (Loxitane)	Dibenzoxazepine	10 mg	Rapid and extensive hepatic metabolism with first-pass effect; $t_{1/2}$=4 hours	N-desmethylloxapine is active; 8-hydroxyloxapine is active	1–2 hours	Widely distributed

FIRST-GENERATION ANTIPSYCHOTICS *(CONTINUED)*

MEDICATION (BRAND NAME)	CHEMICAL CLASS	CHLORPROMAZINE EQUIVALENCE	METABOLISM AND PLASMA HALF-LIFE ($T_{1/2}$)	ACTIVE METABOLITES	TIME TO PEAK PLASMA CONCENTRATION	DISTRIBUTION
Molindone (Moban)	Dihydroindole	10 mg	Rapid and extensive hepatic metabolism	36 recognized metabolites; individual activities are not described	1.5 hours	
Pimozide (Orap)	Diphenylbutylpiperidine	2 mg	Significant hepatic first-pass metabolism; $t_{1/2}$=55 hours on average, but half-lives of up to 150 hours have been reported in some patients	Metabolites exist; activities not reported	6–8 hours, with considerable inter-subject variation in concentration achieved	
Thiothixene (Navane)	Thioxanthene	4 mg	May induce its own metabolism; $t_{1/2}$=34 hours		1–2 hours	

SECOND-GENERATION ANTIPSYCHOTICS

MEDICATION (BRAND NAME)	CHEMICAL CLASS	CHLORPROMAZINE EQUIVALENCE	METABOLISM AND PLASMA HALF-LIFE ($T_{1/2}$)	ACTIVE METABOLITES	TIME TO PEAK PLASMA CONCENTRATION	DISTRIBUTION
Clozapine (Clozaril)	Dibenzodiazepine	50 mg	Extensive extrahepatic presystemic routes of metabolism; $t_{1/2}$=8–12 hours	N-desmethylclozapine is a potent serotonin 5-HT$_{1C}$ receptor antagonist and has affinity for dopamine D$_2$ and serotonin 5-HT receptors and is further metabolized to a compound that is toxic to both myeloid and erythroid lineage precursors	2–3 hours; with significant degree of variation; higher levels in women and increase in age in all patients; clozapine and norclozapine levels should be quantified only in plasma because serum levels underestimate blood levels	95%–97% protein bound

SECOND-GENERATION ANTIPSYCHOTICS *(CONTINUED)*

MEDICATION (BRAND NAME)	CHEMICAL CLASS	CHLORPROMAZINE EQUIVALENCE	METABOLISM AND PLASMA HALF-LIFE ($t_{1/2}$)	ACTIVE METABOLITES	TIME TO PEAK PLASMA CONCENTRATION	DISTRIBUTION
Risperidone (Risperdal)	Benzisoxazole	2 mg	Extensive hepatic metabolism, which is sensitive to the debrisoquine hydroxylation–type genetic polymorphism; $t_{1/2} = 20$–30 hours, with range of 3 hours in extensive metabolizers and 20 hours in poor metabolizers	9-hydroxyrisperidone (paliperidone) and equivalently effective to parent compound; $t_{1/2}$ of 9-hydroxyrisperidone = 21 hours in extensive metabolizers and 30 hours in poor metabolizers	1 hour	90% protein bound

SECOND-GENERATION ANTIPSYCHOTICS (CONTINUED)

MEDICATION (BRAND NAME)	CHEMICAL CLASS	CHLORPROMAZINE EQUIVALENCE	METABOLISM AND PLASMA HALF-LIFE ($T_{1/2}$)	ACTIVE METABOLITES	TIME TO PEAK PLASMA CONCENTRATION	DISTRIBUTION
Risperidone long-acting injectable (Risperdal Consta)	Benzisoxazole	Not available	$t_{1/2}$=3–6 days		Steady-state plasma concentrations are reached after four injections and are maintained for 4–6 weeks after the last injection	
Olanzapine (Zyprexa)	Thienobenzodiazepine	5 mg	Extensive hepatic metabolism; $t_{1/2}$=21–54 hours with longer half-lives in females than in males	Metabolites are inactive	6 hours after ingestion; 15–45 minutes after intramuscular injection	93% protein bound
Quetiapine (Seroquel)	Dibenzothiazepine	75 mg	Extensive first-pass hepatic metabolism; $t_{1/2}$=6 hours	N-desalkyl quetiapine and 7-hydroxylated metabolite are active; 18 other metabolites are inactive	1.5 hours	83% protein bound

Second-Generation Antipsychotics (*CONTINUED*)

Medication (Brand Name)	Chemical Class	Chlorpromazine Equivalence	Metabolism and Plasma Half-Life ($T_{1/2}$)	Active Metabolites	Time to Peak Plasma Concentration	Distribution
Quetiapine slow release (Seroquel XR)	Dibenzothiazepine	Not available	Extensive first-pass hepatic metabolism; $t_{1/2}$=7 hours	N-desalkyl quetiapine and 7-hydroxylated metabolite are active; 18 other metabolites are inactive	6 hours	83% protein bound
Ziprasidone (Geodon)	Benzisothiazolyl	60 mg	Hepatic metabolism; $t_{1/2}$=7 hours (oral); $t_{1/2}$=2–5 hours (intramuscular)	Major metabolite is ziprasidone sulfoxide; metabolites are inactive at 5-HT_{2A}/ D_2 receptors	4–5 hours after ingestion; 1 hour after intramuscular injection	>99% protein bound

SECOND-GENERATION ANTIPSYCHOTICS (CONTINUED)

MEDICATION (BRAND NAME)	CHEMICAL CLASS	CHLORPROMAZINE EQUIVALENCE	METABOLISM AND PLASMA HALF-LIFE ($T_{1/2}$)	ACTIVE METABOLITES	TIME TO PEAK PLASMA CONCENTRATION	DISTRIBUTION
Aripiprazole (Abilify)	Quinolinone	7.5–10 mg	Hepatic, extent unknown; poor metabolizers have about 60% greater exposure to active compounds; $t_{1/2}$=75 hours in extensive metabolizers or about 146 hours in poor metabolizers	Dehydroaripiprazole with a $t_{1/2}$=94 hours	3–5 hours after ingestion or 1–3 hours after intramuscular injection	>99% protein bound

SECOND-GENERATION ANTIPSYCHOTICS (*CONTINUED*)

MEDICATION (BRAND NAME)	CHEMICAL CLASS	CHLORPROMAZINE EQUIVALENCE	METABOLISM AND PLASMA HALF-LIFE ($t_{1/2}$)	ACTIVE METABOLITES	TIME TO PEAK PLASMA CONCENTRATION	DISTRIBUTION
Paliperidone (Invega)	Benzisoxazole	Not available	Limited hepatic metabolism; $t_{1/2}$=21 hours in extensive metabolizers and 30 hours in poor metabolizers; increased $t_{1/2}$ in renal impairment (24–51 hours)	M1, M10, M11, M12, M16; activities not reported	24 hours	74% protein bound
Paliperidone palmitate extended-release injectable suspension (Invega Sustenna)	Benzisoxazole	Not available	Limited hepatic metabolism; $t_{1/2}$=25–49 days	M1, M10, M11, M12, M16	13 days	74% protein bound

SECOND-GENERATION ANTIPSYCHOTICS (CONTINUED)

MEDICATION (BRAND NAME)	CHEMICAL CLASS	CHLORPROMAZINE EQUIVALENCE	METABOLISM AND PLASMA HALF-LIFE ($T_{1/2}$)	ACTIVE METABOLITES	TIME TO PEAK PLASMA CONCENTRATION	DISTRIBUTION
Iloperidone (Fanapt)	Benzisoxazole	Not available	Primarily hepatic metabolism; $t_{1/2}$=18–23 hours in extensive metabolizers and 31–37 hours in poor metabolizers	P95 and P88	3–4 days	95% protein bound
Asenapine (Saphris)	Dibenzo-oxepino pyrrole	Not available	Hepatic glucuronidation and oxidation; $t_{1/2}$=24 hours	Asenapine N+-glucuronide (predominant), N-desmethylasenapine, N-carbamoyl glucuronide	3 days	95% protein bound

Note.   CNS=central nervous system.

APPENDIX 3

Dosing and Administration of First- and Second-Generation Antipsychotics in Schizophrenia

FIRST-GENERATION ANTIPSYCHOTICS

Medication (brand name)	Usual dosing	Dosing in hepatic impairment	Dosing in renal impairment	Dosing in special populations
Chlorpromazine (Thorazine)	*Initial dosage:* 10–25 mg PO bid–qid or 25–50 mg IM q 4–6 hours May increase 20–50 mg/day PO q 3–4 days as indicated clinically *Maximum dosage:* 1 g/day	Caution advised, and dose should be reduced	Not specified; no dose adjustments recommended during dialysis	Elderly patients should be given one-third to one-half the usual adult dosage, and the maintenance dosage is usually less than 300 mg/day
Thioridazine (Mellaril)	*Initial dosage:* 50–100 mg tid with gradual increment *Maximum dosage:* 800 mg/day *Total daily dose:* range of 200–800 mg/day divided bid or qid	Caution advised	Not specified	Caution advised in elderly or frail patients
Fluphenazine (Prolixin)	*Initial dosage:* 2.5–10 mg/day PO in divided doses q 6–8 hours *Maximum dosage:* 40 mg/day *Maintenance dosage:* 1–5 mg/day PO as single daily dose	Contraindicated with hepatic impairment	Not specified	Caution advised in elderly or frail patients

FIRST-GENERATION ANTIPSYCHOTICS *(CONTINUED)*

MEDICATION (BRAND NAME)	USUAL DOSING	DOSING IN HEPATIC IMPAIRMENT	DOSING IN RENAL IMPAIRMENT	DOSING IN SPECIAL POPULATIONS
Fluphenazine decanoate (Prolixin Decanoate)	*Initial dose:* 12.5–25 mg IM or SC, with the dose being repeated or increased as needed and tolerated, usually q 4–6 weeks *Maximum dose:* usually 50 mg IM or SC q 1–4 weeks	Contraindicated with hepatic impairment	Not specified	Caution advised in elderly or frail patients
Perphenazine (Trilafon)	*Initial dosage:* 4–8 mg PO tid in outpatient populations or 8–16 mg PO bid–qid in inpatients *Maximum dosage:* 64 mg/day PO *Alternative dosage:* 5–10 mg IM with additional 5-mg IM doses q 6 hours as needed, with maximum total daily dose of 15 mg IM in outpatients and 30 mg IM in inpatients	Contraindicated with hepatic impairment	Caution advised with renal impairment	Use lower initial doses in the elderly

FIRST-GENERATION ANTIPSYCHOTICS *(CONTINUED)*

MEDICATION (BRAND NAME)	USUAL DOSING	DOSING IN HEPATIC IMPAIRMENT	DOSING IN RENAL IMPAIRMENT	DOSING IN SPECIAL POPULATIONS
Trifluoperazine (Stelazine)	*Initial dosage:* 1–2 mg PO bid *Usual effective dosage:* 15–20 mg/day *Maximum dosage:* 40 mg/day PO *Alternative dosage:* 1–2 mg deep IM q 4–6 hours as needed, with total daily dose of 6 mg IM	Contraindicated with hepatic impairment	Not specified	Use lower initial doses in the elderly: approximately one-half to one-third the usual adult dosage
Prochlorperazine (Compazine)	*Initial dosage:* 5–10 mg PO q 6–8 hours; may increase 5–10 mg q 2–3 days	Not specified	Not specified	Caution advised in elderly or frail patients
Haloperidol (Haldol)	*Initial dosage:* 0.5–2 mg (moderate symptoms) or 3–5 mg (severe symptoms) PO bid–tid *Alternative dosage:* 2–5 mg IM; may repeat q 4–8 hours depending on symptoms; increased to q 1 hour if needed	Caution advised with hepatic impairment	No adjustment	Caution advised in elderly or frail patients

FIRST-GENERATION ANTIPSYCHOTICS (*CONTINUED*)

MEDICATION (BRAND NAME)	USUAL DOSING	DOSING IN HEPATIC IMPAIRMENT	DOSING IN RENAL IMPAIRMENT	DOSING IN SPECIAL POPULATIONS
Haloperidol (Haldol) (*continued*)	*Alternative dosage:* Initial bolus dose of 2–10 mg IV followed by continuous infusion beginning at 10 mg/hour. If control is not achieved, bolus may be repeated every 30 minutes, and infusion rate may be increased by 5 mg/hour. Infusion doses of 2–25 mg/hour by continuous IV infusion, with maximum infusion rate of 40 mg/hour *Oral to IV conversion (approximate):* oral dose×0.625=daily IV dose	Caution advised with hepatic impairment	No adjustment	Caution advised in elderly or frail patients

FIRST-GENERATION ANTIPSYCHOTICS (CONTINUED)

Medication (brand name)	Usual dosing	Dosing in hepatic impairment	Dosing in renal impairment	Dosing in special populations
Haloperidol decanoate (Haldol Decanoate)	*Stabilized at low daily oral dosages (up to 10 mg/day):* use 10–15 times previous daily oral dose IM monthly or q 4 weeks. *Stabilized at high daily oral dosages:* give 20 times previous daily oral dose IM for the first month, then 10–15 times previous daily oral dose IM monthly or every 4 weeks. *Maximum initial dose:* 100 mg IM	Caution advised with hepatic impairment	No adjustment	Caution advised in elderly or frail patients
Loxapine (Loxitane)	*Initial dosage:* 10 mg PO bid. *Maximum dosage:* 250 mg/day in divided doses bid–qid. *Maintenance dosage range:* 60–100 mg/day. *Alternative dosage:* 12.5–50 mg IM q 4–6 hour or longer; most patients use bid dosing	Caution advised with hepatic impairment	Not specified	Caution advised in elderly or frail patients. In geriatric patients with chronic schizophrenia, dosages of 20–80 mg/day have been reported effective

FIRST-GENERATION ANTIPSYCHOTICS *(CONTINUED)*

MEDICATION (BRAND NAME)	USUAL DOSING	DOSING IN HEPATIC IMPAIRMENT	DOSING IN RENAL IMPAIRMENT	DOSING IN SPECIAL POPULATIONS
Molindone (Moban)	*Initial dosage:* 50–75 mg/day PO; may increase to 100 mg/day in 3–4 days *Maintenance dosage:* 5–15 mg tid or qid for mild symptoms; 10–25 mg tid or qid for moderate symptoms; dosages up to 225 mg/day may be required for severe symptoms	Not specified	Not specified	Caution advised in elderly or frail patients
Pimozide (Orap)	*Initial dosage:* 1–2 mg/day PO in divided doses; may increase dose every other day to a maximum of 10 mg/day or 0.2 mg/kg/day, whichever is smaller Effective dosages in chronic schizophrenia range from 2 to 12 mg/day	Reductions in dose should be considered in severe hepatic insufficiency	Caution advised with renal impairment	Caution advised in elderly or frail patients Initial dosage of 1 mg/day is recommended in geriatric patients

FIRST-GENERATION ANTIPSYCHOTICS (*CONTINUED*)

MEDICATION (BRAND NAME)	USUAL DOSING	DOSING IN HEPATIC IMPAIRMENT	DOSING IN RENAL IMPAIRMENT	DOSING IN SPECIAL POPULATIONS
Thiothixene (Navane)	*Initial dosage:* 2 mg PO tid for mild to moderate symptoms; 5 mg PO bid for severe symptoms *Usual effective dosage range:* 20–30 mg PO/day *Maximum dosage:* 60 mg PO/ 24 hours *Alternative dosage:* 4 mg IM bid– qid; usual effective daily dosage range of 16–20 mg IM *Maximum dosage:* 30 mg IM/24 hours	Not specified	Not specified	Caution advised in elderly or frail patients

SECOND-GENERATION ANTIPSYCHOTICS

MEDICATION (BRAND NAME)	USUAL DOSING	DOSING IN HEPATIC IMPAIRMENT	DOSING IN RENAL IMPAIRMENT	DOSING IN SPECIAL POPULATIONS
Clozapine (Clozaril)	*Initial dosage:* 12.5 mg PO daily to bid; increase by 25–50 mg/ day q 3–7 days *Usual effective dosage:* 300–450 mg/day by the end of 2 weeks	Caution advised with hepatic impairment	Caution advised with renal impairment	Caution advised in elderly or frail patients

SECOND-GENERATION ANTIPSYCHOTICS (CONTINUED)

MEDICATION (BRAND NAME)	USUAL DOSING	DOSING IN HEPATIC IMPAIRMENT	DOSING IN RENAL IMPAIRMENT	DOSING IN SPECIAL POPULATIONS
Risperidone (Risperdal)	*Initial dosage:* 2 mg/day PO (given in one dose or two divided doses) Adjust dose at intervals ≥24 hours, in increments of 1–2 mg/day, as tolerated, to recommended dosage of 4–8 mg/day *Maximum dosage:* 16 mg/day	0.5 mg PO bid; may be slowly increased in steps of 0.5 mg bid, if necessary, to a dosage of 1–2 mg bid; for dosages greater than 1.5 mg bid, increases should be made at intervals of at least 1 week	Same dosing as for hepatic impairment	Same dosing as for hepatic impairment
Risperidone long-acting injectable (Risperdal Consta)	*Initial dosage:* 25 mg IM q 2 weeks *Maximum dosage:* 50 mg IM q 2 weeks Give first injection with oral dosage form or other oral antipsychotic and continue for at least 3 weeks, then taper and discontinue oral form	*Initial dosage:* 12.5 mg IM q 2 weeks	Same dosing as for hepatic impairment	Same dosing as for hepatic impairment

SECOND-GENERATION ANTIPSYCHOTICS (CONTINUED)

MEDICATION (BRAND NAME)	USUAL DOSING	DOSING IN HEPATIC IMPAIRMENT	DOSING IN RENAL IMPAIRMENT	DOSING IN SPECIAL POPULATIONS
Olanzapine (Zyprexa)	*Initial dosage:* Daily, without regard to meals, 5–10 mg PO, with target dosage of 10 mg/day within several days; adjust by 5 mg/day at weekly intervals *Maximum dosage:* 20 mg/day; but used clinically up to 50 mg/day	Caution in hepatic impairment; monitor liver function tests	Not specified	*Initial dosage:* 5 mg/day in debilitated patients, those with predisposition to hypotension, or slow metabolizers
Quetiapine immediate release (Seroquel)	*Initial dosage:* 25 mg PO bid, with increases in increments of 25–50 mg bid or tid on the second and third day, as tolerated *Target dosage range:* 300–400 mg/day by fourth day, given in divided doses (bid or tid) When dose adjustment indicated, may increase at intervals ≥48 hours in increments of 25–50 mg bid *Maximum dosage:* 800 mg/day	*Initial dosage:* 25 mg/day; increase in increments of 25–50 mg/day	Not specified	In the elderly, may use same dosing as for hepatic impairment

SECOND-GENERATION ANTIPSYCHOTICS (*CONTINUED*)

MEDICATION (BRAND NAME)	USUAL DOSING	DOSING IN HEPATIC IMPAIRMENT	DOSING IN RENAL IMPAIRMENT	DOSING IN SPECIAL POPULATIONS
Quetiapine slow release (Seroquel XR)	*Initial dosage:* 200–300 mg/day in single dose, preferably in evening without food Dose increases may be made at intervals as short as 1 day and in increments up to 300 mg/day; titrate up to 400–800 mg/day *Maximum dosage:* 800 mg/day	*Initial dosage:* 25 mg/day of quetiapine immediate release; increase in increments of 25–50 mg/day; may switch to Seroquel XR when effective dose is reached	Not specified	In the elderly, may use same dosing as for hepatic impairment
Ziprasidone (Geodon)	*Initial dosage:* 20 mg PO bid with food daily Dose adjustments, if indicated, up to maximum 80 mg bid Adjustments may occur at intervals of ≥48 hours	Generally not indicated	Generally not indicated	Not specified

SECOND-GENERATION ANTIPSYCHOTICS (*CONTINUED*)

Medication (brand name)	Usual dosing	Dosing in hepatic impairment	Dosing in renal impairment	Dosing in special populations
Aripiprazole (Abilify)	*Initial dosage:* 10–15 mg/day PO without regard to meals Dosage should not be increased before 2 weeks' time Dosage range of 10–30 mg/day PO *Maximum dosage:* 30 mg/day	Generally not indicated	Generally not indicated	Not specified
Paliperidone (Invega)	*Initial dosage:* 6 mg once daily in the A.M., without regard to meals Initial dose titration is not required Some patients may benefit from 3–12 mg/day. Increases above 6 mg/day should occur at intervals of more than 5 days and in increments of 3 mg/day *Maximum dosage:* 12 mg/day	For patients with mild to moderate hepatic impairment (Child-Pugh classification A and B), no dose adjustment is recommended	For patients with creatinine clearance 50–79 mL/min, maximum dosage is 6 mg/day For patients with creatinine clearance 10–49 mL/min, maximum dosage is 3 mg/day	In the elderly with normal renal function, no dose adjustment is recommended For patients with creatinine clearance 10–49 mL/min, maximum dosage is 3 mg/day

SECOND-GENERATION ANTIPSYCHOTICS (CONTINUED)

MEDICATION (BRAND NAME)	USUAL DOSING	DOSING IN HEPATIC IMPAIRMENT	DOSING IN RENAL IMPAIRMENT	DOSING IN SPECIAL POPULATIONS
Paliperidone palmitate extended-release injectable suspension (Invega Sustenna)	*Initial dosage:* Begin with dose of 234 mg IM on treatment day 1 and 156 mg IM 1 week later; the monthly maintenance dose is 117 mg IM *Maximum dosage:* Not specified	Not specified	For mild renal impairment (creatinine clearance ≥50 mL/min to <80 mL/min), administer 156 mg IM on treatment day 1 and then 117 mg IM 1 week later for initial dosing For maintenance dosing, use 78 mg IM monthly Not recommended for patients with moderate or severe renal impairment	In elderly, adjust dose according to renal function status

Second-Generation Antipsychotics (CONTINUED)

Medication (Brand Name)	Usual Dosing	Dosing in Hepatic Impairment	Dosing in Renal Impairment	Dosing in Special Populations
Iloperidone (Fanapt)	*Initial dosage:* Begin with 1 mg PO bid and then increase to 2 mg, 4 mg, 6 mg, 8 mg, 10 mg, and 12 mg PO bid on days 2, 3, 4, 5, 6, and 7, respectively Target total daily dose range is 12–24 mg PO	Not recommended for patients with hepatic impairment	Not specified	Caution advised in elderly or frail patients
Asenapine (Saphris)	*Initial and maintenance dosage:* Begin and continue with 5 mg sublingual tablets bid *Maximum dosage:* Not specified	Not recommended in patients with severe hepatic injury (Child-Pugh C); no dose adjustment is recommended for patients with mild or moderate hepatic impairment (Child-Pugh A or B)	No dose adjustment is recommended	In elderly patients, asenapine concentrations were found to be 30%–40% higher compared with younger adults for the same daily dosage

Note.　bid=twice a day; IM=intramuscularly; IV=intravenously; PO=orally; q=every; qid=four times a day; SC=subcutaneously; tid=three times a day.

APPENDIX 4

Medical Workup When Initiating and Continuing First- and Second-Generation Antipsychotics

Measure	Baseline	4 Weeks	8 Weeks	12 Weeks	Quarterly	Every 6 Months	Annually	Every 5 Years	If Signs or Symptoms Arise
Medical history or family medical history of obesity, hypercholesterolemia, diabetes, hypertension, or heart disease	X						X		
Weight and height (body mass index)	X	X	X	X	X		X		
Waist circumference	X	X	X	X	X		X		
Blood pressure	X			X			X		
Fasting glucose Hemoglobin A1c	X	X		X			X		X
Fasting total cholesterol	X			X				X	
Fasting triglycerides	X			X			X[a]	X	
Electrocardiogram	X[a]	X[a]					X[a]		

MEASURE	BASELINE	4 WEEKS	8 WEEKS	12 WEEKS	QUARTERLY	EVERY 6 MONTHS	ANNUALLY	EVERY 5 YEARS	IF SIGNS OR SYMPTOMS ARISE
Prolactin									X
Urine pregnancy test in women of childbearing age	X								X
Basic metabolic panel	X	X					X		X
Liver function tests	X	X					X		X
Thyroid-stimulating hormone	X								X
Drug level									X
Abnormal Involuntary Movement Scale test	X					X			X
Ophthalmological examination	X[a]					X			X

[a]Suggested by authors; not mandatory.
Source. American Diabetes Association et al. 2004; Marder et al. 2004; Muntez and Benjamin 1988.

References

American Diabetes Association, American Psychiatric Association, American Association of Clinical Endocrinologists, et al: North American Association for the Study of Obesity: consensus development conference on antipsychotic drugs and obesity and diabetes. Diabetes Care 27:596–601, 2004

Marder SR, Essock SM, Miller AL, et al: Physical health monitoring of patients with schizophrenia. Am J Psychiatry 161:1134–1349, 2004

Muntez MR, Benjamin S: How to examine patients using the Abnormal Involuntary Movement Scale. Hosp Community Psychiatry 39:1172–1177, 1988

APPENDIX 5

Medical Workup When Initiating and Continuing Clozapine

MEASURE	BASELINE	WEEKLY FOR THE INITIAL 6 MONTHS	12 WEEKS	EVERY OTHER WEEK AFTER 6 MONTHS	EVERY 6 MONTHS	ONCE A MONTH AFTER 1 YEAR	ANNUALLY	IF SIGNS OR SYMPTOMS ARISE
Medical history or family medical history of obesity, diabetes, hypercholesterolemia, hypertension, or heart disease	X						X	
Weight and height (body mass index)	X	X		X		X	X	
Waist circumference	X		X		X			
Blood pressure	X	X					X	
Fasting glucose	X		X				X	Also at week 4
Fasting total cholesterol	X		X				X	
Fasting triglycerides	X		X				X	

MEASURE	BASELINE	WEEKLY FOR THE INITIAL 6 MONTHS	12 WEEKS	EVERY OTHER WEEK AFTER 6 MONTHS	EVERY 6 MONTHS	ONCE A MONTH AFTER 1 YEAR	ANNUALLY	IF SIGNS OR SYMPTOMS ARISE
Electrocardiogram	X						X	Also at week 4
Hemoglobin A1c	X		X				X	X
Urine pregnancy test in women of childbearing age	X							X
Basic metabolic panel	X		X				X	X
Liver function tests	X		X				X	X
Drug level	X		X					X
Abnormal Involuntary Movement Scale test	X						X	
White blood cell count	X	X		X		X		X
Absolute neutrophil count	X	X		X		X		X

Source. Adapted from Magid et al. 2006; Marder et al. 2004.

References

Magid M, Cunningham JL, Netzel PJ: A concise guide to psychotropic medications: laboratory testing, patient warnings and drug interactions. Biological Therapies in Psychiatry 29(9):38–44, 2006

Marder SR, Essock SM, Miller AL, et al: Physical health monitoring of patients with schizophrenia. Am J Psychiatry 161:1334–1349, 2004

APPENDIX 6

Use of First- and Second-Generation Antipsychotics for Agitation Due to Psychosis

DOSING

MEDICATION (BRAND NAME)	ORAL	INTRAMUSCULAR	INTRAVENOUS	NOTES
Chlorpromazine (Thorazine)		25 mg × 1; may repeat 25–50 mg q 1–4 hours as needed. IM formulation can be painful. Switch to PO as soon as possible.	—	Lower risk of EPS but higher risk of hypotension and oversedation compared with haloperidol or atypical antipsychotics
Haloperidol (Haldol)	FDA-approved indication for agitation. *Tablet:* 0.5–10 mg q 1–4 hours. *Maximum dosage:* 100 mg/day for severely refractory cases	0.5–10 mg q 1–4 hours for acute agitation. Switch to PO as soon as possible. PO dose is equivalent to IM dose.	Not FDA approved for agitation. 0.5–2 mg (mild agitation); 2–5 mg (moderate agitation); 5–10 mg (severe agitation). Allow 30 minutes between doses.	Use lower doses in elderly. Check serum K, Mg, Ca, phosphorus, and QTc interval for IV administration. Do not push if QTc≥500. Patient should be receiving telemetry, and QTc should be monitored prior to each IV dose. Clear the IV line with normal saline prior to bolus infusion. Heparin can precipitate IV haloperidol.

		DOSING		
MEDICATION (BRAND NAME)	ORAL	INTRAMUSCULAR	INTRAVENOUS	NOTES
Risperidone (Risperdal)	2 mg; may use different doses of the rapidly dissolving M-tab; may use risperidone solution	—	—	
Olanzapine (Zyprexa)	May use rapidly dissolving olanzapine wafer called Zyprexa Zydis	FDA-approved indication 10 mg; may repeat in 2 hours and 6 hours as needed *Maximum dosage:* 30 mg/day Use 5 mg × 1 in elderly or 2.5 mg × 1 if debilitated. Switch to PO as soon as possible. Peak plasma concentration in 15–45 minutes; elimination half-life = 30 hours	—	Monitor for orthostatic hypotension, especially with repeated IM dosing.
Quetiapine (Seroquel)	Not FDA approved for agitation	—	—	—

DOSING

MEDICATION (BRAND NAME)	ORAL	INTRAMUSCULAR	INTRAVENOUS	NOTES
Ziprasidone (Geodon)	Not FDA approved for agitation	FDA-approved indication 10–20 mg q 2–4 hours *Maximum dosage:* 40 mg/24–72 hours Switch to PO as soon as possible. Peak plasma concentration in 30–45 minutes; elimination half-life is 2–4 hours.	—	Higher dose response 2 hours after dose with 20 mg IM vs. 10 mg IM (90% vs. 57%) Prolongation of QTc appears less common with IM form than with PO form but should be avoided in patients with other QTc-prolonging drugs, recent myocardial infarction, heart failure, etc.
Aripiprazole (Abilify)	Not FDA approved for agitation; oral solution available	FDA-approved indication 9.75 mg × 1 *Maximum dosage:* 30 mg/day *Effective dosage range:* 5.25–15 mg × 1; may repeat q 2 hours or longer if needed. Switch to PO as soon as possible.	—	—

Note. EPS=extrapyramidal symptoms; FDA=U.S. Food and Drug Administration; IM=intramuscular; IV=intravenous; PO=oral.

References

Allen M, Currier G, Hughes D, et al: Treatment of behavioral emergencies: a summary of the Expert Consensus Guidelines. J Psychiatr Pract 9(1):16–38, 2003

Battaglia J, Lindborg SR, Alaka K, et al: Calming versus sedative effects of intramuscular olanzapine in agitated patients. Am J Emerg Med 21:192–198, 2003

Daniel DG, Potkin SG, Reeves KR: Intramuscular (IM) ziprasidone 20 mg is effective in reducing acute agitation associated with psychosis: a double-blind, randomized trial. Psychopharmacology 155:128–134, 2004

Hughes D: Acute psychopharmacological management of the aggressive psychotic patient. Psychiatr Serv 50:1135–1137, 1999

Micromedex Healthcare Series Web site. Available at: http://www.thomsonhc.com/hcs/librarian. Accessed December 2008.

Villari V, Rocca P, Fonzo V, et al: Oral risperidone, olanzapine and quetiapine versus haloperidol in psychotic agitation. Prog Neuropsychopharmacol Biol Psychiatry 32:405–413, 2008

Wise MG, Terrell CD: Neuropsychiatric disorders: delirium, psychotic disorder and anxiety, in Principles of Critical Care, 2nd Edition. Edited by Hall JB, Schmidt GA, Wood LDH. New York, McGraw-Hill, 1998, pp 965–978

Wright P, Birkett M, David SR, et al: Double-blind, placebo-controlled comparison of IM olanzapine and IM haloperidol in the treatment of acute agitation in schizophrenia. Am J Psychiatry 158:1149–1151, 2001

APPENDIX 7

Side Effects of Commonly Used Antipsychotics

	CLOZAPINE	RISPERIDONE	OLANZAPINE	QUETIAPINE	ZIPRASIDONE	ARIPIPRAZOLE	PALIPERIDONE	HALOPERIDOL[a]	PERPHENAZINE
Extrapyramidal symptoms	0	2+	1+	0	1+	1+	2+	3+	2+
Prolactin elevation	0	3+	1+	0	1+	0	3+	3+	2+
Weight gain	3+	2+	3+	2+	0	0	2+	1+	1+
Elevated lipid levels	3+	2+	3+	2+	0	0	2+	0	?1+
Glucose abnormalities	3+	2+	3+	2+	0	0	2+	0	?1+
Prolonged QTc interval	1+	1+	0–1+		2+	0	1+	0	0
Anticholinergic effects	3+	0	2+	1+	0	0	0	0	0–1+
Sedation	3+	1+	2+	2+	1+	1+	1+	1–2+	1+
Hepatic transaminitis	2+	1+	2+	1+	1+	0	1+	0	1+
Hypotension	3+	1+	1–2+	2+	1+	1+	1+	0	1+
Seizures	2+	0	0–1+	0–1+	0–1+	0–1+	0	0	0–1+

Note.   0=no risk or rare effect; 1+=mild or occasional at therapeutic doses (low); 2+=moderate risk at therapeutic doses; 3+=high risk at therapeutic doses.
[a]Oral.

APPENDIX 8

Management of Treatment-Emergent Side Effects of Antipsychotic Medications

In general, treatment-emergent side effects should be addressed first by dose reduction or medication switching. Prescribing medications for side effects may lead to new side effects.

SIDE EFFECT	RECOMMENDATIONS

Tremor	• Enhanced physiological tremor—a fine tremor of approximately 8–10 Hz; made worse with outstretched hands
	  – Check blood levels of medication, if applicable.
	  – Decrease dose, divide dose, or change to slow-release preparation of the medication.
	  – Consider β-blockers (e.g., propranolol can be given at a dosage of 20–30 mg two to three times daily; long-acting propranolol may be given once a day).
	• Parkinsonian tremor—coarse tremor at rest of approximately 4–6 Hz
	  – See treatment recommendations in "Extrapyramidal symptoms" row later in this table.

Sedation	• Perform a thorough evaluation of sleep behaviors, including a patient assessment of sleep quality. • Discontinue sedative-hypnotics. • Try dosing medication at bedtime. • Decrease dose of antipsychotics if possible. • Prescribe a longer-acting version of the same medication (e.g., Seroquel XR). • Substitute a less-sedating alternative medication. • Consider adjunctive medications (e.g., modafinil, amantadine, bupropion, low-dose psychostimulants). However, in patients with psychosis, adjunctive treatment is not recommended or must be used cautiously because it may increase psychosis or worsen the course of the episode.

Side effect	Recommendations

Extrapyramidal symptoms (EPS)— parkinsonian tremor, akathisia, and dystonia	• Usually seen with typical antipsychotics or higher doses of risperidone or paliperidone
	• Parkinsonian tremor—coarse tremor at rest of approximately 4–6 Hz
	  – Decrease dose, divide dose, use bedtime dosing, or switch to alternative medication.
	  – Use pharmacological treatments, including benztropine 1–2 mg twice daily, diphenhydramine 25–50 mg two or three times daily, trihexiphenidyl 2–5 mg two or three times daily, or propranolol 20–30 mg two or three times daily. Long-acting propranolol may be used once a day.
	• Akathisia
	  – May respond to propranolol 20–30 mg two to three times daily. If this is not effective, alternatives include clonidine 0.1 mg three times daily, lorazepam 1 mg two or three times daily, or clonazepam 0.5–1 mg twice daily.
	• Dystonic reactions
	  – Often can be prevented by benztropine 1 mg two or three times daily for the first few days of antipsychotic therapy. Acute dystonic reactions are generally managed with benztropine 1–2 mg intramuscularly or lorazepam 1–2 mg intramuscularly.

Tardive dyskinesia	• Prescribe typical antipsychotics in the lowest dose necessary for the shortest time possible. Midpotency typical agents may be preferred if a typical antipsychotic is selected. • Use atypical antipsychotic medications. • Consider clozapine, which has an extremely low risk of tardive dyskinesia. • Consider other treatment modalities, including electroconvulsive therapy.

SIDE EFFECT	RECOMMENDATIONS
Neuroleptic malignant syndrome (NMS)	• Educate patients with a history of NMS about the need to stay well hydrated and avoid strenuous physical activity when outside during hot weather. • Change to a second-generation antipsychotic if the patient has been taking a first-generation antipsychotic.

Insomnia	• Promote good sleep hygiene:
	  – Encourage regular aerobic exercise at least 4 hours before bedtime.
	  – Avoid alcoholic beverages.
	  – Encourage regular sleep cycles.
	  – Eliminate noises and distracting lights.
	  – Engage in relaxing activities before bed (e.g., reading, sex, meditation).
	  – Try a glass of warm milk.
	• If due to concomitant antidepressant use: reduce the dose of antidepressant, if possible.
	• Try moving the dosing of the medication to the morning.
	• Administer adjunctive medications
	  – Zolpidem 5–10 mg once daily at bedtime
	  – Zaleplon 5–20 mg (10 mg recommended dose) once daily at bedtime
	  – Eszopiclone 2–3 mg once daily at bedtime
	  – Benzodiazepine, such as temazepam 15–30 mg once daily at bedtime or lorazepam 0.5–2 mg once daily at bedtime
	  – Trazodone 25–100 mg once daily at bedtime
	  – Low-dose tricyclic antidepressant, such as amitriptyline 10–50 mg once daily at bedtime
	• Use brief, targeted cognitive therapy.
	• Switch to a more sedating antipsychotic.

SIDE EFFECT	RECOMMENDATIONS

Weight gain	• Exercise (walking, jogging, swimming) at least three times weekly and for at least 30 minutes each time.
	• Diet
	  – Eat smaller portions of three meals per day.
	  – Decrease excess fats (decrease fried foods; eat lean meats; increase vegetables, salads, and fruits).
	  – Decrease excessive low-nutritional-content carbohydrates (soft drinks, desserts, candy, gravies, potatoes, white bread).
	• Avoid snacking and, particularly, no evening snacks.
	• Add medications such as orlistat, sibutramine, amantadine, and topiramate.
	• Switch to another antipsychotic associated with less weight gain.

Source.   Adapted and modified from Miller AL, Chiles JA, Chiles JK, et al.: "The Texas Medication Algorithm Project (TMAP) Schizophrenia Algorithms." *Journal of Clinical Psychiatry* 60:649–657, 1999.

APPENDIX 9

Use of First- and Second-Generation Antipsychotics in Pregnancy and Lactation

MEDICATION (BRAND NAME)	FDA PREGNANCY CATEGORY[a]	ANTENATAL HUMAN DATA
Chlorpromazine (Thorazine)	C	In the Collaborative Perinatal Project, the frequency of congenital abnormalities was no greater than that in control subjects. A separate controlled study found an increased incidence of birth defects in the group exposed to phenothiazines (3.5%) compared with 1.6% in control subjects.
Thioridazine (Mellaril)	Not assigned a pregnancy category by the FDA	There is one case report of infant born with transposition of great vessels, patent foramen ovale, and intact ventricular septum to mother taking thioridazine in combination with fluphenazine. Some controlled human studies do not suggest increase in congenital malformation risk. A separate controlled study found an increased incidence of birth defects in the group exposed to phenothiazines (3.5%) compared with 1.6% in control subjects.

NEONATAL HUMAN DATA	LACTATION DATA[b]	NONHUMAN DATA
Neuroleptic withdrawal symptoms, including extrapyramidal abnormalities, paralytic ileus, necrotizing enterocolitis, fever, cyanotic spells, and transient heart block, have been reported, especially when the drug is used late in pregnancy. It is hypothesized that chlorpromazine might be associated with increased risk of neonatal respiratory distress if used at daily doses greater than 500 mg.	Excreted in small amounts to human milk; reported that a suckling infant may ingest up to 3% of the maternal dose; WHO Working Group on Human Lactation in 1988 did not recommend because of limited data and concerns about developing nervous system unless clinical indications for its use were "compelling." One case of sedation has been reported in an infant who consumed breast milk containing chlorpromazine. RID=0.25%	Cleft palate in mice, skeletal malformations in rats, impaired vascularization and Purkinje cell development in cerebellar cortex in rats.
Neuroleptic withdrawal symptoms, including extrapyramidal abnormalities, have been reported for the phenothiazine class.	One case of sedation has been reported in an infant who consumed breast milk containing another phenothiazine. WHO Working Group on Human Lactation in 1988 did not recommend because of limited data and concerns about developing nervous system unless clinical indications for its use were "compelling."	Cleft palate in rats and mice, treated with 50 times and more than 12 times, respectively, the dose used in humans, but no teratogenicity in rabbits.

MEDICATION (BRAND NAME)	FDA PREGNANCY CATEGORY[a]	ANTENATAL HUMAN DATA
Fluphenazine (Prolixin)	C	There is one case report of hydronephrosis and a separate case of esophageal defects. A separate controlled study found an increased incidence of birth defects in the group exposed to phenothiazines (3.5%) compared with 1.6% in control subjects.

NEONATAL HUMAN DATA	LACTATION DATA[b]	NONHUMAN DATA
Neuroleptic withdrawal symptoms, including extrapyramidal abnormalities, have been reported for the phenothiazine class. Case report of severe rhinorrhea, vomiting, and respiratory distress.	In rats, drug is excreted in milk (milk-to-plasma ratio = 2). One case of sedation has been reported in an infant who consumed breast milk containing another phenothiazine. WHO Working Group on Human Lactation in 1988 did not recommend because of limited data and concerns about developing nervous system unless clinical indications for its use were "compelling."	No teratogenicity in rats or rabbits, but induces cleft palate in mice. Impairs ossification of skull bones and increases the incidence of dilated cerebral ventricles. Rat studies indicate that the drug crosses the placenta and may accumulate in fetal rat liver.

MEDICATION (BRAND NAME)	FDA PREGNANCY CATEGORY[a]	ANTENATAL HUMAN DATA
Perphenazine (Trilafon)	C	A controlled study found an increased incidence of birth defects in the group exposed to phenothiazines (3.5%) compared with 1.6% in control subjects. There are two case reports of infants born with congenital malformations to women treated with perphenazine and other drugs during pregnancy. In the Collaborative Perinatal Project, the frequency of congenital abnormalities was no greater than that in control subjects.

Neonatal human data	Lactation data[b]	Nonhuman data
Neuroleptic withdrawal symptoms, including extrapyramidal abnormalities, have been reported for the phenothiazine class. Hypertonia, tremulousness, and other alterations of neonatal behavior have been observed (especially when treated in third trimester).	In a single human case study, the milk-to-plasma ratio was 1, and the suckling infant would receive about 0.1% of the maternal dose. One case of sedation has been reported in an infant who consumed breast milk containing another phenothiazine. WHO Working Group on Human Lactation in 1988 did not recommend because of limited data and concerns about developing nervous system unless clinical indications for its use were "compelling." RID=0.14%	In mice, drug induces hyperprolactinemia, which can induce uterine adenomyosis. In fetal rats, 40–300 times the human dose produced increased incidence of cleft palate, retrognathia, and micromelia.

MEDICATION (BRAND NAME)	FDA PREGNANCY CATEGORY[a]	ANTENATAL HUMAN DATA
Trifluoperazine (Stelazine)	C	A controlled study found an increased incidence of birth defects in the group exposed to phenothiazines (3.5%) compared with 1.6% in control subjects. Case reports of congenital anomalies include hydrocephalus, phocomelia of all four limbs, reduction defect of the arm, and transposition of the great vessels of the heart. In the Collaborative Perinatal Project, the frequency of congenital abnormalities was no greater than that in control subjects, and no increase in perinatal mortality, birth weight, or IQ scores was seen at age 4. Some evidence indicates that the drug may be a myometrial relaxant.

Neonatal human data	Lactation data[b]	Nonhuman data
Neuroleptic withdrawal symptoms, including extrapyramidal abnormalities, have been reported for the phenothiazine class.	Drug is excreted into human milk. One case of sedation has been reported in an infant who consumed breast milk containing another phenothiazine. Data from fewer than 20 women showed that the drug is transferred in smaller quantities than haloperidol and chlorpromazine and is less likely than those agents to affect infant performance on developmental tasks. WHO Working Group on Human Lactation in 1988 did not recommend because of limited data and concerns about developing nervous system unless clinical indications for its use were "compelling."	Increase in cleft palate in mice, defects of the central nervous system and urogenital system in rats, but no effect on fetal development in rabbits.

MEDICATION (BRAND NAME)	FDA PREGNANCY CATEGORY[a]	ANTENATAL HUMAN DATA
Prochlorperazine (Compazine)	C	A controlled study found an increased incidence of birth defects in the group exposed to phenothiazines (3.5%) compared with 1.6% in control subjects. There are case reports of newborns with cleft palate, micrognathia, congenital heart defects, hip dysplasia, conjoined twinning, and limb anomalies. In the Collaborative Perinatal Project, the frequency of congenital abnormalities was no greater than that in control subjects but suggested a possible association with cardiac septal defects.

NEONATAL HUMAN DATA	LACTATION DATA[b]	NONHUMAN DATA
Neuroleptic withdrawal symptoms, including extrapyramidal abnormalities, have been reported for the phenothiazine class.	One case of sedation has been reported in an infant who consumed breast milk containing another phenothiazine. WHO Working Group on Human Lactation in 1988 did not recommend because of limited data and concerns about developing nervous system unless clinical indications for its use were "compelling."	Increased frequency of cleft palate in offspring of mice and rats treated during pregnancy with drug doses 3–23 times those used in humans.

MEDICATION (BRAND NAME)	FDA PREGNANCY CATEGORY[a]	ANTENATAL HUMAN DATA
Haloperidol (Haldol)	C	Highly lipophilic and easily enters the fetal circulation. There are two case reports of limb defects, but other drugs also were involved. An association is possible between butyrophenone exposure and limb defects. The prospective study from the European Network of Teratogen Information Services found no increased risk of congenital anomalies compared with control subjects. Possible risk of lower birth weight (165 g) and twofold increase in rate of preterm birth were reported. Placental passage may produce fetal concentrations of about 65%.
Loxapine (Loxitane)	C	No epidemiological studies of congenital anomalies in infants born to women who received loxapine during pregnancy have been reported.

NEONATAL HUMAN DATA	LACTATION DATA[b]	NONHUMAN DATA
One case report of withdrawal-emergent syndrome with complete resolution of all symptoms within several days, except for tongue thrust, which persisted until age 6 months. Other case reports of dyskinesia in a neonate and hypothermia and generalized hypotonia in another neonate whose mother had received haloperidol and benztropine mesylate (Cogentin).	Drug is excreted into human milk, and suckling infant will ingest about 3% of maternal dose. Concentrations of the drug have been found in plasma in a few nursing infants but have not been associated with adverse effects. The American Academy of Pediatrics and the WHO Working Group on Human Lactation have expressed some reservation about the use of haloperidol during lactation unless the specific indications are compelling. RID=2.4%	At higher doses, drug can increase resorptions in rat pregnancies and induce cleft palate in mice. At doses of 22 mg/kg or more, can increase neural tube malformations in mucine embryo. Impairs masculine sexual behavior in male rat offspring, and rats given 10 mg/kg dose on gestational days 12–16 or 16–20 had offspring with reductions in whole brain weight.
No reports were located.	No reports were located.	Increase in multiple congenital anomalies in mice but not in rats, rabbits, or dogs when treated with two to three times the human daily dose.

MEDICATION (BRAND NAME)	FDA PREGNANCY CATEGORY[a]	ANTENATAL HUMAN DATA
Molindone (Moban)	C	No reports were located.
Pimozide (Orap)	C	An association is possible between butyrophenone exposure and limb defects, although studies were done with haloperidol and penfluridol.
Thiothixene (Navane)	C	Case report found an association of gestational use of thiothixene along with a phenothiazine and other psychotropic medications with small left colon syndrome in a newborn. One study reported that 1 of 38 newborns whose mothers received thiothixene during the first trimester had a cardiovascular defect.

NEONATAL HUMAN DATA	LACTATION DATA[b]	NONHUMAN DATA
No reports were located.	No reports were located.	No evidence of teratogenicity in rats or mice up to 40 mg/kg/day or in rabbits up to 20 mg/kg/day. The usual human dosage is about 1–3 mg/kg/day.
Extrapyramidal effects may be seen in the newborn after third-trimester maternal exposure.	No reports were located.	Alters gonadotropin levels in fish and rats. No evidence of teratogenicity in rats or rabbits. Fetal growth retardation has been reported in unpublished studies among offspring of rats treated with eight times the human dose.
No reports were located.	No reports were located.	Has not been associated with an increased incidence of malformations in rats, rabbits, or primates.

MEDICATION (BRAND NAME)	FDA PREGNANCY CATEGORY[a]	ANTENATAL HUMAN DATA
Clozapine (Clozaril)	B	Case report of an unexplained seizure in one prenatally exposed infant on postnatal day 8 (mother also received haloperidol and lorazepam concurrently). Case report of infant born at 28 weeks gestation with multiple complications of prematurity. Case report of in utero demise at 32 weeks in a mother taking 50–75 mg/day, but no congenital anomalies were noted. Possible risk of decreased fetal heart rate variability in utero at 34 weeks and during labor and delivery at 37 weeks in case reports. Cohort study in 2005 monitored six women taking clozapine and other concurrent psychotropics during first trimester and reported no statistical difference in the rate of major malformations in the exposed group (0.9%) compared with the control group (1.5%). However, the rate of low birth weight (10%) was higher in the exposed group compared with that in control subjects (2%).

NEONATAL HUMAN DATA	LACTATION DATA[b]	NONHUMAN DATA
Transient floppy infant syndrome in an infant born at 37 weeks' gestation following exposure to clozapine (200–300 mg/day) and high-dose lorazepam during pregnancy (7.5–12.5 mg/day), but no reports of floppy infant syndrome following exposure to clozapine alone.	Possibly unsafe, appears to be concentrated in human breast milk, and the risk of agranulocytosis in the infant is not clear. RID = 1.2%	Teratology studies have been negative in mice, rats, and rabbits at dosages up to 40 mg/kg/day (rabbit and rat studies).

MEDICATION (BRAND NAME)	FDA PREGNANCY CATEGORY[a]	ANTENATAL HUMAN DATA
Risperidone (Risperdal)	C	A single case report of agenesis of corpus callosum in exposed infant. Possible risk of low birth weight based on pooled data from 140 exposures. Potential risk of exaggerated hypotension during spinal anesthesia for cesarean delivery because of α-adrenergic antagonism of drug.

NEONATAL HUMAN DATA	LACTATION DATA[b]	NONHUMAN DATA
Twenty-two infants exposed late in pregnancy have been reported to have transient neonatal withdrawal syndrome symptoms, including jitteriness, tremor, hypertonia or hypotonia, somnolence, poor feeding, and convulsions.	Drug is excreted into human milk, with estimated milk-to-plasma concentration ratio of <0.5 in two lactating women. The calculated relative infant dose was 2.3%–4.7% of the maternal weight-adjusted doses. Measurable levels of the drug and its metabolite 9-hydroxy-risperidone have been measured in the suckling infant's plasma. Manufacturer does not recommend breast-feeding. RID = 2.8%	No teratogenic effects in offspring of rats given up to 10 mg/kg, but some decrease in fetal weight. No increase in congenital malformations in offspring of rabbits and rats treated with six times the human dose, although neonatal mortality was increased. Increase in rat stillbirths in one study. One study reported impaired learning by exposed rats at three times the maximum human dose.

MEDICATION (BRAND NAME)	FDA PREGNANCY CATEGORY[a]	ANTENATAL HUMAN DATA
Olanzapine (Zyprexa)	C	Crosses the placenta. Reported up to the year 2000, from the Lilly Worldwide Pharmacovigilance Safety Database, spontaneous abortion occurred in 13%, stillbirth in 5%, prematurity in 5%, and no occurrence of major malformation. All findings were within the normal limits of those found in unexposed infants. There has been a separate summary report of 96 exposed infants in which 7 infants had perinatal complications, and 1 infant was born with major malformations. Some studies indicate that there may be an increased risk of low birth weight and perinatal complications compared with other antipsychotics. In one study, olanzapine showed a higher amount of placental passage compared with other antipsychotics.

NEONATAL HUMAN DATA	LACTATION DATA[b]	NONHUMAN DATA
No reports were located.	Drug is excreted into human milk. Possible case report of sedation and jaundice in suckling infant of mother prescribed 5 mg/day; other reports of no adverse effect on lactation or child. Mean milk-to-plasma ratio of approximately 0.46 and a median infant dose of 1.6% of the maternal dose. Monitoring of infant is recommended. RID = 1.2%	No increase in congenital malformations in rats and rabbits up to dosages of 18 and 30 mg/kg/day, respectively, but a decrease in fetal viability at high doses in both species.

MEDICATION (BRAND NAME)	FDA PREGNANCY CATEGORY[a]	ANTENATAL HUMAN DATA
Quetiapine (Seroquel)	C	In a cohort study of 36 pregnant women given quetiapine and other psychotropic medications, no statistically significant differences in the rates of major malformations were found in the exposed vs. control group (0.9% vs. 1.5%). There may be an increased risk of low birth weight in exposed infants. In one study, quetiapine had the lowest amount of placental passage compared with that of haloperidol, risperidone, and olanzapine.

NEONATAL HUMAN DATA	LACTATION DATA[b]	NONHUMAN DATA
No reports were located.	Manufacturer does not recommend breast-feeding. Infant exposure has been reported to be about 0.43% of the maternal weight-adjusted dose. At dosages of 100 mg/day, the drug level in human milk is 32 nM, and infant dose is estimated to be <0.01 mg/kg/day; at dosages of 400 mg/day, drug level in human milk is 264 nM, with infant dose of <0.1 mg/kg/day. Neurodevelopmental evaluations done at 9 and 18 months in six infants showed four healthy infants, one with mild motor and mental delay, and one with mental delay, but no causative correlation between delay and drug can be made.	No increase in congenital malformations in offspring of rats and rabbits treated with up to 200 and 100 mg/kg/day, respectively (about 2.4 times the maximum human dose based on surface area). An increase in fetal and pup death was reported at three times the maximum human dose.

MEDICATION (BRAND NAME)	FDA PREGNANCY CATEGORY[a]	ANTENATAL HUMAN DATA
Ziprasidone (Geodon)	C	No reports were located.

NEONATAL HUMAN DATA	LACTATION DATA[b]	NONHUMAN DATA
No reports were located.	No reports were located.	A decrease in rat and rabbit fetal weight and delayed ossification seen at maternal dosages of 10 mg/kg/day and higher (equivalent to half the human dose on surface area basis). Other studies also indicated decreased fetal and pup viability in mothers treated with 10 mg/kg/day. Offspring of rabbits whose mothers were exposed to 30 mg/kg/day had an increase in cardiovascular malformations and kidney changes (equivalent to three times the human dose).

MEDICATION (BRAND NAME)	FDA PREGNANCY CATEGORY[a]	ANTENATAL HUMAN DATA
Aripiprazole (Abilify)	C	No major malformations reported in three case reports of maternal use of 10–20 mg/day.
Paliperidone (Invega)	C	No reports were located.

NEONATAL HUMAN DATA	LACTATION DATA[b]	NONHUMAN DATA
One case report of tachycardia in neonate whose mother received 10 mg/day.	Excreted into rat milk.	In rats, 10 mg/kg/day interferes with rat embryo development. At dosages of 10–30 mg/kg/day, female offspring showed a delay in sexual maturation and impairment of reproductive performance. In rabbits, offspring treated with 100 mg/kg/day (three times the human plasma level) had decreased food intake and increase in abortion.
No reports were located.	Appears in human milk with maternal exposure to risperidone.	No reports were located.

MEDICATION (BRAND NAME)	FDA PREGNANCY CATEGORY[a]	ANTENATAL HUMAN DATA
Paliperidone palmitate extended-release injectable suspension (Invega Sustenna)	C	No reports were located.
Iloperidone (Fanapt)	C	No reports were located.

NEONATAL HUMAN DATA	LACTATION DATA[b]	NONHUMAN DATA
No reports were located.	Appears in human milk with maternal exposure to risperidone, but studies specific to paliperidone palmitate have not been done. Manufacturer does not recommend breastfeeding during paliperidone palmitate usage.	Studies during organogenesis in pregnant rats and rabbits demonstrated no increases in fetal abnormalities, but in rat reproduction studies with risperidone, increases were seen in pup deaths at doses below the maximum daily dose (based on mg/m^2) used in humans.
No reports were located.	It is not known if iloperidone is excreted into human breast milk. However, it is excreted in milk of rats during lactation. The manufacturer does not recommend breastfeeding during iloperidone usage.	Rat and rabbit studies demonstrated developmental toxicity but no teratogenicity. In pregnant rats and rabbits, doses 1–20 times the maximum human dose caused early intrauterine deaths and maternal toxicity.

MEDICATION (BRAND NAME)	FDA PREGNANCY CATEGORY[a]	ANTENATAL HUMAN DATA
Asenapine (Saphris)	C	No reports were located.

NEONATAL HUMAN DATA	LACTATION DATA[b]	NONHUMAN DATA
No reports were located.	It is not known if asenapine is excreted into human breast milk. However, it is excreted in milk of rats during lactation. The manufacturer does not recommend breastfeeding during asenapine usage.	In pregnant rats, asenapine administration was associated with increases in postimplantation loss, early pup death, and decreases in subsequent pup survival. There were no increases seen in structural abnormalities.

Note. FDA=U.S. Food and Drug Administration; WHO=World Health Organization.
[a]See table at end of this appendix for explanation of FDA use-in-pregnancy categories.
[b]Relative infant dose (RID) = (dose of infant mg/kg/day)/(dose of mother mg/kg/day).

U.S. Food and Drug Administration (FDA) use-in-pregnancy categories

A   Adequate, well-controlled studies in pregnant women have not shown an increased risk of fetal abnormalities in any trimester of pregnancy.

B   Animal studies have shown no risk of adverse fetal effects, but no adequate or well-controlled human first-trimester studies are available; *or* animal studies have shown an adverse effect, but adequate and well-controlled studies in pregnant women have not shown a risk to the fetus in any trimester.

C   Animal studies have shown adverse fetal effect(s), but no adequate and well-controlled human studies are available; potential benefits may warrant use of the drug in pregnant women despite potential risks.

D   Positive evidence of human fetal risk; maternal benefit may outweigh fetal risk in serious or life-threatening situations.

X   Product is contraindicated in pregnant women; positive evidence of serious fetal abnormalities in animals, humans, or both; fetal risks clearly outweigh maternal benefit.

References

Burt VK, Suri R, Altshuler L, et al: The use of psychotropic medications during breast feeding. Am J Psychiatry 158:1001–1009, 2001

Committee on Drugs, American Academy of Pediatrics: Use of psychoactive drugs during pregnancy and possible effects on the fetus and newborn. Pediatrics 105:880–887, 2000

Diav-Citrin O, Shechtman S, Ornoy S, et al: Safety of haloperidol and penfluridol in pregnancy: a multicenter, prospective, controlled study. J Clin Psychiatry 66:317–322, 2005

Ernst CL, Goldberg JF: The reproductive safety profile of mood stabilizers, atypical antipsychotics, and broad-spectrum psychotropics. J Clin Psychiatry 63 (suppl 4):42–55, 2002

Gentile S: Antipsychotic therapy during early and late pregnancy: a systematic review [Epub]. Schizophr Bull September 11, 2008; doi:10.1093/schbul/sbn107

Goldstein DJ, Corbin LA, Fung MC: Olanzapine-exposed pregnancies and lactation: early experience. J Clin Psychopharmacol 20:399–403, 2000

Hale TW: Medications and Mothers' Milk. Armarillo, TX, Pharmasoft Publishing, 2004

Hill RC, McIvor RJ, Wojnar-Horton RE, et al: Risperidone distribution and excretion into human milk: case report and estimated infant exposure during breast-feeding. J Clin Psychopharmacol 20:285–286, 2000

Iloperidone [package insert]. Rockville, MD, Vanda, 2009

Invega [package insert]. Titusville, NJ, Janssen, 2009

Lee A GE, Dunn E, Ito S: Excretion of quetiapine in breast milk. Am J Psychiatry 161:1715–1716, 2004

McElhatton PR: The use of phenothiazines during pregnancy and lactation. Reprod Toxicol 6:475–490, 1992

McKenna K, Koren G, Tetelbaum M, et al: Pregnancy outcome of women using atypical antipsychotic drugs: a prospective comparative study. J Clin Psychiatry 66:444–449, 2005

Misri S, Corral M, Wardrop AA, et al: Quetiapine augmentation in lactation: a series of case reports. J Clin Psychopharmacol 26:508–511, 2006

Newham JJ, Thomas SH, MacRitchie K, et al: Birth weight of infants after maternal exposure to typical and atypical antipsychotics: prospective comparison study. Br J Psychiatry 192:333–337, 2008

Newport DJ, Calamaras MR, DeVane CL, et al: Atypical antipsychotic administration during late pregnancy: placental passage and obstetrical outcomes. Am J Psychiatry 164:1214–1220, 2007

Patton SW, Misri S, Corral MR, et al: Antipsychotic medication during pregnancy and lactation in women with schizophrenia: evaluating the risk. Can J Psychiatry 47:959–965, 2002

Paulus W, Sabine S, Karl S, et al: Atypical antipsychotics in early pregnancy. Reprod Toxicol 20:477–478, 2005

Ratnayake T, Libretto SE: No complications with risperidone treatment before and throughout pregnancy and during the nursing period. J Clin Psychiatry 63:76–77, 2002

Reprotox Database Web site. Available at: http://www-thomsonhc-com.ezproxy. umassmed.edu/hcs/librarian. Accessed December 2008.

Saphris [package insert]. Kenilworth, NJ, Schering-Plough, 2009

Stewart RB, Karas B, Springer PK: Haloperidol excretion in human milk. Am J Psychiatry 137:849–850, 1980

Teris Database Web site. Available at: http://www-thomsonhc-com.ezproxy. umassmed.edu/hcs/librarian. Accessed December 2008.

U.S. Food and Drug Administration Web site. Available at: http://www.fda.gov. Accessed December 2008.

WHO Working Group, Bennet PN (ed): Drugs and Human Lactation. Amsterdam, Elsevier, 1988, p 346

Wiles DH, Orr MW, Kolakowska T: Chlorpromazine levels in plasma and milk of nursing mothers. Br J Clin Pharmacol 5:272, 1978

Yaeger D, Smith HG, Altshuler LL: Atypical antipsychotics in the treatment of schizophrenia during pregnancy and the postpartum. Am J Psychiatry 163:2064–2070, 2006

Yonkers KA, Wisner KL, Stowe Z, et al: Management of bipolar disorder during pregnancy and the postpartum period. Am J Psychiatry 161:608–620, 2004

Yoshida K, Smith B, Craggs M, et al: Neuroleptic drugs in breast-milk: a study of pharmacokinetics and of possible adverse effects in breast-fed infants. Psychol Med 28:81–91, 1998

Index

*Page numbers printed in **boldface** type refer to tables or figures.*

Abilify. *See* Aripiprazole
Abnormal Involuntary Movement Scale, **277, 281**
Absolute neutrophil count (ANC), for clozapine use, 11, **281**
Acamprosate, 137
Active metabolites of antipsychotics, **250–260**
Acute intermittent porphyria, 237, **237**
Acute treatment of schizophrenia, 21–22
AD (Alzheimer's disease). *See also* Dementia
behavioral disturbances and psychosis in, 3, 206–210, **207, 209**
ADHD. *See* Attention-deficit/hyperactivity disorder
Adolescents. *See* Children and adolescents
α_1-Adrenergic receptor affinity of antipsychotics
aripiprazole, 16
asenapine, 17, 53
cardiovascular effects of, 222–223
clozapine, 12
iloperidone, 13
olanzapine, 14, 164
paliperidone palmitate, 13
quetiapine, 15, 165
risperidone, 12, 163
ziprasidone, 166
α_2-Adrenergic receptor affinity of antipsychotics
asenapine, 17, 53
clozapine, 12
paliperidone palmitate, 13
quetiapine, 15, 165

risperidone, 12, 163
Affective flattening, 36
Aggression, 3
in borderline personality disorder, 104, 105, 111
in dementia, 3, 209–210, 221, 228
explosive, in children and adolescents, 145, **148,** 149
impulsive, 104–105
management of
benzodiazepines, 22
clozapine, 11, 25
in dementia, 209–210
haloperidol, **148,** 175, 176
in medically ill patients, 221–222
in schizotypal personality disorder, 120
in traumatic brain injury, 231
Agitation, 3
in borderline personality disorder, 111
in delirium, 218–220
in dementia, 3, 209–210, 221, 228
in epilepsy, 233
management of, **284–286**
benzodiazepines, 22, 129, 131
choice of antipsychotic for, 21–22
in dementia, 209–210
droperidol, 10
haloperidol, 175
in medically ill patients, 218, 221 223
burns and trauma, 236
traumatic brain injury, 149
in posttraumatic stress disorder, 81
quetiapine-induced, 15
in schizotypal personality disorder, 120

Agitation *(continued)*
  substance-related, 3, 126–133
    de-escalation techniques for, 126
    due to alcohol intoxication,
      131–132
    due to alcohol withdrawal,
      132–133
    due to phencyclidine
      intoxication, 131
    due to withdrawal, 132–133
    general approach to, 126, 129
    seclusion and restraint for, 126
    stimulants, 130–131
Agranulocytosis, drug-induced, 34
  clozapine, 1, 11, 21, 169, 170, 211
    monitoring for, 11, 169
    patients at risk for, 11
  olanzapine, 234
  in patients with systemic lupus
    erythematosus, 234
Akathisia, 28, 197
  antipsychotics associated with
    aripiprazole, 16, 52, 62, 63
    asenapine, 17
    olanzapine, 14, 15
    paliperidone palmitate, 13
    risperidone, 12
  in geriatric patients, **193,** 197, 213
  prevalence of, 28
  risk factors for, 197
  treatment of, 29, 197, **293**
    benzodiazepines, 22, 197
    beta-blockers, 29, 197
Akinesia, drug-induced, 28
  depression as form of, 27
Alcoholics Anonymous, 137
Alcohol intoxication, 131–132
Alcohol use disorders, **127,** 141–142
  bipolar disorder and, 140
Alcohol withdrawal, 126, 130
  benzodiazepines for, 129, 132
  psychomotor agitation due to,
    132–133
Allergic rhinitis, clozapine-induced, 227
Alogia, 36

Alprazolam, in borderline personality
  disorder, **113**
Altered consciousness, in neuroleptic
  malignant syndrome, 30
Alzheimer's disease (AD). *See also*
  Dementia
  behavioral disturbances and psycho-
    sis in, 3, 206–210, **207, 209**
Amantadine
  for neuroleptic malignant syndrome,
    199
  psychosis induced by, 210
  for weight reduction, **295**
Amenorrhea, 34
American Psychiatric Association
    practice guidelines
  for acute stress disorder and
    posttraumatic stress disorder,
    81, 85
  for bipolar disorder, 46
  for delirium, 220
  for depression, 54
  for obsessive-compulsive disorder,
    64, 70
α-Amino-3-hydroxy-5-methyl-4-
    isoxazole propionic acid (AMPA)
    receptors, 19
Amitriptyline
  in borderline personality disorder,
    108, **112**
  for insomnia, **294**
  interaction with haloperidol, 92
  for pediatric anorexia nervosa, 183
  in psychotic depression, 57, 58, **58**
  in schizotypal personality disorder,
    119
Amotivational syndrome
  cannabis-induced, 136
  in schizophrenia, 36
AMPA (α-amino-3-hydroxy-5-methyl-4-
    isoxazole propionic acid)
    receptors, 19
Amphetamine
  intoxication with, 130–131
  psychosis induced by, 18, 134–135

Analgesic effects of antipsychotics, 236–237
ANC (absolute neutrophil count), for clozapine use, 11, **281**
Anorexia nervosa, pediatric, 3, 183–184
  chlorpromazine for, 183
  haloperidol for, 183–184
  olanzapine for, 184
  pimozide for, 184
Anterior capsulotomy, for obsessive-compulsive disorder, 64
Anterior cingulotomy, for obsessive-compulsive disorder, 64
Anticholinergic agents for extrapyramidal symptoms, 28–29, 129, **293**
  acute dystonia, 28–29, 197–198
  adverse effects in geriatric patients, 196, 197
  parkinsonism, 196
  in pregnancy, 228
  prophylactic, 22, 28, 197
Anticholinergic effects of drugs, 9–10, 34, 172, 196, **290**
  affecting pulmonary system, 226–227
  clozapine, 199
  in geriatric patients, **193**, 196, 197, 199, 213
  monitoring for, **201**
  olanzapine, 199
  psychosis, 210
  in traumatic brain injury patients, 231
Antidepressants, 27. *See also specific drugs and classes*
  antipsychotic interactions with, 72, 90–92
    cytochrome P450–related, 81, 90, **91**, 92
  combined with antipsychotics
    for nonpsychotic depression, 61–63
      in geriatric patients, 204
    for psychotic depression, 54–58, **58**
      in geriatric patients, 205

  for treatment-resistant depression, 59–61
  in frontotemporal dementia, 212
  for generalized anxiety disorder, 72
  for insomnia, **294**
  for obsessive-compulsive disorder, 64
  for schizoaffective disorder, 38
Antiepileptic drugs, 12, 233
Antifungal agents, interaction with pimozide, 177
Antipsychotics, 8–20. *See also specific drugs*
  acute treatment with, 21–22
  adequate trial of, 35
  adverse effects of, 6, 7, 28–34, 110, **290**
    extrapyramidal symptoms, 28–29
    in geriatric patients, 192, **193**, 193–202
    hyperprolactinemia, 34, **35**
    monitoring for, **276–277**
    neuroleptic malignant syndrome, 29–30
    other effects, 34
    in pediatric patients, 170–172, 180, 185
    seizures, 21, 34, 233–234
    sudden cardiac death, 30–31
    tardive dyskinesia, 29
    weight gain and metabolic effects, 31–34, **33**
  atypical (*See* Second-generation antipsychotics)
  background and discovery of, 1, 8
  classification of, 1, 8, 145, **250–260**
  combinations of, 36–37
  cost of, 9, 22, 26
  discontinuation of
    in CATIE study, 25, 26
    in pediatric patients, 185
    in pregnancy, 37
    relapse due to, 21, 22–23
    withdrawal dyskinesia due to, 29

Antipsychotics *(continued)*
  dosage of, 22
    for agitation due to psychosis,
      284–286
    chlorpromazine equivalents, 35,
      250–260
    in hepatic disease, 225
    in renal disease, 224
  drug interactions with, 3, 116
    benzodiazepines, 92
    carbamazepine, 116
    cytochrome P450–related, **91,**
      92
    selective serotonin reuptake
      inhibitors, 72, 81, 90–92,
      116
    valproate, 116
  efficacy of, 1, 8, 21, 25
    CATIE study of, 15, 23, 25–26
    CUtLASS 1 study of, 27
    dopamine D$_2$ receptor occupancy
      and, 18, 20
  first-generation, 1, 8–10, 145
    (See also First-generation
      antipsychotics)
  formulations of, 22, **242–246**
  indications for, 1–2, 104, 125, 145
    bipolar disorder, 2, 46–54, **47,**
      205
    in children and adolescents, 145,
      180–186
    dementia-related behavioral
      disturbances and psychosis,
      207, 208–210, **209,** 229
    dementia with Lewy bodies,
      211–212
    frontotemporal dementia, 212
    generalized anxiety disorder,
      73–81, **77–79**
    in geriatric patients, 203–212
    nonpsychotic depression, 61–63
    obsessive-compulsive disorder,
      65–72, **68**
    Parkinson's disease, 210–211,
      229–230
    personality disorders, 101–123
      borderline personality
        disorder, 110–116,
        112–113
      schizotypal personality
        disorder, 116–121, **119**
    posttraumatic stress disorder,
      82–90, **86–87**
    psychotic depression, 55–58, **58,**
      205
    schizoaffective disorder, 38
    schizophrenia, 1, 8, 20–37,
      39–40, 203–204
    substance abuse disorders,
      125–143, **127–128**
    traumatic brain injury, 231
    treatment-resistant depression,
      2, 59–61, 204
  intramuscular, 22, 216, **217**
  intravenous, 216, **217**
  lipophilicity of, 224
  long-acting preparations of, 23–24, 39
    combined with oral drugs, 37
    for substance-abusing schizo-
      phrenia patients, 138, **139**
  maintenance treatment with, 22–24
  mechanism of action of, 1, 104–105
  medical workup for use of, 20–21,
    276–277
  off-label use of, 2
  onset of action of, 20
  overdose of, 116, 171
  pharmacokinetics of, **250–260**
  plasma concentrations of, 24
    time to peak levels, **250–260**
  polypharmacy with, 36–37
  in pregnancy and lactation, 3, 37,
    227–228, **298–327**
  regulatory approval for use of, 1–2
  resistance to, 34–36
  routes of administration of, 3, 216,
    217, 220, **221**
  second-generation, 1, 8–9, 10–20,
    145 *(See also* Second-
      generation antipsychotics)

selection of, 21–22
switching between, 22, 36, 40
   due to hyperprolactinemia, 34
   due to weight gain, 33–34
typical (*See* First-generation
   antipsychotics)
use in children and adolescents, 3,
   145–186
use in geriatric patients, 3, 191–213
use in long-term care facilities, 3,
   202–203, 208
use in medically ill patients, 3,
   215–238
variability of response to, 21
Antisocial personality disorder, 105
Anxiety
in burn and trauma patients, 236
risperidone-induced, 12
Anxiety disorders, 2, 45, 63–90
benzodiazepines for, 22
generalized anxiety disorder, 2,
   72–81
obsessive-compulsive disorder, 2,
   37, 63–72
pediatric psychosis and, 182
posttraumatic stress disorder, 2,
   81–90
safety and tolerability of
   antipsychotics in, 90–92
Apathy, 36
Appetite effects, of olanzapine-
   fluoxetine combination, 60
Aripiprazole, 16–17
administration of, 16
adverse effects of, 16, 52, 62, 76,
   159, **290**
   cerebrovascular events in
      elderly dementia patients,
      202
   weight gain and metabolic
      effects, 16, 31, **33**, 52, 76,
      159
augmentation for generalized
   anxiety disorder, 75, 76, 80
benefits of, 16

for bipolar disorder, **47**
   acute mania, 46
   in pediatric patients, **147**, 148,
      159–160
   relapse prevention, 51–52, 54
for conduct disorder, 159
for delirium, 220, **221**
for dementia-related behavioral
   disturbances and psychosis,
   209
dosage of, **221, 272**
   for agitation due to psychosis,
      286
   chlorpromazine equivalence, **258**
   for geriatric patients, **192**, 204,
      209
   for pediatric patients, 159, 167
drug interactions with, 17
   carbamazepine, 17
   fluoxetine, 17
   fluvoxamine, 92
efficacy of, 25
formulations of, 17, 167, **217, 246**
intramuscular, 22, **217, 246, 286**
mechanism of action of, 16, 167
for nonpsychotic depression, 62–63
for obsessive-compulsive disorder,
   71
in personality disorders, 108
   borderline personality disorder,
      111, **113**
   symptom response, 107, **109**
pharmacokinetics of, 16, **258**
in pregnancy and lactation, 227,
   322–323
receptor affinity of, 16, 20, 141,
   167
routes of administration of, **217,
   221**
for schizophrenia
   with comorbid substance abuse,
      138
   in geriatric patients, 204
   maintenance treatment, 23
   in pediatric patients, **147**, 148

Aripiprazole *(continued)*
  in substance abuse disorders, **127**
    for agitation, 130
    alcohol dependence, 141
    with bipolar disorder, 140
    with schizophrenia, 138
    stimulant dependence, 142
  for treatment-resistant depression,
    60, 61, 204
    in geriatric patients, 204
  use in children and adolescents,
    146, **147,** 148, 159–160, 167
    for bipolar disorder, 148,
      159–160
    for schizophrenia, 148
  use in medically ill patients, 217
    hepatic disease, 225, **272**
    Parkinson's disease, 211, 230
    renal disease, 224, **272**
Arrhythmias, drug-induced, 30–31. *See*
    also Tachycardia; Torsades de
    points
  stimulants, 130
  thioridazine, 174
Asenapine, 17
  adverse effects of, 17, 31, **33,** 53
  for bipolar disorder, **47**
    relapse prevention, 53
  dosage of, 17, **274**
    in geriatric patients, **274**
  efficacy of, 25
    vs. risperidone, 17
  formulations of, **246**
  pharmacokinetics of, **260**
  in pregnancy and lactation,
    326–327
  receptor affinity of, 17, 53
  sublingual administration of, 17
  use in hepatic disease, **274**
Asenapine N+-glucuronide, **260**
Ataxia, drug-induced
  alcohol, 131
  phencyclidine, 131
  second-generation antipsychotic
    overdose, 171

Attention-deficit/hyperactivity disorder
    (ADHD), 156, 160, 173
  chlorpromazine for, 173, 186
  treatment in pediatric bipolar
    disorder, 181
Autism spectrum disorders, 3, 145,
    146, 149, 184
  haloperidol for, 184
  risperidone for, **147,** 148, **152,** 184,
    237
Autonomic dysfunction, in neuroleptic
    malignant syndrome, 198
Azole antifungal agents, interaction
    with pimozide, 177

Bech-Rafaelson Scale, 57
Behavioral disturbances in dementia,
    206–210, 228–229
  dangerous agitation and aggression,
    3, 209–210
  definitions of, 206
  management of, 206–209, **207, 209**
Behavior therapy, for obsessive-
    compulsive disorder, 64
Behçet's disease, 234
Benzisothiazolyls, 15–16, **257**. *See also*
    Ziprasidone
Benzisoxazoles, 12–14, **255–256,**
    259–260
  iloperidone, 13–14
  paliperidone, 12–13
  risperidone, 12
Benzodiazepines, 22
  for agitation/aggression, 210, 222
  for akathisia, 22, 197, **293**
  for alcohol withdrawal, 129, 132
  antipsychotic interactions with, 92
  in borderline personality disorder,
    113
  for comorbid anxiety and dyspnea, 226
  cytochrome P450 system and, 92
  for generalized anxiety disorder, 72,
    73
    vs. typical antipsychotics, 74,
      77, 78, 80

for insomnia, **294**
for neuroleptic malignant syndrome,
   199
respiratory depression induced by,
   226
for substance-related agitation, 129
   due to phencyclidine
      intoxication, 129, 131
   due to stimulant intoxication,
      129, 131
synergistic effects with alcohol, 131
for tardive dyskinesia, 29
use in geriatric patients, 197, 210
use in medically ill patients, 222
Benztropine
   for acute dystonia, 198, **293**
   for parkinsonism, 196, **293**
   in pregnancy, 228
Beta-blockers
   for akathisia, 29, 197
   use in medically ill patients, 197
   use in stimulant intoxication, 131
Bipolar disorder, 2, 45–54
   age at onset of, 46
   antipsychotics for, 2, 46–54, **47**
      acute mania and mixed states,
         46–48
      bipolar I depression, 48–49
      bipolar II depression, 49–50
      in geriatric patients, 3, 205
      key clinical points regarding,
         53–54
      in patients with comorbid
         substance abuse, 140–141
      relapse prevention, **47**, 50–53
   bipolar I and II disorders, 46
   in children and adolescents, 3, 145
   psychosis and, 182
   treatment of, **147**, 148, 149,
      150–151, 153, 180–181
      aripiprazole, 148, 159–160
      in attention-deficit/hyper-
         activity disorder, 181
      duration of, 181
      olanzapine, 155, 157

quetiapine, 158–159
risperidone, 148, 155–156
ziprasidone, 160–161
comorbid with substance abuse, 3,
   138–141
   assessment for, 140
   integrative approach to, 140
   medication selection for, 140
   treatment recommendations for,
      141
incidence of, 45
practice guideline for treatment of,
   46
with rapid cycling, 46
recurrences of, 46
suicide and, 181
Birth defects and antipsychotic use in
   pregnancy, 227–228, **298–327**
Black-box warnings
   for antipsychotic use in elderly
      dementia patients, 200–201
   for clozapine, 11
   for droperidol, 31
   for mesoridazine, 31
   for thioridazine, 10, 31, 174
Bleuler, Eugen, 5
Blood pressure effects of drugs, 21,
   194, **290**
   aripiprazole, 52
   chlorpromazine, 194, 222
   clozapine, 1, 12, 149, 194, 211, 222,
      224, **280**
   in geriatric patients, **193**, 194
   iloperidone, 13–14
   monitoring for, 194, **276, 280**
   in neuroleptic malignant syndrome,
      30
   olanzapine, 15, 194, 223
   phencyclidine, 131
   phenothiazines, 9–10
   quetiapine, 15, 223
   risperidone, 12, 223
   stimulants, 130
   thioridazine, 194
   ziprasidone, 16

Borderline personality disorder (BPD),
2, 102, 110–116
adverse effects of antipsychotics in,
110, 116
antipsychotic indications and
efficacy in, 105–106, 111,
112–113, 122
for agitation/aggression, 111,
122
clinical features of, 104
clinical use of antipsychotics in,
106–108, 111, 114
dosage, 106–107, 114, 122
symptom response, 107–108,
109, 111, 114, **115,** 122
guidelines for antipsychotic
selection and use in, 108–110,
110, 114–115
history of antipsychotic use in, 103
key clinical points regarding
antipsychotics in, 122–123
long-term antipsychotic use in,
108–109, 110, 123
medical workup for antipsychotic
use in, 115–116, 123–124
neurobiology of, 104–105
typical vs. atypical antipsychotics
in, 110–111
BPRS (Brief Psychiatric Rating Scale),
14, 53, 57, 118, 158
Bradykinesia, 28
Breast-feeding and antipsychotic use,
3, 37, 228, **298–327**
Brief Psychiatric Rating Scale (BPRS),
14, 53, 57, 118, 158
Bromazepam, for generalized anxiety
disorder, **78**
Bromocriptine, for neuroleptic
malignant syndrome, 30, 199
Buprenorphine, 137
Burn patients, 3, 236
Buspirone, for generalized anxiety
disorder, 72
Butyrophenones, 10, **252.** *See also*
First-generation antipsychotics

Calcium channel blockers, for tardive
dyskinesia, 29
Cannabis-associated psychosis,
135–136
CAPS (Clinician-Administered PTSD
Scale), 83, 84, 85, **86, 87,** 88, 89
Part 2, 82, 85, **86**
Carbamazepine, 161
in borderline personality disorder,
113
drug interactions with, 116
aripiprazole, 17
clozapine, 168
N-Carbamoyl glucuronide, **260**
Cardiovascular disease, 3, 222–224
clozapine use in, 224
schizophrenia and, 5, 6
thioridazine use in, 175
ziprasidone use in, 16, 195
Cardiovascular effects of drugs, 34,
222–224. *See also* Orthostatic
hypotension; QTc interval
prolongation; Tachycardia
chlorpromazine, 31, 194, 222
clozapine, 1, 11, 12, 21, 149, 168,
170, 194, 211, 223–224
droperidol, 10, 31
fluphenazine, 31
in geriatric patients, **193,** 194–195,
199
haloperidol, 31, 129, 220, 223, **224**
iloperidone, 13–14
mesoridazine, 31
monitoring for, 194, **201**
in neuroleptic malignant syndrome,
30
olanzapine, 15, 194, **224**
paliperidone, 13
phencyclidine, 131
phenothiazines, 9–10
pimozide, 10, 31, 172, 177
prochlorperazine, 31
QTc interval prolongation, 30–31,
166, 194–195, 220, 222, 223,
224

quetiapine, 15, **224**
risperidone, 12, 13, **224**
second-generation antipsychotic
overdose, 171
stimulants, 130
sudden cardiac death, 10, 11, 30–31
thioridazine, 10, 31, 171, 172, 174,
175, 194, 195, 223, **224**
trifluoperazine, 31
ziprasidone, 16, 166, 171, 195, 223,
224, 225, **286**
Cataract, quetiapine-induced, 15
Catatonia, 21, 22
CATIE (Clinical Antipsychotic Trials of
Intervention Effectiveness), 15,
23, 25–26, 32–33
CBT. *See* Cognitive-behavioral therapy
Center for Epidemiologic Studies
Depression Scale (CES-D Scale), 83
Central nervous system (CNS)
depression, drug-induced, 171
Cerebrovascular events related to
antipsychotic use in elderly
dementia patients, 202, 229
CES-D Scale (Center for Epidemiologic
Studies Depression Scale), 83
CGI-S (Clinical Global Improvement–
Severity scale), 53, 69, 75, 76, **77**,
79, 89, 158, 160, 184
Child Mania Rating Scale—Parent
Version, 160
Child-Pugh score of liver dysfunction,
225–226
Children and adolescents, 3, 145–186
antipsychotic treatment in, 180–186
for anorexia nervosa, 183–184
for autism spectrum disorders
and pervasive
developmental delay, 184
for bipolar disorder, 180–181
discontinuation of, 185
key clinical points regarding,
185–186
for psychosis, 182–183
for Tourette syndrome, 185

first-generation antipsychotics for,
146, 172–180
adverse effects of, 172, 180,
185
chlorpromazine, 173–174
clinical use of, 172
fluphenazine, 178
haloperidol, 175–176
indications for, **147–148**
molindone, 178–179
pimozide, 176–178
vs. second-generation
antipsychotics, 161–162,
186
thioridazine, 174–175
trifluoperazine, 179–180
increase in antipsychotic
prescriptions for, 146
second-generation antipsychotics
for, 146–171, **150–153**
adverse effects of, 170–171, 185
aripiprazole, 146, **147**, 148,
159–160, 167
clozapine, 149, 154–155,
168–170
vs. first-generation antipsychotics, 161–162, 186
guidelines for selection and use
of, 162–163
indications for, 146–148, **147**
medical workup before initiation
of, 162–163
monitoring during treatment
with, 163
olanzapine, 156–157, 164–165
other uses of, 149
overdose of, 171
quetiapine, 157–159, 165
risperidone, 146, **147, 148**,
155–156, 163–164
ziprasidone, 160–161, 165–167
Chlordiazepoxide
for alcohol withdrawal, 132
for generalized anxiety disorder,
77

Chlorpromazine, 9
  adverse effects of
    lupus, 235
    orthostatic hypotension, 194
    QTc interval prolongation, 31
    seizures, 173, 233
    weight gain, **33**
  for anxiety, 74
  augmentation for generalized
    anxiety disorder, **77**
  background and discovery of, 1, 8
  for bipolar mania, **47**
  contraindications to, 173
  for delirium, **221**
  dosage of, **221, 262**
    for agitation due to psychosis,
      284
    for geriatric patients, **262**
    for pediatric patients, 174
  efficacy of, 21
  formulations of, 173, 216, **217, 242**
  interaction with ziprasidone, 166
  intravenous, 216, **217, 242**
  in personality disorders, 108
    borderline personality disorder,
      111, **112**
    symptom response, **109**
  pharmacokinetics of, **250**
  in pregnancy and lactation,
    298–299
  routes of administration of, **217,
    221**
  for steroid-induced psychiatric
    symptoms, 235
  use in children and adolescents,
    147, 173–174
    for anorexia nervosa, 183
    for attention-deficit/hyperactivity
      disorder, 173, 186
  use in medically ill patients
    hepatic disease, **262**
    other medical disorders, **237,**
      237–238
    renal disease, 224, **262**
Nor-2-Chlorpromazine, **250**

Chlorpromazine-equivalent drug
    dosages, 35, **250–260**
Nor-2-Chlorpromazine sulfate, **250**
Chlorprothixene, for generalized
    anxiety disorder, **78**
Cholestasis, 226
Cholesterol. *See* Hyperlipidemia
Cholinergic receptor affinity of
    antipsychotics
  clozapine, 12
  olanzapine, 14, 164
Cholinesterase inhibitors, 208
  in dementia with Lewy bodies, 212
  in Parkinson's disease, 211
Citalopram, for behavioral disturbances
    in dementia, 208
Classification of antipsychotics, 1, 8,
    145, **250–260**
Clinical Antipsychotic Trials of
    Intervention Effectiveness
    (CATIE), 15, 23, 25–26, 32–33
Clinical Global Improvement–Severity
    scale (CGI-S), 53, 69, 75, 76, **77,
    79,** 89, 158, 160, 184
Clinician-Administered PTSD Scale
    (CAPS), 83, 84, 85, **86, 87,** 88, 89
  Part 2, 82, 85, **86**
Clomipramine
  interaction with haloperidol, 92
  for obsessive-compulsive disorder,
    64
Clonazepam
  for akathisia, **293**
  for weaning from mechanical
    ventilation, 226
Clonidine
  for akathisia, **293**
  for tardive dyskinesia, 29
Clozapine, 10–12, 39–40
  administration of, 12
  adverse effects of, 1, 11–12, 21,
    168, 170, **290**
    agranulocytosis, 11, 21, 169,
      170, 211, 223, 234
    allergic rhinitis, 227

anticholinergic effects, 199
cardiac effects, 11–12, 21, 168,
    170, 223–224
in geriatric patients, 211
hepatotoxicity, 226
lupus, 235
monitoring for, 11, **280–281**
orthostatic hypotension, 194
in pediatric patients, 149
seizures, 1, 12, 21, 168, 170, 234
weight gain and metabolic
    effects, 12, 21, 31, **33**
augmentation for posttraumatic
    stress disorder, 83
background and discovery of, 1, 10
CATIE study of, 26
contraindications to, 168
for dementia-related behavioral
    disturbances and psychosis,
    209
discontinuation of, 11
dosage of, **268**
    chlorpromazine equivalence, **254**
    for geriatric patients, **192, 209**
    for pediatric patients, 149,
        169–170
drug interactions with
    carbamazepine, 168
    fluvoxamine, 92
efficacy of, 1, 8, 10–11, 18, 21, 24–25
formulations of, 12, 168, **217, 245**
indications for, 11, 24–25
maintenance treatment with, 23
mechanism of action of, 12, 168
medical workup for use of, 11,
    168–169, **280–281**
for obsessive-compulsive disorder, 71
pharmacokinetics of, **254**
in pregnancy and lactation, 227,
    312–313
receptor affinity of, 12, 18, 168
for schizoaffective disorder, 38
for schizophrenia, 168
    with comorbid substance abuse,
        127, 138

negative symptoms, 11, 36
in pediatric patients, 149, **151,
    152,** 154–155
to reduce suicide risk, 11, 23, 25
treatment-resistant, 1, 11, 21,
    23, 24, 35–36
in substance abuse disorders
    with bipolar disorder, 141
    with schizophrenia, **127,** 138
for tardive dyskinesia, 11, 29, 168
use in children and adolescents,
    147, 148, 149, **151–152,**
    154–155, 168–170
    for schizophrenia, 149, 154–155
    therapeutic serum levels of, 171
use in medically ill patients, 217
    cardiac disease, 224
    hepatic disease, **268**
    Parkinson's disease, 210–211, 230
    renal disease, 224, **268**
    respiratory failure, 227
    traumatic brain injury, 231
Clozaril. *See* Clozapine
CNS (central nervous system)
    depression, drug-induced, 171
Cocaine dependence, 125, **127–128,**
    142
    bipolar disorder and, 140
Cocaine intoxication, 130–131
Cognitive-behavioral therapy (CBT)
    for generalized anxiety disorder, 72
    for obsessive-compulsive disorder,
        69
    for posttraumatic stress disorder, 81
Cognitive disorders
    delirium, 218–220, **221**
    dementia, 228–229
        antipsychotic risks in elderly
            patients with, 200–202
        with behavioral disturbances and
            psychosis, 206–210, **207,
            209,** 228–229
        frontotemporal, 3, 212
        with Lewy bodies, 3, 196,
            211–212

Cognitive effects of drugs
    anticholinergic agents, 196, 199
    antiparkinsonian drugs, 210
    benzodiazepines, 197
    in geriatric patients, 196, 199
    in neuroleptic malignant syndrome,
        198
    stimulants, 130
Cogwheel rigidity, 28, 171
Compazine. *See* Prochlorperazine
Compliance with treatment, 6, 7, 23,
    37, 39, 40, 137
Conduct disorder, 145, 146, 149,
    158
    aripiprazole for, 159
    risperidone for, **150**
Congenital malformations and
    antipsychotic use in pregnancy,
    227–228, **298–327**
Constipation, drug-induced, 34
    anticholinergic agents, 196
    aripiprazole, 76
    in geriatric patients, 199
    olanzapine, 15
    risperidone, 12
Coordination of care, 7
Coronary artery disease, 6, 217.
    See also Cardiovascular disease
Corticosteroids
    psychiatric symptoms induced by, 3,
        235–236
    for rheumatologic disorders, 234
Cortico-striatal-thalamic circuit, in
    obsessive-compulsive disorder,
    65
Cost of antipsychotics, 9, 22, 26
Cost Utility of the Latest Antipsychotic
    Drugs in Schizophrenia Study
    (CUtLASS 1), 27
Creatine kinase, in neuroleptic
    malignant syndrome, 30
CUtLASS 1 (Cost Utility of the Latest
    Antipsychotic Drugs in
    Schizophrenia Study), 27
Cymbalta. *See* Duloxetine

Cytochrome P450 (CYP) enzyme
    system, 225
    antipsychotics and, **91,** 92
        aripiprazole, 16–17
        haloperidol, 92
        quetiapine, 233
    benzodiazepines and, 92
    selective serotonin reuptake
        inhibitors and, 72, 81, 90, 92

Dantrolene, for neuroleptic malignant
    syndrome, 30, 199
Davidson Trauma Scale, 85, **87**
DBS (deep brain stimulation), for
    obsessive-compulsive disorder, 64
DBT (dialectical behavior therapy), for
    borderline personality disorder,
    113
Deep brain stimulation (DBS), for
    obsessive-compulsive disorder, 64
Dehydroaripiprazole, **258**
Deinstitutionalization, 8
Delirium, 3, 199, 218–221
    in burn and trauma patients, 236
    environmental interventions for, 219
    etiologies of, 219
    pharmacotherapy for, 219–220, **221**
    practice guideline for treatment of, 220
    prevalence in medically ill patients, 219
    in pulmonary disease patients, 226
Delusions, 21, 102
    in dementia, 228
    in epilepsy, 233
    in psychotic depression, 54
    in schizophrenia, 7
    substance-induced, 133
Dementia, 3, 191, 228–229
    antipsychotic risks in elderly
        patients with, 200–202, 229
        cerebrovascular events, 202
        death, 200–202
    with behavioral disturbances and
        psychosis, 206–210, 228–229
    dangerous agitation and
        aggression, 3, 209–210, 221

definitions of, 206
management of, 206–209, **207,
209**
frontotemporal (FTD), 3, 212
with Lewy bodies (DLB), 3, 196,
211–212
Depersonalization, in personality
disorders, 102, **103**
Depression, 54–63
bipolar, 45–46 (*See also* Bipolar
disorder)
bipolar I depression, 48–49
olanzapine-fluoxetine
combination for, 49
quetiapine, **47,** 48–49, 52
bipolar II depression, 49–50, 52
in geriatric patients, 205
comorbidity with
generalized anxiety disorder, 72
obsessive-compulsive disorder,
64
pediatric psychosis, 182
schizophrenia, 5, 27
in geriatric patients, 3
nonpsychotic, 61–63
aripiprazole for, 62–63
in geriatric patients, 204
key clinical points regarding, 63
postpsychotic, 27
psychotic, 2, 27, 54–58
combination of antipsychotic and
antidepressant for, 55–58,
58
electroconvulsive therapy for, 54,
58
in geriatric patients, 54, 205
key clinical points regarding, 58
prevalence of, **5**4
in schizoaffective disorder, 38
steroid-induced, 235
suicide and, 27
treatment-resistant (TRD), 2, 59–61
key clinical points regarding, 61
olanzapine-fluoxetine
combination for, 59–60

other atypical antipsychotics for,
2, 60–61
Derealization, in personality disorders,
102, **103**
N-Desalkyl quetiapine, **256, 257**
Desipramine, interaction with
haloperidol, 92
N-Desmethylasenapine, **260**
N-Desmethylclozapine, **254**
N-Desmethylloxapine, **252**
N-Desmethylprochlorperazine, **252**
Diabetes mellitus, 224. *See also*
Hyperglycemia
drug-induced, 32–33
clozapine, 32, **280**
in geriatric patients, **193,** 199
monitoring for, **276**
olanzapine, 32
quetiapine, 32
risperidone, 32
gestational, 227
schizophrenia and, 5, 31
use of antipsychotics in, 109, 217
Diabetic ketoacidosis, 32
Dialectical behavior therapy (DBT), for
borderline personality disorder,
113
Dialysis patients, 224
Diaphoresis
in neuroleptic malignant syndrome, 30
stimulant-induced, 130
Dibenzodiazepines, 10–12, **254.** *See
also* Clozapine
Dibenzo-oxepino pyrroles, 17, **260.** *See
also* Asenapine
Dibenzothiazepines, 15, **256.** *See also*
Quetiapine
Dibenzoxazepines, 10, **252.** *See also*
First-generation antipsychotics
Dihydroindoles, 10, **253.** *See also* First-
generation antipsychotics
Diphenhydramine
for acute dystonia, 28–29, 198
for parkinsonism, **293**
in pregnancy, 228

Diphenylbutylpiperidines, 10, **253**.
    See also First-generation
    antipsychotics
Discontinuation of antipsychotics
    in CATIE study, 25, 26
    clozapine, 11
    in pregnancy, 37
    relapse due to, 21, 22–23
    withdrawal dyskinesia due to, 29
Disruptive behavior disorders,
    pediatric, 149
    psychosis and, 182
    risperidone for, **147**, 148, **150, 152,
    153**
Dissociation, in posttraumatic stress
    disorder, 81
Distribution of antipsychotics,
    250–260
Disulfiram, 137
Divalproex. *See* Valproate
Dizziness, drug-induced
    asenapine, 53
    clozapine, 223
    iloperidone, 13
    olanzapine, 15, 223
    paliperidone palmitate, 13
    quetiapine, 15, 223
    risperidone, 75, 223
    second-generation antipsychotic
        overdose, 171
    ziprasidone, 16
DLB (dementia with Lewy bodies), 3,
    196, 211–212
L-Dopa, 210
Dopamine
    in generalized anxiety disorder,
        73–74, 80
    in obsessive-compulsive disorder,
        65
    in phencyclidine intoxication, 131
    in posttraumatic stress disorder, 82,
        83, 90
    in schizophrenia, 17–18, 104
    in schizotypal personality disorder,
        104

Dopamine receptor affinity of
    antipsychotics, 1, 17–20, 104
    efficacy and D_2 occupancy, 18, 20
    extrapyramidal symptoms and D_2
        occupancy, 20
    partial agonism of D_2 receptors, 20
    relative to serotonin receptor
        affinity, 18, 19
    specific drugs
        aripiprazole, 16, 20, 141, 167
        asenapine, 17, 53
        clozapine, 12, 18, 20, 168
        haloperidol, 10, 18, 20
        iloperidone, 13
        olanzapine, 14, 20, 164
        paliperidone, 12
        paliperidone palmitate, 13
        quetiapine, 15, 20, 142, 165
        risperidone, 12, 20, 163
        ziprasidone, 16, 165
    tardive dyskinesia and, 29
Dopamine receptor subtypes, 18
Droperidol, 10
    for agitation, 10
    cardiovascular effects of, 10, 31
    interaction with ziprasidone, 166
Drowsiness, drug-induced, 10
    asenapine, 53
    risperidone, 12
Drug-drug interactions, 3, 116
    with aripiprazole, 17
    with benzodiazepines, 92
    with carbamazepine, 116
    cytochrome P450–related, **91,** 92
    in medically ill patients, 216, 238
    with paliperidone, 12
    with pimozide, 177
    with selective serotonin reuptake
        inhibitors, 72, 81, 90–92, 116
    with thioridazine, 175
    with valproate, 116
    with ziprasidone, 16, 166
Dry mouth, drug-induced
    aripiprazole, 52, 76
    in geriatric patients, 199

iloperidone, 13
olanzapine, 15
olanzapine-fluoxetine combination,
  60
quetiapine, 15
Duloxetine
  antipsychotic interactions with, 92
  for generalized anxiety disorder, 72
Dysarthria, phencyclidine-induced, 131
Dyskinesia. *See also* Tardive dyskinesia
  stimulant-induced, 130
Dyspepsia, drug-induced
  aripiprazole, 76, 159
  quetiapine, 159
  ziprasidone, 16
Dysphagia, clozapine-induced, 12
Dystonia, drug-induced, 28, 197
  drugs associated with, 28
    haloperidol, 10, 129
    paliperidone, 13
    prevalence of, 28
    stimulants, 130
  due to second-generation
    antipsychotic overdose, 171
  in geriatric patients, **193**, 197–198
  laryngeal, 28, 226
  tardive, 11
  treatment of, 28–29, 198, **293**

Eating Attitudes Test, 184
Eating Disorder Inventory, 183
ECG. *See* Electrocardiogram
ECT. *See* Electroconvulsive therapy
Effexor. *See* Venlafaxine
Elderly persons. *See* Geriatric patients
Electrocardiogram (ECG). *See also* QTc
    interval prolongation
  effects of second-generation
    antipsychotic overdose, 171
  monitoring for antipsychotic use,
    276
    clozapine, 11, **281**
    in geriatric patients, 195
    haloperidol, 129
    intravenous antipsychotics, 220

  in medically ill patients, 223
  pimozide, 178
  thioridazine, 10
  ziprasidone, 166, 195
  QTc interval prolongation on, 30–31,
    166, 194–195, 223
Electroconvulsive therapy (ECT), **293**
  for geriatric mania, 205
  for obsessive-compulsive disorder,
    64
  for psychotic depression, 54, 58,
    205
  for treatment-resistant depression,
    204
Epidemiologic Catchment Area Study,
    136, 138
Epilepsy, 3, 183, 233–234. *See also*
    Seizures
EPS. *See* Extrapyramidal symptoms
ERP (exposure and response
    prevention), for obsessive-
    compulsive disorder, 64, 70
Escitalopram
  for generalized anxiety disorder,
    72
  for nonpsychotic depression, 62–63
Eszopiclone, **294**
Exposure and response prevention
    (ERP), for obsessive-compulsive
    disorder, 64, 70
Extrapyramidal symptoms (EPS),
    28–29
  antipsychotics associated with, 172,
    290
    aripiprazole, 16, 20
    asenapine, 17
    fluphenazine, 22, 178
    haloperidol, 10, 22, 129, 175
    olanzapine, 14, 20
    paliperidone, 13
    paliperidone palmitate, 13
    piperazine phenothiazines, 10
    risperidone, 12, 20
    trifluoperazine, 179
  in children and adolescents, 180

Extrapyramidal symptoms (EPS)
    (continued)
    dopamine D$_2$ receptor occupancy
        and, 20
    drug efficacy and, 8
    due to second-generation
        antipsychotic overdose, 171
    in geriatric patients, **193**, 195–198,
        200
    in medically ill patients, 3, 218
        traumatic brain injury, 231
    monitoring for, 200, **201**
    treatment of, 28–29, 129, **293**
        acute dystonia, 28–29, 197–198
        adverse effects in geriatric
            patients, 196, 197
        parkinsonism, 196
        in pregnancy, 228
        prophylactic, 22, 28, 197
    types of, 28
Eye movement desensitization and
    reprocessing therapy, for
    posttraumatic stress disorder, 81

Falls, in geriatric patients, 198
    parkinsonism and, 196
    tardive dyskinesia and, 196
Fanapt. See Iloperidone
Fatigue, iloperidone-induced, 13
First-generation antipsychotics (FGAs),
    1, 8–10, 145. See also
    Antipsychotics; specific drugs
    adverse effects of, 9–10
    classes of, 9–10
        butyrophenones, 10
        dibenzoxazepines, 10
        dihydroindoles, 10
        diphenylbutylpiperidines, 10
        phenothiazines, 9–10
        thioxanthenes, 10
    compared with second-generation
        antipsychotics, 9, 24–27
    in pediatric patients, 161–162,
        186
    depression and, 27

dosage of, **262–268**
efficacy of, 21
formulations of, **242–244**
high-potency vs. low-potency, 21–22
intramuscular, 22
pharmacokinetics of, **250–253**
in pregnancy and lactation,
    298–311
selection of, 21–22
use in children and adolescents,
    146, 172–180
    adverse effects of, 172, 180, 185
    chlorpromazine, 173–174
    clinical use of, 172
    fluphenazine, 178
    haloperidol, 175–176
    indications for, **147–148**
    molindone, 178–179
    pimozide, 176–178
    thioridazine, 174–175
    trifluoperazine, 179–180
Flat affect, 36
Fluoxetine
    combined with aripiprazole for
        nonpsychotic depression,
        62–63
    combined with olanzapine
        for bipolar depression, 49, 52,
            54
        in borderline personality
            disorder, **113**
        for psychotic depression, 55, 58,
            58
        for treatment-resistant
            depression, 59–60
    drug interactions with, 92
        aripiprazole, 17
        thioridazine, 175
    for generalized anxiety disorder,
        74
    for obsessive-compulsive disorder,
        64
    for pediatric anorexia nervosa, 183
    for treatment-resistant depression,
        59–60

Fluphenazine, 10, 22
adverse effects of, 31, 178
dosage of, **262**
chlorpromazine equivalence, **250**
for pediatric patients, 178
formulations of, 178, **242**
vs. olanzapine for posttraumatic
stress disorder, 89
pharmacokinetics of, **250**
in pregnancy and lactation,
300–301
for Tourette syndrome, **237**
use in children and adolescents,
148, 178
use in hepatic disease, **262**
Fluphenazine decanoate, 23–24, 178, **243**
dosage of, 24, **263**
chlorpromazine equivalence, **251**
pharmacokinetics of, **251**
for substance-abusing schizophrenia
patients, 138, **139**
use in hepatic disease, **263**
Fluphenazine enanthate, 178, **243, 251**
Flushing, stimulant-induced, 130
Fluspirilene, for generalized anxiety
disorder, 74, **78**
Flu syndrome, aripiprazole-induced, 52
Fluvoxamine
drug interactions with
aripiprazole, 92
clozapine, 92
thioridazine, 175
for obsessive-compulsive disorder,
64, 65, 69
Folate, for alcohol intoxication, 131
Food and antipsychotic administration
aripiprazole, 16
asenapine, 17
ziprasidone, 16, 167
Frontotemporal dementia (FTD), 3, 212

GAD. *See* Generalized anxiety disorder
GAF (Global Assessment of
Functioning), 118
Galactorrhea, 34, 200

Gambling addiction, in Parkinson's
disease, 211
Gastrointestinal effects of drugs
anticholinergic agents, 196
aripiprazole, 16, 76, 159
in geriatric patients, 199
olanzapine, 15
quetiapine, 159
risperidone, 12, 13
stimulants, 130
ziprasidone, 16, 160
Generalized anxiety disorder (GAD), 2,
72–81
comorbidity with, 72
initial treatment options for, 72–73
neurobiology of, 73
prevalence of, 72
relapses of, 73
somatic symptoms of, 72
treatment-resistant, 73, 80
antipsychotic augmentation for,
73–80, **77–79**
acute treatment, 74–76
dosing strategies, 76
maintenance treatment, 76
rationale for, 73–74
antipsychotic monotherapy for, 80
key clinical points regarding,
80–81
Geodon. *See* Ziprasidone
Geriatric patients, 3, 191–213
adverse effects of antipsychotics in,
3, 192, **193**, 193–202,
212–213
anticholinergic effects, 199
cardiovascular effects, 194–195
orthostatic hypotension, 194
QTc interval prolongation,
194–195
clozapine-induced
agranulocytosis, 11
in dementia patients, 200–202,
212
cerebrovascular events, 202
risk of death, 200–202

Geriatric patients *(continued)*
　adverse effects of antipsychotics in
　　(continued)
　　extrapyramidal symptoms,
　　　195–198
　　　acute dystonia, 197–198
　　　akathisia, 197
　　　parkinsonism, 195–196
　　　tardive dyskinesia, 196–197
　　falls, 198
　　hyperprolactinemia, 199–200
　　management of, 194
　　metabolic effects, 199
　　monitoring for, 200, **201**
　　neuroleptic malignant syndrome,
　　　198–199
　antipsychotic dosage for, 192, **192,**
　　204, **209,** 212
　antipsychotic treatment in, 203–212
　　for bipolar disorder, 205
　　for dementia with behavioral
　　　disturbances and psychosis,
　　　206–210, **207, 209,** 229
　　for dementia with Lewy bodies,
　　　211–212
　　for frontotemporal dementia, 212
　　informed consent for, 209, 210
　　key clinical points regarding,
　　　212–213
　　for nonpsychotic depression, 204
　　for Parkinson's disease,
　　　210–211, 212, 229–230
　　for psychotic depression, 54,
　　　205
　　for schizophrenia, 203–204
　antipsychotic use in long-term care
　　facilities, 3, 202–203, 208
　principles of medication
　　management for, 192, 212
Glaucoma, 199
Global Assessment of Functioning
　(GAF), 118
Glutamate, 18–19
Glutamate receptors, 19
Gynecomastia, 34, 200

H_1 receptor. *See* Histamine receptor
　affinity of antipsychotics
Haldol. *See* Haloperidol
Haldol Decanoate. *See* Haloperidol
　decanoate
Half-lives of antipsychotics, **250–260**
Hallucinations, 7, 21, 102
　in dementia, 228
　in dementia with Lewy bodies, 211
　in epilepsy, 233
　in Parkinson's disease, 210
　in personality disorders, 102–103,
　　103
　in posttraumatic stress disorder, 81
　substance-induced, 133
　　stimulants, 130
Haloperidol, 8, 10
　adverse effects of, 10, 22, 129, 172,
　　175, 184, **290**
　　extrapyramidal symptoms, 10,
　　　22, 129, 175
　　hyperprolactinemia, **35**
　　QTc interval prolongation, 31,
　　　129, 220, 223, **224**
　　weight gain, **33**
　augmentation for obsessive-
　　compulsive disorder, 66, 67,
　　　68, 70, 72
　　with tic disorder, 66
　for delirium, 220, **221**
　for dementia-related behavioral
　　disturbances and psychosis,
　　　209, 210
　dosage of, 22, **221, 264–265**
　　for agitation due to psychosis,
　　　284
　　chlorpromazine equivalence, **251**
　　for geriatric patients, **192, 209,**
　　　210
　　for pediatric patients, 172, 176
　efficacy of, 21–22
　　vs. iloperidone, 14
　formulations of, 175, 176, 216, **217,**
　　244
　interaction with antidepressants, 92

intramuscular, 22, **217**, **244**, **284**
intravenous, 216, **217**, 220, 236,
   244, 284
maintenance treatment with, 23
in personality disorders, 103, 108
   borderline personality disorder,
      111, **112**
   schizotypal personality disorder,
      117, **119,** 120
   symptom response, 107, 108,
      109
pharmacokinetics of, **252**
in pregnancy and lactation, 228,
   308–309
for psychotic depression, 57
receptor affinity of, 10, 18
routes of administration of, 216,
   217, 220, **221**
for steroid-induced psychiatric
   symptoms, 235
in substance abuse disorders, **127**
   for agitation, 129
   amphetamine psychosis, 135
   cocaine dependence, 142
use in children and adolescents,
   148, 151, 172, 175–176
   for agitation/aggression, 175
   for anorexia nervosa, 183–184
   for autism spectrum disorders,
      184
   vs. second-generation antipsy-
      chotics, 154, 161–162
   for Tourette syndrome, 175, 176,
      237
use in medically ill patients
   burns and trauma, 236
   epilepsy, 233
   hepatic disease, 225, **264**
   Huntington's disease, **237,** 238
   other medical disorders, **237**
Haloperidol decanoate, 23–24, 176,
   244
dosage of, **266**
   chlorpromazine equivalence, **251**
pharmacokinetics of, **252**

for substance-abusing schizophrenic
   patients, 138, **139**
Hamilton Rating Scale for Anxiety
   (Ham-A), 53, 74, 75, 76, **77–79,**
   80, **86,** 88
Hamilton Rating Scale for Depression
   (Ham-D), 50, 51, 53, 55, 56, 69,
   88, 117, 118
Headache, drug-induced
   aripiprazole, 62, 63
   olanzapine, 15
   quetiapine, 158, 159
   ziprasidone, 160
Hepatic disease, 3, 225–226, **262–274**
Hepatic drug metabolism, 225,
   250–260
Hepatic effects of drugs, 226, **290**
Hepatic encephalopathy, 226
Hiccups, **237**
Histamine (H_1) receptor affinity of

   antipsychotics
   aripiprazole, 16
   asenapine, 17, 53
   clozapine, 12
   olanzapine, 14
   paliperidone palmitate, 13
   quetiapine, 165
   risperidone, 12, 163
   ziprasidone, 166
HIV (human immunodeficiency virus)
   disease, 3, 231–232
Hostility, in posttraumatic stress
   disorder, 81
5-HT receptor. *See* Serotonin receptor
   affinity of antipsychotics
Human immunodeficiency virus (HIV)
   disease, 3, 231–232
Huntington's disease, 203, **237,** 238
3-Hydroxychlorpromazine, **250**
8-Hydroxyloxapine, **252**
7-Hydroxyperphenazine, **251**
7-Hydroxyquetiapine, **256, 257**
9-Hydroxyrisperidone, 12, **255.** *See also*
   Paliperidone
7-Hydroxytrifluoperazine, **251**

Hyperactivity. *See also* Attention-deficit/
   hyperactivity disorder
   paliperidone-induced, 13
   stimulant-induced, 130
Hyperacusis, phencyclidine-induced,
   131
Hyperglycemia, drug-induced, 32, **290**
   chlorpromazine, 217
   clozapine, 12, 32, 155, **280**
   in geriatric patients, **193**
   haloperidol, 217
   in medically ill patients, 217
   monitoring for, **276**
   olanzapine, 15, 26, 32
   in pregnancy, 227
   quetiapine, 32, 217
   risperidone, 32, 217
   thioridazine, 217
Hyperlipidemia, drug-induced, 32–33,
   290
   clozapine, 12, 21, 155, **280**
   in geriatric patients, **193,** 199
   in medically ill patients, 217
   monitoring for, **276**
   olanzapine, 15, 21, 26
Hyperprolactinemia, drug-induced, 12,
   34, **35,** 50, **290**
   dopamine D_2 receptor occupancy
      and, 20
   in geriatric patients, **193,** 199–200
   iloperidone, 34, **35**
   monitoring for, **276**
   olanzapine, 157
   paliperidone, 13, 34, **35**
   risperidone, 12, 17, 34, **35,** 156,
      200
Hypersexuality, in Parkinson's disease,
   211
Hypersomnia, induced by olanzapine-
   fluoxetine combination, 60
Hypertension, drug-induced
   aripiprazole, 52
   clozapine, 149
   phencyclidine, 131
   stimulants, 130

Hyperthermia
   drug-induced
      clozapine, 12
      in neuroleptic malignant
         syndrome, 30, 198–199
      stimulants, 130
   psychomotor agitation with, 131
Hypomania, 46
Hypotension. *See* Orthostatic
   hypotension

Illusions, 102
   in personality disorders, 102, **103**
   in posttraumatic stress disorder, 81
Iloperidone, 13–14
   adverse effects of, 13–14
      hyperprolactinemia, 34, **35**
      weight gain and metabolic
         effects, 14, 31, **33**
   dosage of, 13, 14, **274**
   efficacy of, 14, 25
   formulations of, **246**
   maintenance treatment with, 14
   pharmacokinetics of, **260**
   in pregnancy and lactation, **324–325**
   receptor affinity of, 13
   use in hepatic disease, **274**
Imipramine
   interaction with haloperidol, 92
   for psychotic depression, 55–56
Impulse-control disorders, in
   Parkinson's disease, 211
Impulsive aggression, 105
   in borderline personality disorder,
      104
   neurobiology of, 104–105
Incoordination, alcohol-induced, 131
Informed consent for antipsychotic use
   in elderly patients, 209, 210
   rechallenge after neuroleptic
      malignant syndrome, 30
Insomnia
   drug-induced
      aripiprazole, 76
      management of, **294**

ziprasidone, 16
in medically ill patients, 217
Institutionalization, 1, 8
Insulin resistance, 32
Intoxication-related psychomotor
agitation, 126, 130–132
alcohol, 131–132
phencyclidine, 131
stimulants, 130–131
Intraocular pressure elevation, 199
Invega. *See* Paliperidone
Invega Sustenna. *See* Paliperidone
palmitate extended-release
injectable suspension
Ionotropic glutamate receptors, 19
Irritability, drug-induced
aripiprazoles, 76
steroids, 235
stimulants, 130

Jitteriness, aripiprazole-induced, 76

Kainate receptors, 19

Lactation and antipsychotic use, 3, 37,
228, **298–327**
Lamotrigine
for bipolar depression, 52
for bipolar disorder relapse
prevention, 50
Laryngeal dystonia, 28, 226
Lenticular opacity, quetiapine-induced, 15
Leukocytosis, in neuroleptic malignant
syndrome, 30
Leukopenia, clozapine-induced, 149
Lexapro. *See* Escitalopram
Lightheadedness, drug-induced
aripiprazole, 159
olanzapine, 15
risperidone, 12
Lithium
for bipolar disorder, 46, 53
in children and adolescents
aripiprazole and, **147**
risperidone and, 156

with comorbid substance abuse,
140
relapse prevention, 48, 50
for treatment-resistant depression, 204
Long-acting antipsychotics, 23–24, 39,
40
combined with oral drugs, 37
for substance-abusing schizophrenia
patients, 138, **139**
Long-term care facilities, guidelines for
antipsychotic use in, 3, 202–203,
208
Lorazepam
for agitation/aggression, 22
in elderly dementia patients, 210
for akathisia, **293**
for alcohol withdrawal, 132
for dystonic reactions, **293**
for insomnia, **294**
for substance-related agitation, 129
for weaning from mechanical
ventilation, 226
Loxapine, 10
dosage of, **266**
chlorpromazine equivalence, **251**
for geriatric patients, **266**
formulations of, **244**
in personality disorders, 108
borderline personality disorder,
111, **112**
symptom response, 107, **109**
pharmacokinetics of, **252**
in pregnancy and lactation, **308–309**
use in children and adolescents, 172
Loxitane. *See* Loxapine
LSD (lysergic acid diethylamide), 18
Lupus, drug-induced, 234–235
Luvox. *See* Fluvoxamine
Lysergic acid diethylamide (LSD), 18

Macrolide antibiotics, interaction with
pimozide, 177
MADRS (Montgomery-Åsberg
Depression Rating Scale), 48, 49,
50, 51, 53, 60, 62

Maintenance treatment
    of bipolar disorder, **47,** 50–53
    of generalized anxiety disorder, 76
    of obsessive-compulsive disorder,
        70–71, 72
    of schizophrenia, 22–24
        aripiprazole, 23
        clozapine, 23
        fluphenazine decanoate, 23–24
        haloperidol, 23
        haloperidol decanoate, 23–24
        iloperidone, 14
        olanzapine, 23
        paliperidone palmitate, 13, 24
        quetiapine, 13, 23
        risperidone, 23
        ziprasidone, 23
Mania, 45–46. *See also* Bipolar disorder
    antipsychotics for, 46–48, **47**
    electroconvulsive therapy for, 205
    in schizoaffective disorder, 38
    steroid-induced, 235
Masked facies, 28
Mechanical ventilation, weaning from,
    226
Medically ill patients, 3, 215–238
    agitation/aggression in, 221–222
    with burns or trauma, 236
    with cardiovascular disease,
        222–224, **224**
    considerations for antipsychotic use
        in, 216–218
        drug-drug interactions, 216,
            238
        electrocardiogram monitoring,
            223
        extrapyramidal symptoms, 218
        metabolic effects, 217
        pharmacokinetics, 3, 216
        routes of administration, 3, 216,
            217
        sedation, 217–218
    delirium in, 218–220, **221**
    with dementia, 228–229
    with epilepsy, 233–234
    with hepatic insufficiency, 225–226,
        262–274
    with HIV disease, 231–233
    key clinical points regarding
        antipsychotic use in, 238
    with other medical disorders, **237,**
        237–238
    with pain, 236–237
    with Parkinson's disease, 210–211,
        229–230
    with pulmonary disease, 226–227
    with renal disease, 224–225,
        262–274
    with rheumatologic disorders,
        234–235
    role of antipsychotic treatment in,
        215
    schizophrenia in, 5
    steroid-induced psychiatric
        symptoms in, 235–236
    with traumatic brain injury, 231
    use of beta-blockers in, 197
Medical workup for antipsychotic use,
    20–21, **276–277**
    in borderline personality disorder,
        115–116, 123–124
    clozapine, 168–169, **280–281**
    in pediatric patients, 162–163
    in schizotypal personality disorder,
        121, 122–123
Mefloquine, interaction with
    ziprasidone, 166
Mellaril. *See* Thioridazine
Melperone, for generalized anxiety
    disorder, 74, **77**
Mesoridazine, 31, **250**
    interaction with ziprasidone, 166
Metabolic effects of drugs, 31–34.
    See also Hyperglycemia;
        Hyperlipidemia; Weight gain
    chlorpromazine, 217
    clozapine, 12, 21, 32, 155, 217
        monitoring for, **280–281**
    in geriatric patients, **193,** 199
    haloperidol, 217

in medically ill patients, 217
molindone for patients with, 102
monitoring for, **127–128**, 199, **201,
    276–277, 280–281**
olanzapine, 15, 21, 26, 32, 33, 217
quetiapine, 32, 217
risperidone, 32, 217
thioridazine, 217
Metabolic syndrome, 33
Metabolism of antipsychotics, **250–260**
Metabotropic glutamate receptors, 19
Methadone, 137
Methamphetamine psychosis, 134–135
Methotrimeprazine, 236
N-Methyl-D-aspartate (NMDA)
    receptors, 19
Methylphenidate, 18
Migraine, 237, **237,** 238
Moban. *See* Molindone
Molindone, 10
    adverse effects of, **35**
    dosage of, **267**
        chlorpromazine equivalence, **253**
        for pediatric patients, 179
    formulations of, 179, **244**
    pharmacokinetics of, **253**
    in pregnancy and lactation,
        310–311
    use in children and adolescents,
        148, 153, 178–179
    vs. second-generation
        antipsychotics, 162
Monoamine oxidase inhibitors, 210
Montgomery-Åsberg Depression Rating
    Scale (MADRS), 48, 49, 50, 51,
    53, 60, 62
Mood disorders, 2, 45–63
    bipolar disorder, 45–54
    nonpsychotic depression, 61–63
    pediatric psychosis and, 182
    psychotic depression, 54–58
    safety and tolerability of
        antipsychotics in, 90–92
    treatment-resistant depression,
        59–61

Mood stabilizers
    for bipolar disorder
        with comorbid attention-deficit/
            hyperactivity disorder, 181
        with comorbid substance abuse,
            140, 141
        mania, 46, 53
        relapse prevention, 48, 50
    for schizoaffective disorder, 38, 40
Mortality
    antipsychotic-related risk in elderly
        dementia patients, 200–202,
        229
    antipsychotic-related sudden
        cardiac death, 30–31
    clozapine, 11
    droperidol, 10
    delirium and, 219
    in schizophrenia, 5–6
Moxifloxacin, interaction with
    ziprasidone, 166
Muscarinic receptor affinity of
    antipsychotics
    anticholinergic side effects due to,
        199
    clozapine, 12
    olanzapine, 14
Musculoskeletal pain, quetiapine-
    induced, 159
Mydriasis, stimulant-induced, 130
Myocarditis, clozapine-induced, 11, 21,
    168, 170, 224

Naltrexone, 137
NanoCrystal® technology, 13, 24
Nasal congestion, drug-induced
    iloperidone, 13
    risperidone, 12
Nasal discharge, ziprasidone-induced,
    16
National Institute of Mental Health
    (NIMH)
    Clinical Antipsychotic Trials of
        Intervention Effectiveness
        (CATIE), 15, 23, 25–26, 32–33

National Institute of Mental Health
(NIMH) *(continued)*
studies of second-generation
antipsychotics in pediatric
patients, 154, 161
Study of Pharmacotherapy of
Psychotic Depression
(STOP-PD), 56–57
Nausea/vomiting
antipsychotic treatment for, 173,
237, **237**
drug-induced
aripiprazole, 16, 76, 159
olanzapine, 15
risperidone, 12
stimulants, 130
ziprasidone, 16, 160
Navane. *See* Thiothixene
Nefazodone, interaction with pimozide,
177
Negative symptoms of schizophrenia,
21, 36
clozapine for, 11, 36
dopamine dysregulation and, 18
selective serotonin reuptake
inhibitors for, 36
Neonatal effects of antipsychotics,
227–228, **298–327**
Neurobiology
of borderline personality disorder,
104–105
of cocaine abuse, 130
of generalized anxiety disorder,
73–74, 80
of impulsive aggression, 104–105
of obsessive-compulsive disorder, 65
of phencyclidine intoxication, 131
of posttraumatic stress disorder, 82,
83, 90
of schizophrenia, 17–18, 104
of schizotypal personality disorder,
104
Neuroimaging
in borderline personality disorder,
105

of clozapine dopamine D_2 receptor
occupancy, 18
in obsessive-compulsive disorder,
65
of serotonin and dopamine receptor
affinities of antipsychotics, 19
Neuroleptic malignant syndrome
(NMS), 15, 29–30, 198
clinical features of, 30
in geriatric patients, **193,** 198–199
informed consent for antipsychotic
rechallenge after, 30
prevalence of, 15
with rhabdomyolysis, 30
risk factors for, 198
treatment of, 30, 198–199, **294**
Neuroleptics, 8. *See also* Antipsychotics
Neurosurgery, for obsessive-compulsive
disorder, 64
Nicotine replacement therapy, 137
Nicotinic receptor affinity, of clozapine,
12
NIMH. *See* National Institute of Mental
Health
NMDA (*N*-methyl-D-aspartate)
receptors, 19
NMS. *See* Neuroleptic malignant
syndrome
Norepinephrine
clozapine effects on, 12
in cocaine abuse, 130
in phencyclidine intoxication, 131
ziprasidone effects on, 16
Nystagmus, drug-induced
alcohol, 131
phencyclidine, 131

OAS-M (Overt Aggression Scale—
Modified for Outpatients), 84, **86**
Obesity/overweight, 31–33, 217.
See also Weight gain
OBRA (Omnibus Budget Reconciliation
Act) guidelines for antipsychotic
use in long-term care facilities, 3,
202–203, 208

Obsessive-compulsive disorder (OCD), 2, 37, 63–72
  comorbidity with, 64
    pediatric psychosis, 182
    tic disorder, 64
  cortico-striatal-thalamic circuit dysfunction in, 65
  course of, 64
  initial treatment options for, 63–64
    exposure and response prevention, 64
    selective serotonin reuptake inhibitors, 64
  neurobiology of, 65
  practice guideline for treatment of, 64, 70
  prevalence of, 63
  treatment-resistant, 64–72
    antipsychotic augmentation for, 65–72, **68**
      acute treatment, 65–70
      dosing strategies, 70, 72
      drug interactions with, 72
      maintenance treatment, 70–71, 72
      in patients with tic disorders, 66
      rationale for, 65
      in schizophrenia, 71
    antipsychotic monotherapy for, 71, 72
    other biological treatments for, 64
Ocular effects of drugs, 34
  monitoring for, **277**
  oculogyric crisis, 28
  quetiapine, 15
Off-label use of antipsychotics, 2
Olanzapine, 14–15
  adverse effects of, 14, 15, 74, **290**
    anticholinergic effects, 199
    cerebrovascular events in elderly dementia patients, 202
    extrapyramidal symptoms, 14, 20, 196

hepatotoxicity, 226
    hyperprolactinemia, 34, **35**
    orthostatic hypotension, 194
    QTc interval prolongation, **224**
    weight gain and metabolic effects, 15, 21, 26, 31, 33, **33**, 51
  augmentation for generalized anxiety disorder, 74, **78**, 80, 85
  augmentation for obsessive-compulsive disorder, 66, **68**, 69, 70, 72
  augmentation for posttraumatic stress disorder, 83, **86**, 90
  for bipolar disorder, **47**
    acute mania, 46
    in pediatric patients, **153**, 155, 157
    relapse prevention, 50–51, 54
  dosage of, 15, 46, **221**, **270**
    for agitation due to psychosis, **285**
    chlorpromazine equivalence, **256**
    for geriatric patients, **192**, 204, **209**, 210
    for pediatric patients, 155, 157, 164–165
  efficacy of, 21, 25
  formulations of, 14, 164, **217**, **245**
    intramuscular, 14–15, 22, **245**
    monotherapy for posttraumatic stress disorder, 88–89
  in personality disorders, 108
    borderline personality disorder, 111, **113**
    schizotypal personality disorder, 118, 120
    symptom response, 107, **109**
  pharmacokinetics of, **256**
    in pediatric patients, 156–157
  in pregnancy and lactation, 227, **316–317**
  for psychotic depression
    combined with fluoxetine, 55
    combined with sertraline, 56–57, 58, **58**

Olanzapine *(continued)*
  receptor affinity of, 14, 20, 164
  routes of administration of, **217,
    221**
  for schizophrenia
    CATIE study of, 25–26
    with comorbid substance abuse,
      138
    in geriatric patients, 204
    maintenance treatment, 23
    negative symptoms, 36
    in pediatric patients, **151–153,**
      157
    positive symptoms, 14
    treatment-resistant, 35–36
  for steroid-induced psychiatric
    symptoms, 235–236
  in substance abuse disorders, **127**
    for agitation, 130
    amphetamine psychosis, 135
    cocaine dependence, 142
    with schizophrenia, 138
  for tardive dyskinesia, 29
  for treatment-resistant depression,
    59–60
  use in children and adolescents,
    147, 148, **151–153,** 156–157,
    164–165
    for anorexia nervosa, 184
    for autism spectrum disorders
      and developmental delay,
      184
    for bipolar disorder, 155, 157
    vs. clozapine, 154–155
    vs. first-generation
      antipsychotics, 161–162
    for schizophrenia, 157
  use in medically ill patients, 217,
    270
    delirium, 220, **221**
    dementia-related behavioral
      disturbances and psychosis,
      209, 210
    dementia with Lewy bodies,
      212
    hepatic disease, 225, **270**
    other medical conditions, **237**
    for pain, 237, **237**
    Parkinson's disease, 211, 230
    renal disease, 224
    systemic lupus erythematosus,
      234
    traumatic brain injury, 231
Olanzapine-fluoxetine combination
  adverse effects of, 60
  for bipolar depression, 49, 52, 54
  in borderline personality disorder,
    113
  for psychotic depression, 55
  for treatment-resistant depression,
    59–60, 61
Omnibus Budget Reconciliation Act
    (OBRA) guidelines for
    antipsychotic use in long-term
    care facilities, 3, 202–203, 208
Oppositional defiant disorder, 158
Oral hypoesthesia, asenapine-induced,
    17
Orap. *See* Pimozide
Orlistat, **295**
OROS (osmotic-controlled release oral
    delivery system) paliperidone, 12
Orthostatic hypotension, drug-induced,
    21, 194, **290**
  chlorpromazine, 194, 222
  clozapine, 1, 12, 194, 211, 222, 224
  in geriatric patients, **193,** 194
  iloperidone, 13–14
  monitoring for, 194
  olanzapine, 15, 194, 223
  phenothiazines, 9–10
  quetiapine, 15, 223
  risperidone, 12, 223
  thioridazine, 194
  ziprasidone, 16
Osmotic-controlled release oral delivery
    system (OROS) paliperidone, 12
Overdose of antipsychotics, 116, 171
Overt Aggression Scale—Modified for
    Outpatients (OAS-M), 84, **86**

Pain management, 3, 235–237, **237**
Paliperidone, 12–13
  adverse effects of, 13, **290**
    hyperprolactinemia, 13, 34, **35**
    weight gain and metabolic
      effects, 31, **33**
  dosage of, 12, **272**
  drug interactions with, 12
  efficacy of, 12–13, 25
  extended-release, 12
  formulations of, **246**
  mechanism of action of, 12
  osmotic-controlled release oral
    delivery system (OROS) for, 12
  pharmacokinetics of, **255, 259**
  in pregnancy and lactation,
    322–323
  for schizoaffective disorder, 38
  use in hepatic or renal disease, **272**
Paliperidone palmitate extended-
  release injectable suspension, 13,
  24, **246**
  adverse effects of, 13
  dosage of, 13, **273**
  pharmacokinetics of, **259**
  in pregnancy and lactation, **324–325**
  use in renal disease, **273**
Pancreatitis, 33
Panic attacks, in posttraumatic stress
  disorder, 81
Panic disorder
  generalized anxiety disorder and, 72
  risperidone for, 75
PANSS (Positive and Negative
  Syndrome Scale), 14, 17, 57, 84,
  85, **86, 87,** 89, 118, 120, 158
Parkinsonism, drug-induced, 28
  in geriatric patients, **193,** 195–196
  management of, 196, **293**
  olanzapine, 196
  risperidone, 196
Parkinson's disease, 3, 210–211, 212,
  229–230
  impulse-control disorders in, 211
  psychosis in, 210–211, 229–230

Paroxetine
  for bipolar depression, 49
  combined with aripiprazole for
    nonpsychotic depression,
    62–63
  drug interactions with, 92
    haloperidol, 92
    thioridazine, 175
  for generalized anxiety disorder, 72,
    75
  for obsessive-compulsive disorder,
    64, 69
  for posttraumatic stress disorder, 81
Pathological gambling, in Parkinson's
  disease, 211
Patient Checklist for PTSD—Military
  Version (PCL-M), 84, **86**
Patient Global Improvement Scale
  (PGI-I), 89
Paxil. *See* Paroxetine
PCL-M (Patient Checklist for PTSD—
  Military Version), 84, **86**
PCP (phencyclidine) intoxication, 19,
  129, 131
Pediatric patients. *See* Children and
  adolescents
Pentamidine, interaction with
  ziprasidone, 166
Peripheral edema, induced by
  olanzapine-fluoxetine combination,
  60
Perphenazine, 10
  adverse effects of, **290**
  augmentation for posttraumatic
    stress disorder, 83
  CATIE study of, 25–26
  combined with amitriptyline for
    psychotic depression, 58, **58**
  dosage of, **263**
    chlorpromazine equivalence, **251**
    for geriatric patients, **263**
  formulations of, **243**
  pharmacokinetics of, **251**
  in pregnancy and lactation, **302–303**
  use in renal or hepatic disease, **263**

Perphenazine sulfoxide, **251**
Personality disorders, 2, 101–123.
    See also Borderline personality
    disorder; Schizotypal personality
    disorder
    adverse effects of antipsychotics in,
        110, 122
    antipsychotic indications and
        efficacy in, 105–106, 122
    borderline personality disorder,
        110–116, **112–113**
    clinical use of antipsychotics in,
        106–108
        dosage, 106–107, 122
        symptom response, 107–108,
            109, 122
    guidelines for antipsychotic
        selection and use in, 108–110,
        110
    history of antipsychotic use in, 103
    key clinical points regarding
        antipsychotics in, 122–123
    long-term antipsychotic use in,
        108–109, 110
    mechanism of antipsychotic action
        in, 104–105
    other types of, 121–122
    psychosis in, 102–103, **103**
    role of antipsychotics in, 101–102
    schizotypal personality disorder,
        116–121, **119**
Pervasive developmental delay, 3, 145,
    146, 149, 184
PET (positron emission tomography)
    in obsessive-compulsive disorder, 65
    of serotonin and dopamine receptor
        affinities of antipsychotics, 19,
        20
PGI-I (Patient Global Improvement
    Scale), 89
Pharmacokinetics, **250–260**
    in medically ill patients, 3, 216
    of olanzapine in pediatric patients,
        156–157
    renal failure and, 224–225

Pharyngitis, drug-induced
    aripiprazole, 52
    quetiapine, 158
Phencyclidine (PCP) intoxication, 19,
    129, 131
Phenothiazines, 9–10. *See also* First-
    generation antipsychotics
    adverse effects of, 9–10, 226
    aliphatic, 9
    for burn and trauma patients, 236
    classification of, 9
    pharmacokinetics of, **250–252**
    piperazine, 10
    piperidine, 10
    in pregnancy, 227
Pimozide, 10
    adverse effects of, 10, 31, 172, 177
    cardiac monitoring during treatment
        with, 178
    contraindications to, 177
    for delusions, 10
    dosage of, **267**
        chlorpromazine equivalence, **253**
        for geriatric patients, **267**
        for pediatric patients, 177
    drug interactions with, 177
        ziprasidone, 166
    formulations of, **244**
    pharmacokinetics of, **253**
    in pregnancy and lactation,
        310–311
    in schizotypal personality disorder,
        117
    use in children and adolescents,
        148, 176–178
        for anorexia nervosa, 184
        for Tourette syndrome, 176–177,
            237
    use in hepatic or renal disease, **267**
Pindolol, interaction with thioridazine,
    175
Pittsburgh Sleep Quality Index, 8383
Plasma drug concentrations, 24
    time to peak levels, **250–260**
Polyarteritis nodosa, 234

Polydipsia, psychogenic, clozapine for, 11
Polypharmacy, 36–37
Positive and Negative Syndrome Scale (PANSS), 14, 17, 57, 84, 85, **86, 87,** 89, 118, 120, 158
Positive symptoms of schizophrenia, 21
dopamine dysregulation and, 18
olanzapine for, 14
Positron emission tomography (PET)
in obsessive-compulsive disorder, 65
of serotonin and dopamine receptor affinities of antipsychotics, 19, 20
Postictal psychosis, 233
Postpsychotic depression, 27
Posttraumatic stress disorder (PTSD), 2, 81–90
antipsychotic augmentation for, 82–88, **86–87,** 90
acute treatment, 83–88
dosing strategies, 88, 90
maintenance treatment, 88
rationale for, 82–83
antipsychotic monotherapy for, 88–89
clinical features of, 81, 83
comorbidity with, 81
initial treatment options for, 81–82
neurobiology of, 82–83, 90
practice guideline for treatment of, 82, 85
prevalence of, 81, 90
"Practice Guideline for the Treatment of Patients With Acute Stress Disorder and Posttraumatic Stress Disorder," 81, 85
"Practice Guideline for the Treatment of Patients With Bipolar Disorder," 46
"Practice Guideline for the Treatment of Patients With Delirium," 220
"Practice Guideline for the Treatment of Patients With Major Depressive Disorder (Revision)," 54

Practice Guideline for the Treatment of Patients With Obsessive-Compulsive Disorder," 64, 70
Pregnancy
antipsychotic use in, 3, 37, 227–228, **298–327**
FDA drug categories in, 327
testing for, **277**
Prochlorperazine, 10, 31
dosage of, **264**
chlorpromazine equivalence, **252**
formulations of, **243**
for nausea/vomiting, 237, **237**
pharmacokinetics of, **252**
in pregnancy and lactation, **306–307**
Prolactin. *See* Hyperprolactinemia
Prolixin. *See* Fluphenazine
Prolixin Decanoate. *See* Fluphenazine decanoate
Prolixin Enanthate. *See* Fluphenazine enanthate
Promethazine, 235
Propranolol
for akathisia, 29, **293**
interaction with thioridazine, 175
for parkinsonism, **293**
Protease inhibitors, interaction with pimozide, 177
Protein binding of antipsychotics, **250–260**
Pseudoparkinsonism, drug-induced, 28
in geriatric patients, **193,** 195–196
management of, 196, **293**
olanzapine, 196
risperidone, 196
Psychoeducation, 39
Psychosis, 102. *See also* Schizophrenia
antipsychotics for agitation due to, **284–286**
in dementia, 206–209, **207, 209,** 228–229
with Lewy bodies, 211–212
in epilepsy, 233

Psychosis *(continued)*
in Parkinson's disease, 210–211, 229–230
in personality disorders, 2, 102–103, **103**
in posttraumatic stress disorder, 81
in rheumatologic diseases, 234
steroid-induced, 235
substance-induced, 3, 18, 133–136, 142, 143
cannabis, 135–136
general approach to, 133–134
phencyclidine, 19, 131
stimulants, 18, 130, 134–135
in traumatic brain injury, 231
treatment in long-term care facilities, 3, 202–203, 208
Psychosis in children and adolescents, 3, 145, 146, 149, 182–183
anxiety disorders and, 182
disruptive behavior disorders and, 182
first-generation antipsychotics for, **147–148,** 172–180
chlorpromazine, 173
fluphenazine, 178
haloperidol, 176
molindone, 179
thioridazine, 174
trifluoperazine, 179
mood disorders and, 182
neurological disease and, 183
second-generation antipsychotics for, **147,** 149, **151–153,** 183
aripiprazole, 159
clozapine, 149, 154–155
olanzapine, 157
quetiapine, 158
substance abuse and, 182
Psychosocial interventions, 39
Psychotic depression, 2, 27, 54–58
in children and adolescents, 54, 145, 149
combination of antipsychotic and antidepressant for, 55–58

drug selection for, 57–58, **58**
inadequate use of, 54–55
key clinical points related to, 58
electroconvulsive therapy for, 54, 58, 205
in geriatric patients, 54, 205
posttraumatic stress disorder and, 81
practice guideline for treatment of, 54
prevalence of, 54
PTSD. *See* Posttraumatic stress disorder
PTSD Interview (PTSD-I) scale, 89
Pulmonary disease, 3, 226–227

QTc interval prolongation, drug-induced, 30–31, 166, 194–195, 220, 222, 223, **224, 290**
chlorpromazine, 31
droperidol, 10, 31
fluphenazine, 31
in geriatric patients, **193,** 194–195
haloperidol, 31, 129, 220, 223, **224**
mesoridazine, 31
monitoring for, **201**
olanzapine, **224**
pimozide, 10, 31, 172, 177
prochlorperazine, 31
quetiapine, **224**
risperidone, **224**
second-generation antipsychotic overdose, 171
thioridazine, 10, 31, 172, 174, 175, 195, 223, **224**
trifluoperazine, 31
ziprasidone, 16, 166, 171, 195, 223, **224,** 225, **286**
Quetiapine, 15
abuse potential of, 142
administration of, 15
adverse effects of, 15, 158, 159, **290**
hepatotoxicity, 226
QTc interval prolongation, **224**

weight gain and metabolic
effects, 15, 31, **33,** 158
augmentation for generalized
anxiety disorder, 75, **79**
augmentation for obsessive-
compulsive disorder, 66, **68,**
69, 72
augmentation for posttraumatic
stress disorder, 83–84
for bipolar disorder, **47**
bipolar I depression, 48–49, 52,
54
bipolar II depression, 50, 52
in pediatric patients, **150,**
158–159
relapse prevention, 52, 54
combined with venlafaxine for
psychotic depression, 56, 58,
58
for delirium, 220, **221**
for dementia-related behavioral
disturbances and psychosis,
209
dosage of, 15, **221, 270**
for bipolar depression, 48–49,
50, 52
chlorpromazine equivalence, **256**
for geriatric patients, **192,** 204,
209, 270
in hepatic disease, 225
for pediatric patients, 158, 165
efficacy of, 15, 25
formulations of, 15, 165, **217, 245**
interaction with antiepileptic drugs,
233
monotherapy for posttraumatic
stress disorder, 89
pharmacokinetics of, **256**
in pregnancy and lactation, 227,
318–319
receptor affinity of, 15, 20, 142, 165
for schizophrenia
CATIE study of, 25–26
with comorbid substance abuse,
138

in geriatric patients, 204
maintenance treatment, 13, 23
in pediatric patients, **152,** 158
in substance abuse disorders, **127**
alcohol dependence, 142
with bipolar disorder, 140
cocaine dependence, 142
with schizophrenia, 138
for tardive dyskinesia, 29
for treatment-resistant depression,
60, 61
use in children and adolescents,
147, 148, **150, 152,** 157–159,
165
for bipolar disorder, 158–159
for schizophrenia, 158
for Tourette syndrome, 157–158,
185
use in medically ill patients
dementia with Lewy bodies, 212
epilepsy, 233
hepatic disease, 225, **270**
Huntington's disease, **237,** 238
migraine, 237, **237**
Parkinson's disease, 211, 230
renal disease, 224
traumatic brain injury, 231
for weaning from mechanical
ventilation, 226
Quetiapine slow-release, 15, **245**
dosage of, **271**
pharmacokinetics of, **257**
use in hepatic disease, **271**
Quinidine, interaction with ziprasidone,
166
Quinolinones, 16–17, **258.** *See also*
Aripiprazole

Race/ethnicity, and risk of clozapine-
induced agranulocytosis, 11
Receptor affinity of antipsychotics
aripiprazole, 16, 20, 141, 167
asenapine, 17, 53
clozapine, 12, 18, 20, 168
haloperidol, 10, 18, 20

Receptor affinity of antipsychotics
    (continued)
  iloperidone, 13
  olanzapine, 14, 20, 164
  paliperidone, 12
  paliperidone palmitate, 13
  quetiapine, 15, 20, 142, 165
  risperidone, 12, 18, 20, 163
  ziprasidone, 15–16, 16, 165–166, 166
Renal disease, 3, 224–225, **262–274**
Repetitive transcranial magnetic
    stimulation, for obsessive-
    compulsive disorder, 64
Reserpine, for tardive dyskinesia, 29
Respiratory depression, drug-induced,
    226–227
Respiratory dyskinesias, 29
Restlessness, drug-induced, 28.
    See also Akathisia
Rhabdomyolysis, 30
Rheumatologic disorders, 3, 234–235
Rigidity, drug-induced, 28, 195
  in neuroleptic malignant syndrome,
    30, 198–199
  phencyclidine, 131
  second-generation antipsychotic
    overdose, 171
Risperdal. *See* Risperidone
Risperdal Consta. *See* Risperidone long-
    acting injectable
Risperidone, 12
  administration of, 12
  adverse effects of, 12, 75, **290**
    cerebrovascular events in elderly
      dementia patients, 202
    extrapyramidal symptoms, 12,
      20, 196
    hepatotoxicity, 226
    hyperprolactinemia, 12, 17, 34,
      35, 156, 200
    QTc interval prolongation, **224**
    weight gain and metabolic
      effects, 12, 17, 31, **33**
  augmentation for generalized
    anxiety disorder, 75, **79,** 80

augmentation for obsessive-
    compulsive disorder, 66–69,
    68, 70, 72
  with tic disorder, 66
augmentation for posttraumatic
    stress disorder, 84–85, **86–87,**
    88, 90
for bipolar disorder, **47**
  mania and mixed states, 46
  in pediatric patients, **147,** 148,
    155–156
  relapse prevention, 48, 52–53, 54
dosage of, 88, **221, 269**
  for agitation due to psychosis,
    285
  chlorpromazine equivalence, **255**
  for geriatric patients, **192,** 204,
    209, 210
  in hepatic disease, 225
  for pediatric patients, 155, 164
  in renal disease, 225
efficacy of, 12, 25
  vs. asenapine, 17
  vs. iloperidone, 14
formulations of, 12, 163, **217, 245**
generic, 12
mechanism of action of, 12
in personality disorders, 108
  schizotypal personality disorder,
    118, **119,** 120
  symptom response, 107, **109**
pharmacokinetics of, **255**
for posttraumatic stress disorder, 89
in pregnancy and lactation, 227,
    314–315
for psychotic depression, 57
receptor affinity of, 12, 18, 20, 163
for schizophrenia
  CATIE study of, 25–26
  with comorbid substance abuse,
    138
  in geriatric patients, 204
  maintenance treatment, 23
  negative symptoms, 36
  treatment-resistant, 35

for steroid-induced psychiatric symptoms, 235
in substance abuse disorders, **128**
cocaine dependence, 142
with schizophrenia, 138
for tic disorder, **152**
for treatment-resistant depression, 60, 61
use in children and adolescents, 146, **147,** 148, **150–153,** 155–156, 163–164
for autism spectrum disorders and developmental delay, **147,** 148, **150, 152, 153,** 184, 185, **237**
for bipolar disorder, 148, 155–156
vs. first-generation antipsychotics, 161–162
use in medically ill patients
burns and trauma, 236
delirium, 220, **221**
dementia-related behavioral disturbances and psychosis, **209,** 210
epilepsy, 233
hepatic disease, 225, **269**
Huntington's disease, **237,** 238
Parkinson's disease, 230
renal disease, 225, **269**
systemic lupus erythematosus, 234
traumatic brain injury, 231
Risperidone long-acting injectable, 12, 24, 163, **245**
for bipolar disorder relapse prevention, **47,** 48, 52–53, 54
for comorbid bipolar disorder and substance abuse, 141
for comorbid schizophrenia and substance abuse, 138, **139**
dosage of, 163, **269**
pharmacokinetics of, **256**
use in renal or hepatic disease, **269**
Routes of antipsychotic administration, 3, 216, **217**

SANS (Scale for the Assessment of Negative Symptoms), 158
Saphris. *See* Asenapine
Scale for the Assessment of Negative Symptoms (SANS), 158
Schedule for Affective Disorders and Schizophrenia, 56
Schizoaffective disorder, 2, 37–38
antipsychotics for pediatric patients with, **153**
diagnostic criteria for, 37–38
posttraumatic stress disorder and, 81
prognosis for, 38
treatment of, 38, 40
Schizophrenia, 2, 5–40. *See also* Psychosis
brain structural changes in, 104
cannabis use as risk factor for, 135–136
clinical course of, 5
clinician-patient relationship in, 7
comorbidity with, 5
depression, 5, 27
medical illness, 5
posttraumatic stress disorder, 81
substance abuse, 2–3, 5, **127–128,** 136–138
dopamine hypothesis of, 17–18
in geriatric patients, 3, 191
glutamate and NMDA receptors in, 19
mortality in, 5–6
neurobiology of, 17–18
obesity and, 31–33
overlap between schizotypal personality disorder and, 104, 117
pregnancy and, 227
quality of life in, 7
relapses of, 6, 21, 22–23
remission of, 7
smoking and, 5
suicide in, 5, 6
symptoms of, 21
dopamine dysregulation and, 18

Schizophrenia treatment, 20–37, 39–40
    acute treatment, 21–22
    adequate trial of, 35
    adherence to, 6, 7, 23, 37, 39, 40,
        137
    adverse effects of, 6, 7, 28–34
        extrapyramidal symptoms and
            neurological effects, 28–29
        hyperprolactinemia, 34, **35**
        neuroleptic malignant syndrome,
            29–30
        other effects, 34
        sudden death, 30–31
        weight gain and metabolic
            effects, 31–34, **33**
    antipsychotic polypharmacy for,
        36–37
    in children and adolescents,
        147–148, 151–153, 183
    coordination of care for, 7
    depression and, 27
    efficacy of antipsychotics for, 6, 7, 8,
        20
    first- vs. second-generation
        antipsychotics for, 9, 24–27
    in geriatric patients, 203–204
    goals of, 6–7, 21
    key clinical points regarding, 39–40
    in long-term care facilities, 2,
        202–203, 208
    maintenance treatment, 22–24
    medical workup for antipsychotic
        use, 20–21
    for negative symptoms, 36
    for obsessive-compulsive symptoms,
        71
    in pregnancy, 37
    resistance to, 34–36
        clozapine for, 1, 11, 21, 23, 24,
            35–36
        definition of, 34–35
        olanzapine for, 35–36
        risperidone for, 35
    in substance-abusing patients,
        127–128, 136–138

    integrative treatment, 136–137
    noncompliance with, 137
    selection of antipsychotics for,
        137–138, **139**
    switching antipsychotics for, 22, 36,
        40
Schizotypal personality disorder
    (STPD), 2, 102, 116–121
    adverse effects of antipsychotics in,
        110, 121
    antipsychotic indications and
        efficacy in, **112,** 118, **119,**
        122
        agitation and aggression, 120,
            122
        prophylaxis to delay onset of
            overt psychosis, 118
    brain structural changes in, 104
    clinical features of, 104
    clinical use of antipsychotics in,
        106–108, 120
        dosage, 106–107, 120, 122
        symptom response, 107–108,
            109, 117, 122
    diagnostic category of, 116–117
    guidelines for antipsychotic
        selection and use in, 108–110,
        110, 120–121
    history of antipsychotic use in,
        103
    key clinical points regarding
        antipsychotics in, 122–123
    long-term antipsychotic use in,
        108–109, 110, 123
    medical workup for antipsychotic
        treatment in, 121, 122–123
    neurobiology of, 104
    overlap between schizophrenia and,
        104, 117
    rationale for antipsychotic use in,
        117
    typical vs. atypical antipsychotics
        in, 117–118
Scleroderma, 234
Seclusion and restraint, 126

Second-generation antipsychotics
(SGAs), 1, 8–9, 10–20, 145. *See
also* Antipsychotics; *specific drugs*
adverse effects of, **290**
classes of, 10–17
benzisothiazolyls: ziprasidone,
15–16
benzisoxazoles, 12–14
iloperidone, 13–14
paliperidone, 12–13
risperidone, 12
dibenzodiazepines: clozapine,
10–12
dibenzo-oxepino pyrroles:
asenapine, 17
dibenzothiazepines: quetiapine,
15
quinolinones: aripiprazole, 16–17
thienobenzodiazepines:
olanzapine, 14–15
compared with first-generation
antipsychotics, 9, 24–27
in pediatric patients, 161–162,
186
cost of, 9, 22, 26
dosage of, **268–274**
for agitation due to psychosis,
285–286
chlorpromazine equivalents,
254–260
efficacy of, 25
CATIE study of, 25–26
CUtLASS 1 study of, 27
formulations of, **245–246**
maintenance treatment with, 23, 25
mechanism of action of, 17–20
dopamine, 17–18
glutamate and NMDA, 18–19
issues underlying, 19–20
partial agonism of D_2 receptors,
20
serotonin, 18
onset of action of, 22
overdose of, 171
pharmacokinetics of, **254–260**

preferential use of, 9, 22
in pregnancy and lactation, 227,
312–327
for schizoaffective disorder, 38, 40
for treatment-resistant depression,
59–60
use in children and adolescents,
146–171
adverse effects of, 170–171, 185
aripiprazole, 146, **147**, 148,
159–160, 167
clozapine, 149, 154–155,
168–170
controlled trials of, **150–153**
vs. first-generation
antipsychotics, 161–162
guidelines for selection and use
of, 162–163
indications for, 146–148, **147**
medical workup for, 162–163
monitoring during treatment
with, 163
olanzapine, 156–157, 164–165
other uses of, 149
overdose of, 171
quetiapine, 157–159, 165
risperidone, 146, **147**, 148,
155–156, 163–164
ziprasidone, 160–161, 165–167
Sedation, drug-induced, 34, **290**
aripiprazole, 16, 76, 218
benzodiazepines, 22
clozapine, 12
in geriatric patients, 199
haloperidol, 184
management of, **292**
in medically ill patients, 3, 217–218
olanzapine, 15, 74, 218
paliperidone palmitate, 13
in pediatric patients, 170–171
phenothiazines, 9–10
quetiapine, 218
ziprasidone, 16, 160, 218
Sedative-hypnotic withdrawal, 126,
130

Seizures, drug-induced, 21, 34,
    233–234, **290**. *See also* Epilepsy
chlorpromazine, 173, 233
clozapine, 1, 12, 21, 168, 170, 233
phencyclidine, 131
pimozide, 177
stimulants, 130, 131
Selective serotonin reuptake inhibitors
    (SSRIs). *See also specific drugs*
antipsychotic interactions with,
    90–92, 116
    cytochrome P450–related, 72,
        81, 90, **91,** 92
combined with aripiprazole for
    nonpsychotic depression, 62
in frontotemporal dementia, 212
for generalized anxiety disorder,
    72–73
    antipsychotic augmentation of,
        73–81, **77–79**
for obsessive-compulsive disorder,
    37, 64
    antipsychotic augmentation of,
        65–72, **68**
    inadequate response to, 64, 71
for posttraumatic stress disorder,
    81–83
    antipsychotic augmentation of,
        82–88, **86–87,** 90
for psychotic depression, 55, 56–57
for schizophrenia
    negative symptoms, 36
    obsessive-compulsive symptoms,
        71
Seroquel. *See* Quetiapine
Seroquel XR. *See* Quetiapine slow-
    release
Serotonin
    in borderline personality disorder,
        104–105
    in cocaine abuse, 130
    in generalized anxiety disorder, 73,
        80
    in impulsive aggression, 104–105
    in obsessive-compulsive disorder, 65

in posttraumatic stress disorder,
    82–83, 90
Serotonin-dopamine antagonists, 8, 18,
    19. *See also* Second-generation
    antipsychotics
Serotonin-norepinephrine reuptake
    inhibitors (SNRIs), 92
Serotonin (5-HT) receptor affinity of
    antipsychotics, 18
    aripiprazole, 16, 141, 167
    asenapine, 17, 53
    clozapine, 12, 18
    iloperidone, 13
    olanzapine, 14, 164
    paliperidone, 12
    paliperidone palmitate, 13
    quetiapine, 15, 142, 165
    relative to dopamine receptor
        affinity, 18, 19
    risperidone, 12, 18, 163
    ziprasidone, 15–16, 166
Sertraline
    combined with aripiprazole for
        nonpsychotic depression,
        62–63
    combined with olanzapine for
        psychotic depression, 56–57,
        58, **58**
    for obsessive-compulsive disorder,
        64
    for pediatric anorexia nervosa, 183
    for posttraumatic stress disorder,
        81, 85
Sexual behaviors, in Parkinson's
    disease, 211
Sexual dysfunction, 34, 200
SGAs. *See* Second-generation
    antipsychotics
Sialorrhea, clozapine-induced, 12
Sibutramine, **295**
SLE (systemic lupus erythematosus),
    234–235
Sleep disturbances
    in delirium, 218
    drug-related

aripiprazole, 76
  management of, **294**
  olanzapine-fluoxetine
    combination, 60
  ziprasidone, 16
  in medically ill patients, 217–218
Smoking
  clozapine for, 11
  metabolic syndrome and, 33
  schizophrenia and, 5
SNRIs (serotonin-norepinephrine
  reuptake inhibitors), 92
Social phobia
  generalized anxiety disorder and, 72
  obsessive-compulsive disorder and, 64
  risperidone for, 75
Somnolence, drug-induced
  aripiprazole, 159
  asenapine, 17
  iloperidone, 14
  olanzapine-fluoxetine combination,
    60
  quetiapine, 15, 158, 159
  risperidone, 75
  second-generation antipsychotic
    overdose, 171
  ziprasidone, 16, 160
Specific phobia, 72
Speech
  disorganized, 21
  slurred, due to antipsychotic
    overdose, 171
SSRIs. *See* Selective serotonin
  reuptake inhibitors
Stelazine. *See* Trifluoperazine
Steroid-induced psychiatric symptoms,
  3, 235–236
Stimulants
  for attention deficit/hyperactivity
    disorder in pediatric bipolar
    disorder, 181
  intoxication with, 130–131
    benzodiazepines for, 129, 131
  psychosis induced by, 18, 130,
    134–135

Stimulant use disorders, 141–142
STOP-PD (Study of Pharmacotherapy
  of Psychotic Depression), 56–57
STPD. *See* Schizotypal personality
  disorder
Stroke
  antipsychotic-related risk in elderly
    dementia patients, 202, 229
  schizophrenia and, 6
Study of Pharmacotherapy of Psychotic
  Depression (STOP-PD), 56–57
Substance abuse disorders, 2–3,
  125–143
  clozapine for, 11
  comorbidity with, 2–3, 136–141
    agitation, 3
    bipolar disorder, 3, 138–141
    depression, 3
    pediatric psychosis, 182
    schizophrenia, 2–3, 5, 136–138
  indications for antipsychotics in,
    125–126, **127–128**
  key clinical points regarding
    antipsychotic use in, 142–143
  psychomotor agitation in, 126–133
    antipsychotics for, 129–130,
      142
    benzodiazepines for, 129
    due to intoxication, 130–132
      with alcohol, 131–132
      with phencyclidine, 131
      with stimulants, 130–131
    due to withdrawal, 132
      from alcohol, 132–133
    general approach to, 126, 129
  substance-induced psychosis,
    133–136, 142, 143
    cannabis, 135–136
    general approach to, 133–134
    stimulants, 130, 134–135
  urine toxicology testing in,
    127–128, 130
Substance use disorders, 141–142
  alcohol, 141–142
  stimulants, 141–142

Sudden cardiac death, drug-related,
    30–31, 223
  clozapine, 11
  droperidol, 10
  thioridazine, 223
Suicide
  bipolar disorder and, 181
  clozapine to reduce risk of, 11, 23,
      25
  depression and, 27
  schizophrenia and, 5, 6
  treatment noncompliance and, 39
Sundowning, 206
Switching between antipsychotics, 22,
    36, 40
  due to hyperprolactinemia, 34
  due to weight gain, 33–34
Systemic lupus erythematosus (SLE),
    234–235

Tachycardia, drug-induced, 34
  clozapine, 12, 149, 211, 224
  in geriatric patients, 199
  iloperidone, 14
  in neuroleptic malignant syndrome,
      30
  paliperidone, 13
  phencyclidine, 131
  second-generation antipsychotic
      overdose, 171
  stimulants, 130
  ziprasidone, 16
Tachypnea, in neuroleptic malignant
    syndrome, 30
Tardive dyskinesia (TD), 29, 50, 196
  in children and adolescents, 180
  drugs associated with, 172
    fluphenazine, 178
    haloperidol, 10, 175
    olanzapine, 15
    risperidone, 12
    trifluoperazine, 179
  in geriatric patients, **193,** 196–197
  management of, 29, 196–197, **293**
    clozapine, 11, 29, 168

monitoring for, 29
in patients with personality
    disorders, 108–109, 110
prevalence of, 29
with respiratory muscle
    involvement, 226
risk factors for, 29
Tardive dystonia, clozapine for, 11
TBI (traumatic brain injury), 3, 149,
    183, 218, 231
TD. *See* Tardive dyskinesia
Teratogenic effects of drugs, 227–228,
    298–327
Tetanus, **237,** 238
Texas Consensus Conference Panel on
    Medication Treatment of Bipolar
    Disorder, 46
Therapeutic relationship, 7
Thiamine, for alcohol intoxication, 131
Thienobenzodiazepines, 14–15, **256.**
    See also Olanzapine
Thioridazine, 10
  adverse effects of
    orthostatic hypotension, 194
    QTc interval prolongation, 10,
        31, 172, 174, 175, 195, 223,
        224
    weight gain, **33**
  augmentation for generalized
      anxiety disorder, **77**
  contraindications to, 175
  dosage of, **262**
    chlorpromazine equivalence, **250**
    in pediatric patients, 175
  drug interactions with, 175
    pimozide, 177
    ziprasidone, 166
  formulations of, 175, **242**
  in personality disorders, 108
    borderline personality disorder,
        111
    symptom response, 107, **109**
  pharmacokinetics of, **250**
  in pregnancy and lactation,
      298–299

for steroid-induced psychiatric
symptoms, 235
use in children and adolescents,
147, 172, 174–175
use in hepatic disease, **262**
Thiothixene, 8, 10
augmentation for generalized
anxiety disorder, **77**
dosage of, **268**
chlorpromazine equivalence, **253**
formulations of, **244**
in personality disorders, 108
borderline personality disorder,
111, **112**
schizotypal personality disorder,
119, 120
symptom response, 107, **109**
pharmacokinetics of, **253**
in pregnancy and lactation,
310–311
use in children and adolescents, 172
Thioxanthenes, 10, **253.** *See also* First-
generation antipsychotics
Thorazine. *See* chlorpromazine
Tiapride, 236
Tic disorders, 145
antipsychotics for pediatric patients
with, **148,** 149, **152**
obsessive-compulsive disorder and,
64
antipsychotic augmentation for,
66–67
Topiramate, **295**
Torsades de pointes, drug-induced,
30–31, 194–195, 223. *See also* QTc
interval prolongation
droperidol, 10
haloperidol, 223
risk factors for, 223
thioridazine, 174, 223
Tourette syndrome, 237, **237**
pediatric, 3, **148,** 149, 185
haloperidol for, 175
pimozide for, 176–177
quetiapine for, 157–158, 185

treatment in long-term care
facilities, 203
Transient ischemic attack, 202
Tranylcypromine, in borderline
personality disorder, **113**
Trauma patients, 3, 236
Traumatic brain injury (TBI), 3, 149,
183, 218, 231
Trazodone
in frontotemporal dementia, 212
for insomnia, **294**
TRD. *See* Depression, treatment-
resistant
Treatment adherence, 6, 7, 23, 37, 39,
40, 137
Tremor, drug-induced, 28, 195
aripiprazole, 52
management of, **292, 293**
second-generation antipsychotic
overdose, 171
Trifluoperazine
adverse effects of, 31
augmentation for generalized
anxiety disorder, 74, 75, **78,** 80
dosage of, 76, **264**
chlorpromazine equivalence, **251**
for geriatric patients, **264**
for pediatric patients, 179–180
formulations of, 179, **243**
in personality disorders, 108
borderline personality disorder,
111, **113**
symptom response, 107, **109**
pharmacokinetics of, **251**
in pregnancy and lactation,
304–305
use in children and adolescents,
148, 179–180
use in hepatic disease, **264**
Trifluoperazine sulfoxide, **251**
Triflupromazine, 9
Triglycerides. *See* Hyperlipidemia
Trihexyphenidyl
for parkinsonism, **293**
in pregnancy, 228

Trilafon. *See* Perphenazine
Trismus, 171

Urinary hesitancy/retention, drug-
    induced, 34
    anticholinergic agents, 196
    in geriatric patients, 199
Urine toxicology testing, **127–128,** 130

Vaginitis, aripiprazole-induced, 52
Valproate
    for bipolar disorder, 46, 53
        with comorbid substance abuse,
            140
        in pediatric patients
            aripiprazole and, **147**
            quetiapine and, **150,** 158
            risperidone and, 156
        relapse prevention, 48, 50
    drug interactions with, 116
    for tardive dyskinesia, 29
Varenicline, 137
Venlafaxine
    combined with aripiprazole for
        nonpsychotic depression,
        62–63
    for generalized anxiety disorder, 72
    interaction with haloperidol, 92
    for psychotic depression, 55–56
        combined with quetiapine,
            55–56, 58, **58**
Visiting Nurse Association (VNA)
    services, 39
Visual blurring, drug-induced, 34
    anticholinergic agents, 196
    risperidone, 75
Vitamin E, for tardive dyskinesia, 29
VNA (Visiting Nurse Association)
    services, 39

Wandering behaviors, 206, 208
Watson's PTSD Scale, 89
WBC (white blood cell) monitoring, for
    clozapine use, 11, **281**
Weakness, ziprasidone-induced, 16

Weight gain, drug-induced, 15, 21, 26,
    31–34, **33, 290**
    aripiprazole, 16, 31, **33,** 52, 76, 159
    asenapine, 17, 31, **33,** 53
    chlorpromazine, 217
    clozapine, 12, 21, 31, **33, 151,** 217,
        280
    in geriatric patients, **193,** 199
    haloperidol, 217
    iloperidone, 14, 31, **33**
    management of, 33–34, **295**
    in medically ill patients, 217
    monitoring for, **276, 280**
    olanzapine, 15, 21, 26, 31, 33, **33,**
        51, 74, **151,** 157, 217
    olanzapine-fluoxetine combination,
        60
    paliperidone, 31, **33**
    in pediatric patients, **151,** 170, 185
    quetiapine, 15, 31, **33,** 158, 217
    risperidone, 12, 17, 31, **33, 151,**
        156, 217
    thioridazine, 217
    ziprasidone, 16, 31, **33**
White blood cell (WBC) monitoring, for
    clozapine use, 11, **281**
Withdrawal dyskinesia, 29

Yale-Brown Obsessive Compulsive
    Scale (Y-BOCS), 64, 65, 67, 69,
    70–71
Yale Global Tic Severity Scale, 158, 185
Y-BOCS (Yale-Brown Obsessive
    Compulsive Scale), 64, 65, 67, 69,
    70–71
Young Mania Rating Scale (YMRS**),**
    49, 50, 51, 52, 155–156, 157,
    159–160, 161

Zaleplon, **294**
Zileuton, interaction with pimozide, 177
Ziprasidone, 15–16
    administration of, 16
    adverse effects of, 16, 160–161,
        290

hyperprolactinemia, 34, **35**
lupus, 235
QTc interval prolongation, 16,
166, 171, 195, 223, **224,**
225, **286**
weight gain and metabolic
effects, 16, 31, **33**
for bipolar disorder, **47**
in pediatric patients, 160–161
contraindications to, 16, 195
for delirium, 220, **221**
dosage of, 16, **221, 271**
for agitation due to psychosis, **286**
chlorpromazine equivalence, **257**
for pediatric patients, 160–161,
166–167
drug interactions with, 16, 166
pimozide, 177
efficacy of, 25
electrocardiogram monitoring for,
166, 195
formulations of, 16, 166, **217, 246**
for generalized anxiety disorder, 80
intramuscular, 16, 22, 166, **286**
mechanism of action of, 16
overdose of, 171
pharmacokinetics of, **257**
precautions for use of, 166, 195
in pregnancy and lactation, 227,
320–321

receptor affinity of, 15–16,
165–166
routes of administration of, **217,
221**
for schizophrenia
CATIE study of, 25–26
with comorbid substance abuse,
138
maintenance treatment, 23
in substance abuse disorders, **128**
for agitation, 130
with schizophrenia, 138
for tic disorder, **152, 237**
for treatment-resistant depression,
60, 61
use in children and adolescents,
147, 148, **152,** 160–161,
165–167
for autism spectrum disorders
and developmental delay,
184
for bipolar disorder, 160–161
use in medically ill patients, 217
cardiac disease, 16, 195
hepatic disease, 225, **271**
Parkinson's disease, 211
renal disease, 225, **271**
Ziprasidone sulfoxide, **257**
Zolpidem, **294**
Zyprexa; Zyprexa Zydis. *See* Olanzapine